PSYCHOLOGY FOR HEALTH CARE

PSYCHOLOGY FOR HEALTH CARE
Key Terms and Concepts

Bridget Adams and Barbara Bromley

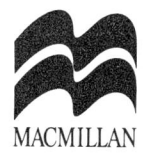

MACMILLAN

© Bridget Adams and Barbara Bromley 1998

Foreword © Sally Kendall

All rights reserved. No reproduction, copy or transmission of this publication may be made without written permission.

No paragraph of this publication may be reproduced, copied or transmitted save with written permission or in accordance with the provisions of the Copyright, Designs and Patents Act 1988, or under the terms of any licence permitting limited copying issued by the Copyright Licensing Agency, 90 Tottenham Court Road, London W1P 9HE.

Any person who does any unauthorised act in relation to this publication may be liable to criminal prosectuion and civil claims for damages.

The authors have asserted their rights to be identified as the authors of this work in accordance with the Copyright, Designs and Patents Act 1988.

First published 1998 by
MACMILLAN PRESS LTD
Houndmills, Basingstoke, Hampshire RG21 6XS
and London
Companies and representatives
throughout the world

ISBN 0-333-64808-0 hardcover
ISBN 0-333-64809-9 paperback

A catalogue record for this book is available from the British Library.

This book is printed on paper suitable for recycling and made from fully managed and sustained forest sources.

10 9 8 7 6 5 4 3 2 1
06 05 04 03 02 01 00 99 98

Editing and origination by
Aardvark Editorial, Mendham, Suffolk

Printed in Hong Kong

Contents

List of figures and tables — vii
Acknowledgements — ix
Foreword — x
Preface — xii
Using this book — xiv
Handy headings — xvii
Historical background — xviii

1	Aggression and agression management	1
2	Anxiety and depression	15
3	Attitudes, attitude change and persuasion	28
4	Behaviourism and behaviour therapies	40
5	Biopsychology and physical interventions	56
6	Cognitive psychology and cognitive therapies	78
7	Health beliefs, lifestyle and health promotion	95
8	Humanistic psychology and counselling	115
9	Language and therapeutic communication	128
10	Loss and grief therapy	147
11	Memory and response to memory changes	160
12	Mind and altered states of consciousness	174
13	Pain and pain management	192
14	Perception and response to perceptual changes	208
15	Perception of self and others	226
16	Planning, playing and problem-solving	246

17	Psychodynamic psychology and psychotherapies	263
18	Research, statistics and psychometrics	279
19	Social psychology, groups and social skills	298
20	Stress and stress management	317
Appendix: Using a library		336
Bibliography		339
Index		360

List of Figures and Tables

Figures

1.1	Model of variables and processes in affective aggression	5
1.2	Determinants of anger arousal	5
1.3	Aggression in hospital: a case example for discussion	11
1.4	Reciprocity negotiation	13
3.1	Three-component model of attitude	29
3.2	Labelling	32
3.3	Communication variables	34
3.4	Persuasion	35
4.1	Behaviour modification programme: a case example for discussion	44
4.2	Modelling	49
4.3	Operant conditioning: reinforcement of the stimulus–response (S–R) unit	52
4.4	Social learning theory	54
5.1	Left hemisphere of brain	58
5.2	Inside the brain	59
5.3	Inheritance of eye colour or other single-gene characteristic	65
5.4	Motor and sensory pathways	67
5.5	Visual pathways	68
5.6	Auditory pathways	69
5.7	The nervous system	72
6.1	Catastrophising	83
6.2	Cognitive appraisal model	85
7.1	Health belief model	99
7.2	Protection motivation theory	100
7.3	Theory of reasoned action	100
7.4	Theory of planned behaviour	100
7.5	Health action process approach	101
8.1	Styles of therapy	117

9.1	Facial expressions	134
10.1	Poems of loss and grief	154
12.1	EEG wave traces in sleep	188
14.1	The colours of the spectrum and the relative sensitivity curves believed to be typical of the three main types of cone found in the human retina	212
14.2	Colour vision: colour of objects	213
14.3	Figure-ground reversal	216
15.1	Self-concept	240
15.2	Sexuality – a poem for discussion	243
17.1	Penis envy	275
18.1	Normal (Gaussian) distribution curve	288
19.1	Sociograms	314
20.1	Factors in stress	319
20.2	Physiological arousal systems	324
20.3	Stress and performance	328
A.1	Outline of the Dewey Decimal Classification	337

Tables

1.1	Ethological classification of aggression	8
4.1	Reinforcement schedules	53
7.1	Dimensions of health	97
12.1	Stages of a normal sleep cycle	189

Acknowledgements

The authors would like to thank the following for giving permission to use their material: Jacky Fleming for two cartoons from *Be a Bloody Train Driver* (Penguin, 1991), Stephen Parr for his poem 'Dad', Judith Thwaite for her poem 'For Mark', New Victoria Publishers for N. Leigh Dunlap's cartoon from *Morgan Calabrese*, Steven Appleby for his cartoon of cats' facial expressions from *The Box of Secret Thoughts* published by Bloomsbury Publishing (1996) and Little, Brown and Company for Grace Nichols' poem 'Invitation' from *The Fat Black Women's Poems*, published by Virago.

Special thanks go to Professor Sally Kendall for writing the Foreword and to Bill O'Neill for the cartoons he drew for us to illustrate the concepts of labelling and modelling.

Many thanks are due to those students who eagerly read through chunks of text as the manuscript was nearing completion – and their assignments were due. Their comments were perceptive and enlightening. Thanks also to all those students who knowingly or inadvertently contributed ideas as we watched them wrestle with unfamiliar terms and concepts during their seminar presentations.

Thanks to all family and friends who took sole responsibility for tasks that are normally shared, and supported us throughout, and those who read, proofread and made helpful suggestions. Special thanks to one particular 'apple polisher' who wishes to remain anonymous, and to colleagues Crys Oldman, Ann White and Nasim Kanji who read chapters, corrected errors, contributed items and pointed out fresh sources of material.

Finally, we would like to thank Frances Arnold and Houri Alavi at Macmillan for their continuous support and patience.

Every effort has been made to trace all the copyright holders but if any have been inadvertently overlooked the publishers will be pleased to make the necessary arrangement at the first opportunity.

Foreword

Health-care practitioners, managers, researchers and educationalists are all engaging in their field of practice during a period in which the health service itself has been undergoing turbulent change. The changes have resulted from policy decisions that have emphasised issues such as cost-efficiency, clinical effectiveness, care in the community and evidence-based practice. Within these very broad based issues are specific implications for quality improvement (such as the introduction of the named nurse concept and the increase in audit-based activity), all of which have taken place within an evolving organisational context.

Coupled with complex service delivery issues is the way in which health itself has been defined and refined. Health is no longer perceived to be merely the absence of disease but rather a much more holistic understanding of the integration of physical, social and psychological factors that interplay with the individual in society, families and communities. These relationships are increasingly recognised and understood by users as well as health practitioners, so that appropriate and effective health care has become as much a matter of conceptual and theoretical interpretation within the context of health care as the application and implementation of knowledge.

It is against this background that users of the health service come with their health needs seeking health advice, treatment for disease, counselling or rehabilitation to mention but a few. Health-care professionals are expected to provide, and be accountable for, the most clinically effective and cost-effective care for which they have research evidence, in order to meet user's needs swiftly and appropriately – what has been termed doing the right thing in the right way. It is clearly evident that health practitioners in the twenty-first century and beyond require a wide and expanding knowledge base in order to plan and deliver care that is of demonstrably high quality.

In order better to understand issues of health, illness, disability, death, dying and so on, there is no doubt that health practitioners require a sound knowledge base in psychology. It is, however, both impractical and inappropriate for all health professionals to undertake diplomas and degrees in psychology. This volume provides the means by which any health practitioner can either learn for the first time, undertake revision or extend her knowledge in relation to psychology for health care. For example, for the health visitor who is engaged in health promotion, there is a complete chapter on health beliefs, lifestyle and health promotion. This chapter enables her to revise the major models of health promotion and to consider their relative limitations, to appreciate the relative merits of teaching and learning approaches, to understand the relationship between different psychological schools and health behaviour, and to engage in further reading if necessary.

A further example is the junior doctor dealing with death and dying with relatively little experience. The chapter on loss and grief helps him to understand the significance of attachment behaviour and loss, the different staging models that have been developed to understand the process of dying, the limitations of these and what it really means for patients and their relatives.

Likewise, the chapter on research provides both the novice and the more experienced researcher with definitions of research terms, which are often confusingly presented in the research literature, as well as examples of tools to measure psychological constructs such as attitudes.

Using this book, these health professionals can access the information they require easily and extend and expand their knowledge base rapidly. While the authors would encourage readers to follow up the extensive references and deepen their knowledge of health-care psychology, the book nevertheless provides well-organised discussion on a wide range of psychology topics that will be meaningful to most health practitioners.

In conclusion, this volume will be an extremely valuable tool for the development of high-quality health care. As technological advance in medicine extends our capability to prolong life and to prevent the onset of many major diseases, the psychological aspects of care will take on an increasingly important role. In the past, there have been complaints from the public, and research studies demonstrate that the people delivering health care have not paid sufficient attention to psychological need, especially in such domains as communication, anxiety and pain management. It is already obvious that simply to 'reassure the patient' is not enough, but within this era of evidence-based practice it is surely incumbent on health professionals to utilise the knowledge in volumes such as this in order to ensure that the quality of practice meets the highest expectations.

PROFESSOR SALLY KENDALL
Buckinghamshire College

PREFACE

> I keep six honest serving-men
> (They taught me all I knew);
> Their names are What and Why and When
> And How and Where and Who
>
> from *The Elephant's Child*
> by Rudyard Kipling

This book is for new students and experienced professionals who are undertaking a course of study in health care that includes psychology, health psychology, counselling or interpersonal skills. No previous knowledge of psychology is assumed.

The 'human condition' is examined in the research and practice of psychology, which requires many disciplines and has produced a myriad of reports. Approaches are often complex and may be contradictory. A person looking for information on any of the branches of the subject may have a hard time tracking it down and then taking in what is written.

We have devised this book as an introduction to some of the main discoveries and thoughts that are relevant to health care. We have tried to guide readers in finding where to look for information and define, where we can, the terms used by the pioneers in this vast study, and the meanings of what seem at first difficult concepts. The text is as simple and plain as we can make it and illustrates applications to practice with examples.

Many concepts in psychology are named using invented words. These are sometimes common words to which a special meaning applies. Examples are 'complex' used as a noun in psychodynamic literature and 'iconic' to refer to a style of thinking. Others may be derived by combining words or parts of words, from Greek, Latin or other languages. For example, the word PSYCHOLOGY combines *psyche*, the Latin for soul, spirit or mind (from a similar Greek word), with *logos*, the Greek for word, study or reasoning. The pronunciation or stresses may not be obvious, and we have shown these when we think it may help. Psyche, for example, when used on its own, is pronounced with two syllables as 'sigh-key'.

Some sources that we cite may be difficult to obtain. We include references where the subject may be found in more readily accessible secondary sources, if we think that this will be helpful or where criticisms and applications are included, but readers are encouraged to unearth the primary sources when undertaking an in-depth study.

Psychology for Health Care: Key Terms and Concepts will be useful for nurses, midwives, health visitors, occupational therapists, physiotherapists, medical students, doctors, ambulance personnel, psychologists, psychotherapists, counsellors and all other health-care professionals. It may also be of interest to patients and clients and their relatives, friends and helpers.

This book will additionally have a useful contribution to make to access, diploma and degree level courses in psychology, health psychology and health studies.

Using this book

This book can be used as an introductory text that will provide a stepping stone to psychology, health psychology and specialist textbooks and journals. It can also serve as a glossary for a quick reference to individual terms or as a comprehensive revision aid. The content is not restricted to health psychology in its usual mainstream sense but includes a wide range of terms and concepts that all contribute to an understanding of the psychological needs of people requiring health care.

The table of contents shows that there are 20 main chapters relating to how the main approaches or perspectives within psychology contribute to an understanding of the terms and concepts. Six main perspectives of behavioural, biological, cognitive, humanistic, psychodynamic and social psychology represent fundamentally different ways of looking at the human condition. A number of other perspectives can be seen to be related to these or to have been derived from them. These perspectives can be defined as follows.

Behaviourism aims to explain, predict and control behaviour by exploring the extent to which environment determines behaviour. The key assumption of the school of behaviourism is that learning takes place by conditioning and that this learned behaviour can be described in terms of stimulus–response units (S–R units). A related approach is **social learning theory**, which is an extension and development of behavioural principles that takes social interaction into consideration (see Chapter 4).

Biopsychology combines biology and psychology and is the perspective that helps us to understand behaviour and mental experience by examining what is happening physiologically in the body, particularly in the brain and nervous system (see Chapter 5). A related approach is **ethology**, which is the study of animals in their natural habitat. Also related to this is **comparative psychology**, which uses laboratory studies of animals in order to reveal underlying principles of behaviour. Biopsychology may also be combined with social psychology to give a **biosocial** or **biopsychosocial** perspective, often referred to in relation to health care.

Cognitive psychology is chiefly concerned with the experimental investigation of those mental processes to do with knowing and understanding. Areas for enquiry include attention, perception, memory, thinking, problem-solving and language. A related field is **cybernetics**, which is the science of systems of control and communications that uses special-purpose models, most of which can be applied by computer programs (see Chapter 6).

Humanistic (or phenomenological) psychology focuses on the wholeness of experience and emphasises the searching for personal meanings and essences of experience as they appear to an individual (see Chapter 8).

Psychodynamic psychology is based on the belief that it is possible to interpret what is going on in the unconscious mind, based on elaborate schematic theories of the structure and dynamics of emotional development (see Chapter 17).

Social psychology covers all those areas of human behaviour concerned with interaction and communication in everyday social settings and can be considered to be an academic discipline in its own right as well as a subdivision of psychology. The main topics are language and communication, interpersonal perception and attributions, attitudes and attitude change, conformity and obedience, group structures and processes, and organisations (see Chapter 19). Social psychology may also be combined with biology to give a **biosocial** or **biopsychosocial** approach. Allied to this is **ethnography**, the qualitative study of a group of people including the language and cultural norms. This kind of study aims to describe and analyse the ways in which these people use their language to represent concepts and categorise the meaning of their world in a cultural context.

Other approaches, such as **lifespan development, developmental psychology** or **the psychology of individual differences**, have developed from the basic perspectives and integrate relevant themes.

Each chapter in this book opens with a note to introduce the area, followed by a selection of published definitions. These show how opinions differ and how definitions have changed with time. In psychology, it is important to realise that there may be no definite answers but sometimes only suggestions.

A summary is given of some of the more important arguments in each area, with indications of where these might be relevant to practice. We hope that this will give an appropriate context to the individual terms and concepts that follow. The key terms and concepts are then arranged alphabetically in each chapter, with a brief definition in most cases and a fuller account where this is needed to explain a particular concept. Cross-references are given where the same, or a similar, item appears in another chapter. Terms that are defined elsewhere in the book are given in italics if their meaning is not obvious.

Also included is a page of 'Handy headings', which gives a short summary of some of the most useful terms. The historical background sets the scene for all that follows.

Different pathways through the text may be useful for different purposes.

Overview of the different perspectives: Historical background – Research, statistics and psychometrics – Behaviourism and behaviour therapies – Biopsychology and physical interventions – Cognitive psychology and cognitive therapies – Humanistic psychology and counselling – Psychodynamic psychology and psychotherapies – Social psychology, groups and social skills – Handy headings.

Sections with a strong biological basis: Biopsychology and physical interventions – Mind and altered states of consciousness – Aggression and aggression management – Anxiety and depression – Pain and pain management – Stress and stress management.

Sections with a strong cognitive basis: Cognitive psychology and cognitive therapies – Memory and response to memory changes – Perception and response to perceptual changes – Planning, playing and problem-solving.

Sections with a strong social basis: Social psychology, groups and social skills – Attitudes, attitude change and persuasion – Health beliefs, lifestyle and health promotion – Language and therapeutic communication – Perception of self and others.

Main therapeutic approaches: Language and therapeutic communication – Behaviourism and behaviour therapies – Biopsychology and physical interventions – Cognitive psychology and cognitive therapies – Humanistic psychology and counselling – Psychodynamic psychology and psychotherapies – Social psychology, groups and social skills – Loss and grief therapy.

Index: All terms are also listed in the index. This may be a useful place to start when seeking information about a particular word or locating cross-references.

A guide to using a library has been included to indicate where psychology texts may be located (see Appendix).

Handy Headings

PURE PSYCHOLOGY IS DEFINED AS:
- *the scientific study of behaviour and experience*

APPLIED PSYCHOLOGY FOR HEALTH CARE IS:
- *a vast collection of individual studies*
- *a rich mixture of contrasting and contradictory approaches, often integrative, eclectic or multimodal*

Influenced by:
- arts • magic • superstition • myth • religion • science • philosophy • healing • medicine

Following or integrating different schools, approaches or perspectives:
- Behaviourism and social learning theory
- Biopsychology and biopsychosocial approaches
- Cognitive psychology and cognitive-behavioural approaches
- Humanistic (phenomenological) psychology
- Psychodynamic (including psychoanalytic) psychology
- Social psychology

Using quantitative and qualitative research methods
- project justification • choice of paradigm
- general, pilot or preliminary work • detailing and categorising
- selection of variables • formation of hypotheses or research questions
- project design • collection of data
- analysis of data • theories, laws and models
- publication and debate • application

Meeting the criteria of:
RELIABILITY AND VALIDITY

In order to:
DESCRIBE – EXPLAIN – PREDICT – CONTROL

Involving analysis and integration of the domains of the:
- AFFECTIVE – feelings and emotions
- COGNITIVE – beliefs and understanding
- CONATIVE – intentions, will

and concerned with issues such as:
- lifespan development • mind–body interaction, integration and reductionism
- free will and determinism • nature–nurture interaction and integration
- the individual within society • language and communication
- mental and physical health and illness • death and dying

HISTORICAL BACKGROUND

Early Philosophy, Mind and Reason

Modern psychology has many strands, all of which are influenced in one way or another by early ideas of magic, superstition, myth, religion, science, philosophy, healing and medicine.

In the Western world, the first written accounts of significant influence were those of Hippocrates, Plato, and Aristotle in the fifth and fourth centuries BC. These were in turn based on early Egyptian, other North African, Indian and other influences.

Hippocrates, remembered now in the Hippocratic oath of modern medicine, was a physician who described temperament in medical terms and was among the first to think of epilepsy as an illness resulting from natural causes rather than divine inspiration. This idea was later suppressed during the dark ages and was not fully appreciated until the twentieth century.

Plato (427–347 BC) was concerned with the teaching of philosophy in order to achieve the ideal state. He emphasised that the purpose of education was not to put knowledge or thoughts into the pupils' minds but to make them think for themselves. He demonstrated that conventional morality was often muddled and inadequate, and he attempted to analyse the elements of the human mind to show that its well-being, full development and happiness are to be secured by doing right and not doing wrong. He distinguished between doing right through deliberate choice, generous impulse and acting on animal appetite. He outlined the various arguments concerning whether we do something right because we know it is right or because there is some sort of reward. Plato followed Socrates' teaching that doubt was the most important feature of human thought and that knowledge of one's own doubts and limitations was the basis of real wisdom. These ideas are periodically lost and re-established throughout history.

Aristotle ($c.384$–322 BC) was interested in the relationship between mind and reason. He was concerned with the concept of the association of ideas in the mind, and notions of similarities and differences. He distinguished between our knowledge of the world derived from the senses and the power of rational thought, explaining desire in terms of the pleasure, or its reverse, gained from the senses. He defined five senses: sight, hearing, taste, smell and touch. Aristotle's ideas are derived from intuition and are often unsupported by observation (what we call armchair philosophising). They have remained largely unchallenged for centuries and have profoundly influenced thinking. Much of what Aristotle described is similar to what people today tend intuitively to believe until introduced to more rigorous and scientific education.

The Stoic philosophers overrode Aristotle's neutral stance towards our biology by distinguishing between universal reason, which they considered to be pure and good, and man's often irrational nature, which by definition must be impure and bad. This led to passions and feelings being regarded as vile. Early Christian teachings, notably those of St Augustine (AD 354–430), took this further and thought of man as a pure rational soul temporarily using an impure, mortal, earthly body. They denounced the senses as evil sources of satisfaction and desire, while continuing to teach that all knowledge derives from them. Sexual feelings were particularly condemned and, more often than not, women were blamed for leading men astray, as is portrayed in the Biblical story contained in the Book of Genesis.

The Reformation, the Inquisition and Witchcraft; The Separation of Mind and Body, and the Suppression of Doubt

Confusion between mind and reason, and value judgements of mind versus body, coloured late Roman and medieval thought. For hundreds of years, theology was inextricably drawn into the psychological strands of philosophy, and new ideas were suppressed.

Not until the thirteenth century did new ideas begin to emerge. St Thomas Aquinas (1224–1274) revived Aristotelian philosophy. He regarded the soul as immortal but made respectable and non-heretical the revival of Aristotle's biological intellectualism, which did not condemn the senses and biological functions.

Over the next three centuries, the deadening influence of religious orthodoxy was beginning to be challenged in many spheres: political, economic, medical and philosophical. Important advances in medicine, notably Harvey's demonstration of the circulation of the blood, were made. The supreme authority of the Church to sway people's minds regarding all questions of moral conduct and personal responsibility was challenged.

In a desperate attempt by religious orthodoxy to hold onto its power, the Inquisition and its teachings about witchcraft and heresy led to extensive witch-hunts and purges. Until doubt and enquiry could be acknowledged as legitimate human responses to times of profound change, doubt was logically regarded as the ultimate of all heretical evils and must therefore be due to demonic possession. The body was seen as something gross that could be inhabited by any spirit craving a lodging. Witches, mostly women, were recognisable as those who expressed or led others to express excessive sexual appetite or who were hysterical or psychotic people. Burning and other inhuman treatment of the mere body was justified in terms of the purifying effect on the soul.

Johannis Weyer (1515–1588), city physician at Arnhem, deserves credit for insight and moral courage in asserting that the illnesses attributed to witchcraft came from natural causes. Weyer has been called the first clinical psychiatrist, both for his humanity and for his factual approach to psychological phenomena.

René Descartes (1596–1650) attempted to resolve the mind–body dilemma by postulating that the body worked on mechanical, physical lines but was controlled by the soul, which he thought had its seat in the pineal gland in the middle of the brain. The soul, operating via the pineal, regulated the flow of 'animal spirits' along the nerves and blood vessels like an elaborate plumbing system. Descartes' (or Cartesian) theory is of mind–body interaction, with a firm distinction drawn between the two entities. Thenceforth, philosophers and theologians could mostly devote themselves to the problem of mind, leaving it to the physical scientists to puzzle out the relationship between the mind and the nervous system.

The empiricist philosophers of the late seventeenth and eighteenth centuries (Locke, Hume, Berkeley and others) again revived the Aristotelian concept of the association of ideas, which seemed to fit the increased knowledge of the nervous system and its connection with mental phenomena. Immanuel Kant (1724–1804) proposed the division of mental faculties into knowing, feeling and willing (cognition, affection and conation). Kant insisted on the unity of perception and on the experience of an active self that organises experience.

Positivism, the Brain, and the Beginnings of Scientific Psychology

Auguste Comte (1798–1857), who is also credited with the founding of sociology, introduced a style of philosophy known as positivism, which advocates the study of man by the methods of science, marking the beginning of the demise of armchair philosophising and the start of systematic observation.

Concurrently with all these advances, physiologists had been busy adding knowledge about the nervous system and the brain. Thomas Willis (1621–1675) studied brain structures and postulated that the nerves were not tubes through which animal spirits flowed but fibres by which some influence passed from brain to body. In the 1790s Galvani found that muscle contraction in frogs resulted from electrical discharge. In the early 1800s Bell and Magendie showed that the motor and sensory nerves were distinct and that each individual nerve fibre served only one function. Bell added a sixth sense – muscle or kinaesthetic sensation – to Aristotle's original five. Pierre Flourens, c.1824, published evidence that there existed in pigeons a general correspondence between certain major divisions of the brain and various levels of bodily activity.

The stimulus given to experimental work on the animal brain, and its possible application to the human brain, was largely derived from Charles

Darwin's theory of evolution published in 1859. It was gradually becoming clear that man's pre-eminence was due to the greater growth and complexity of the cortex of the brain.

In 1861 Pierre Broca discovered the site of the centre for speech in the left hemisphere of the human brain. Hughlings Jackson in 1775 described the function of the nervous system as hierarchical, and the concept of levels of mental functioning was developed. Marshall Hall (1790–1857) described the difference between voluntary action and reflex action in the nervous system. Hermann Helmholtz (1821–1894) measured the speed of the nerve impulse and later developed his theories of vision and hearing. Gustav Fechner (1801–1887) can be considered to be the founder of experimental psychology through his attempts to apply the laws of mathematics to the physiology of sensation and develop psychology as a science with a mathematical base.

The appearance of psychology as a subject discipline in its own right is generally dated at 1879, when Wilhelm Wundt (1832–1920) founded the first laboratory for experimental psychology at Leipzig. Wundt's institute's researches added to knowledge about problems of sensation and reaction time. Wundt also attempted to develop a psychological theory that, while acknowledging the importance of introspection as a method of direct observation of oneself, laid stress upon the importance of experimentation and measurement in psychology.

Oswald Kulpe began work on imageless thought using introspection in a systematically controlled fashion. The technique of introspection in its purest form was carried over to America by E.B. Titchener (1867–1927), a student of Wundt and Kulpe. Experimental studies of behaviour then became popular. By 1882 Stanley Hall had founded America's first psychological laboratory at Johns Hopkins University, and 10 years later there were 15 such laboratories in the USA. In Britain, after some smaller beginnings, a psychological laboratory was founded at Cambridge in 1913 under the direction of C.S. Myers.

Psychoanalysis, Behaviourism and Humanistic Psychology

At the same time, new discoveries were being made in psychological medicine. Ancient ideas of divine and demoniacal possession had persisted despite attempts to contradict them, and it was still largely believed that the abnormal behaviour of the mentally ill was the product of some external influence or physical agent. Jean Charcot (1825–1893) was the first to demonstrate that hysterical phenomena could be induced and even relieved by suggestion. Further work by Pierre Janet, Bernheim and Liebeault began to uncover the mind's unconscious dynamics but these early discoveries were soon overshadowed by the work of Sigmund Freud (1856–1939).

Freud used the methods of hypnosis and free association and the study of his own dreams to evolve his theories about unconscious mental striving, largely based on sexual repression and defence mechanisms. Psychoanalysis became both a mode of treating patients and a system of psychology. Carl Gustav Jung (1875–1962) differed from Freud in rejecting the theory of infantile sexuality, introducing the notion of collective unconscious and considering all people as a mixture of masculine and feminine characteristics. He considered the libido not as exclusively sexual but as a generalised life energy or will to live.

By the 1920s introspection as a method of enquiry was being seriously questioned. Observation and measurement of behaviour was considered more reliable, in particular by John B. Watson (1878–1958). A new brand of psychology – behaviourism – emerged. Watson believed that, to be a science, psychology must adopt only objective methods. The study of inaccessible, private, mental processes was to have no place in a truly scientific psychology. Behaviourism (in one form or another) was to remain the dominant force within psychology for the next 30 years or so, especially in the USA and to a lesser extent in Britain. The emphasis on learning, in the form of conditioning, was to make that topic one of the central areas of research in psychology as a whole. Behaviourist theories of learning are often referred to as stimulus–response or S–R theories because of their attempt to analyse all behaviour into stimulus–response units, no matter how complex the behaviour. In contrast to Freudian analysis, behaviourism gave rise to a form of therapy for neuroses based on a use of conditioning and deconditioning to the relevant stimuli.

Purposive or hormic psychology developed as a reaction to behaviourism. William McDougall (1871–1944) rejected the mechanistic views of behaviourism and held that the mind has an element of free will and that purposive striving played a decisive role in mental activity, behaviour being the resultant of mind–body interaction. Like Freud, however, McDougall believed that social organisation developed from inborn drives or instincts.

Carl Rogers (1902–1987) and Abraham Maslow (1908–1970) rejected both the psychoanalytic and the behaviourist approaches. They emphasised that the individual's uniqueness and freedom to choose a particular course of action and are the leading proponents of humanistic or phenomenological psychology. Central themes of the theory and psychotherapy are self-concept and self-actualisation. The psychodynamics of the individual are not considered to have fixed or generalised interpretations. Humanistic therapy is client centred or person centred (rather than analyst centred): the therapist does not offer any explanations or interpretations but instead assists clients in exploring and finding their own meanings.

Gestalt Psychology, Cognitive Development and Social Learning Theory

Another reaction against behaviourism came in the form of the Gestalt school of psychology, which emerged in the 1920s and 1930s in Austria and Germany. The Gestalt view is that 'the whole is more than the sum of its parts' and focuses attention on the organising functions of the nervous system. Gestalt principles can also be applied to learning, showing that insight is often more important than trial and error. After 1920 the Gestalt movement spread to America, where Kurt Lewin (1890–1947) developed his field theory, in which he viewed the mind as a dynamic tension system and behaviour as the means of reducing or abolishing tension. The aim of the individual is to attain a tension-free state of equilibrium. This links with the homeostatic principles of the time, in which the ideal state is seen as quiescent and free from disturbance.

Freud's dynamic concept of the mind links up with educational theories from Plato to Rousseau (1712–1778) and Froebel (1782–1852) that the child is an individual in his or her own right and that education should develop innate qualities and not merely be an implanting of adult precepts.

The work of Freud and the evolutionary theories of Darwin combined to bring about the growth of interest in child development. Sir Francis Galton (1822–1911) is usually regarded as the father of the mental test, using statistical methods in correlating mental traits. His work was continued in Britain by Karl Pearson, Cyril Burt, Godfrey Thomson, William Brown and C.E. Spearman. In the USA, J.M. Cattell (1860–1944) carried out independent studies, while in Paris, Alfred Binet (1857–1911) studied the problem of backwardness in schoolchildren. Mental testing of all sorts became widespread in schools, in the armed forces and for job selection.

Jean Piaget (1896–1980), working on various tests, became concerned with underlying mental structures and outlined his theory of cognitive development. Piaget believed that children think in a way (concrete operations) that is fundamentally different from that of adults and that they have to develop through a series of stages before they can reach adult thinking (formal operations). This was later disputed by, for example, Peter Bryant and Margaret Donaldson, who believed that adults and children alike use a mixture of concrete and abstract thinking, according to context and individual interests, and that differences are due more to differing concepts, memory and concentration span.

A development of behaviourism arose in social learning theory, in the USA in the 1940s and 1950s, as an attempt to reinterpret certain aspects of Freud's psychoanalytic theory in terms of conditioning theory. This was carried on in the 1960s and 1970s, notably by Albert Bandura, who emphasised learning through watching and imitating others.

Jerome Bruner was greatly influenced both by Piaget and social leaning theory; rather than describing stages of growth, he was concerned with ways of representing the world (enactive, iconic and symbolic), the need for language for the development of logical thought and the ways in which social interaction lead to the acquisition of language. These theories of cognitive development and social learning have led to significant changes in education and health-care practice, the emphasis now being on providing plenty of concrete examples and the opportunity to explore concepts through play and the age-appropriate use of language.

Brain Scans, Cybernetics and Modern Psychology

Fresh lines of investigation into the mode of brain functioning were opened up in the 1960s in the use of the electroencephalogram (EEG). Together with newer forms of brain imaging – computerised axial tomography (CAT), positron-emission tomography (PET) and magnetic resonance imaging (MRI) – this allows study of the structure and activity of the brain without interference or damage. Another modern approach to investigating brain function is the science of cybernetics, which attempts to explain human thinking and behaviour using artificial intelligence, feedback and communication systems.

Although many definitions can be found, modern psychology is best defined as the scientific study of behaviour and experience. Psychology is not a single subject but a complex mosaic: a vast collection of individual studies with the common aim of using scientific methods to describe, understand, predict and (if appropriate) influence or control human behaviour and experience.

Underlying all modern psychology is the still unresolved relationship between mind (or consciousness) and neurological processes, in particular brain activity. Many psychologists recognise the importance of the brain and nervous system but are inclined to think of physiological activity as being separate from mental experience. Others regard psychology and physiology as fully integrated. Those who believe that all mental experience will eventually be explained in terms of the brain and nervous system are referred to as reductionists.

Health Psychology and Health Care

The emergence of health psychology as a rapidly growing discipline in its own right offers health-care professionals a vehicle with which to explore the concept of health and the many factors that influence health along the continuum from wellness to impaired health to dysfunctional health and ultimately to death.

There are various definitions of or approaches to health psychology. The following one by Matarazzo (1980), cited in Pitts and Phillips (1991: 3), is perhaps the most comprehensive:

> Health psychology is the aggregate of the specific educational, scientific and professional contributions of the discipline of psychology to
>
> - the promotion and maintenance of health
> - the prevention and treatment of illness
> - the identification of etiologic and diagnostic correlates of health, illness and related dysfunction
> - and the analysis and improvement of the health care system and health policy formation.

Health psychology is a new section within the British Psychological Society and, at the time of writing, is asking to be formally recognised as a division.

By emphasising health promotion and illness prevention through the identification of health risk factors and the development of strategies to cope with life crises, health psychology provides health care professionals with a supplement to the traditional medical approach to health problems.

1 AGGRESSION AND AGGRESSION MANAGEMENT

Aggression may be regarded as any form of behaviour that is directed at living or inanimate objects with the intention of causing physical or psychological harm or to gain an advantage. It is often thought of as taking the form of a physical and violent attack upon someone. However, it is more commonly expressed as a verbal outpouring of emotion towards a person. Its manifestation can be direct or indirect, active or passive, instrumental or hostile, impulsive or planned, overt or subtle.

Definitions	
Dollard et al. (1939)	An act whose goal-response is to injure an organism.
Buss (1961)	A response that delivers noxious stimuli to another organism.
Argyle (1983)	Behaviour which is intended to harm, physically or verbally, people (or animals) who want to avoid such treatment.
Berkowitz (1993)	Any form of behaviour that is intended to injure someone physically or psychologically.

Approaches, Arguments and Applications

The frequency with which aggression is reported in the workplace and the community is increasing. More than half of all nurses report encountering aggression, particularly in accident and emergency departments. Randall (1997) quotes statistics showing that, in the USA, physical assaults are the third largest cause of death at work for men and the primary cause for women. In the UK, the rate is about one tenth, but still high. Many people, when interviewed for research, report being harassed or attacked by neighbours, but most do not seek help from the police for fear of repercussion. A recent addition to our language is the concept of 'road rage'.

The nature–nurture debate considers whether aggression is a biologically determined instinct that derives from an innate drive or urge compelling the individual to seek a particular goal or whether it stems from the process of socialisation and is a learned response to environmental stimuli. Early studies were divided between seeing aggression as either wholly internally generated or wholly externally triggered. Freudian psychoanalysis regards aggression as an unavoidable internally generated conflict between biological urges and social constraints. Lorenz (1966) also proposes that aggression is not a reaction to external factors but a spontaneous urge that continually seeks expression. Karen Horney's psychodynamic interpretation saw aggression as socially determined and hence avoidable (Horney, 1967, cited by Ryckman, 1989). Distinctions have been made between spontaneous energy, hormonally triggered behaviour, emotional response to frustration, overcrowding, intergroup conflict and response to pain or fear.

Current research is concerned with a range of internal and external factors involving an individual's past and present experience and relating predisposition to physiological arousal in response to social and environmental conditions.

Ethological approaches: ethology is the study of animals in their natural habitat. Such approaches suggest that aggressive urges are instinctual and innate responses in all species. They allow the individual to adapt to the environment and hence survive. The application of these theories to human behaviour has been largely superseded by studies involving a wider consideration of social and cultural factors.

Biopsychological approaches: biological explanations of aggression tend to focus upon either finding an aggression centre in the brain (see *limbic system*, Chapter 5) or describing biochemical changes. Biochemical studies tend to link aggression to male *hormones* or to the effects of drugs and alcohol. A link may exist between aggression and neurological changes in Alzheimer's disease. The nerve pathways responsible for controlling aggression are thought to relate to acetylcholine, and patients with Alzheimer's disease are deficient in the enzyme responsible for the production of acetylcholine. The findings of biopsychological studies are generally inconclusive and take little account of motivation, personal values and the social context in which aggression occurs.

Behavioural approaches: these argue that aggression is a learned or conditioned response to frustration that is maintained through reinforcement.

Social learning theory approaches: these propose that all behaviour is learned in a social context through observation, imitation and reinforcement. Bandura (1965) demonstrated that young children learned to be aggressive through watching the behaviour of older role models. *Modelling* may be an important factor in aggression by reducing *inhibitions* and *desensitising* the individual. The more the child is exposed to aggressive behaviour and the more this is rewarded, the more aggressive the child may become. The most effective role models are the family and *peer group*, although 'distance' *modelling* via television plays a part. Kelleher (1995), cited by Randall (1997), argues that the 'entertainment culture', with a constant exposure to violence on television, is one of the most potent forces making society more aggressive. In the USA, children of 13 or 14 years old may have been exposed to as many as 100 000 acts of violence on television, of which approximately 8000 are murders (Randall, 1997: 2).

Cognitive approaches: here the assumption is that aggression is controlled by cognitive processes. If an individual experiences arousal and attributes this to an outside force, the *cognitive appraisal* may be hostile and antagonistic. This facilitates the labelling of the emotion as anger rather than as some other emotion such as fear. The consequences of responding aggressively will then be weighed up in deciding how to act.

Psychodynamic approaches: these deal with the hidden, unconscious factors that influence the way in which we respond to situations and events. Freud argued that aggression is a natural biological instinct, which he related both to ethological approaches and to his notions of the conflict between the *Eros* and *Thanatos* forces within us all, which drive us to act when we feel threatened. Proponents of psychodynamic approaches, such as Horney (1942), argue that aggression is not innate but an unconsciously learned response to a hostile environment. Whatever the cause, most psychodynamic approaches agree that if direct expression is blocked, *indirect expression* may result, the individual directing the aggression inwards towards the self. Primitive *defences* such as aggression may provide a patient with a means of *catharsis* and act as a safety valve as the patient attempts to come to terms with health problems.

Key Terms and Concepts

Adult bullying: as yet, there is no agreed definition of bullying. Like other new or abstract concepts, it is mainly described in terms of examples. These range from being ridiculed in front of others, being subjected to bad language and having 'dog muck' posted through the letter box to actual physical assault. Where definitions are given, these indicate that bullying is considered to be the systematic or repeated use of aggression and may involve an abuse of power. Randall (1997) uses the principle of *reinforcement* to explain why bullying may be maintained. He also describes the formation of a bullying and a *victim* personality (see also Chapters 8 and 19). It is suggested that bullying at work may be reduced by:

- taking all conflict seriously
- not confusing aggression with competition, which may be healthy and motivating
- developing a culture of assertiveness
- promoting communication skills such as active listening
- confronting the bullies
- increasing management and supervision training
- promoting teamwork
- providing employee assistance programmes.

Bullying in the community can be addressed by:

- the empowerment of individuals
- the recognition of learned helplessness
- the provision of community support
- the improved use of local media resources for raising awareness
- giving information about support systems.

Affect: mood or feeling. See Chapter 6.

Affective or hostile aggression: often associated with anger, this is the most common form of aggression, its purpose being to inflict injury on persons or property. Geen's (1990) model of affective aggression suggests that aggression stems from the appraisal of two variables:

- background variables, which may predispose an individual to behave aggressively, such as biological inheritance, learning history and social norms
- situation variables, which elicit aggressive behaviour as a response to conditions of stress, arousal and anger (Figure 1.1).

This can be compared with the model of anger arousal adapted from Hollin and Howells (1989) (Figure 1.2).

Agonistic: involving conflict or dispute, controversial, combative.

Amygdala: part of the *limbic system* thought to be related to inhibiting aggressive responses (see Chapter 5).

Anger: a natural human emotion of displeasure, often passionately felt, which can be expressed in a variety of ways, including aggressive ones, or not at all. Anger is thought to be important in health- and illness-related conditions, particularly when it is repressed or inhibited (Eysenck, 1985, 1994; Spielberger *et al.*, 1988) (see Chapter 7). Anger is usually considered to be one of the basic emotions (see Chapter 6), which is associated with characteristic facial expressions and postures and linked to fundamental physiological processes, in particular via the *hypothalamus* of the brain (see Chapter 5). During evolutionary processes, basic emotions would have formed a useful set of response patterns, directing an animal towards or away from situations with varying degrees of urgency. Anger may be a response to confusion, frustration or fear, all of which may be associated with other health problems.

Anger management: a range of activities including controlled expression of anger, *relaxation exercises*, *cognitive appraisal*, *stress inoculation* and displacement activities may be used to enable an individual to manage provoking situations. Anger management training may be helpful both for people who find it impossible to show their anger and for those who flare up too easily. Techniques include cognitive and behaviour therapies, psychodynamic therapy, group therapy, relaxation, exercise and creative arts. See Chapters 4, 6, 8 and 17.

Most techniques involve talking through what triggers or sustains anger and trying to work out ways of preventing it or of lessening the effects through more acceptable forms of expression. Painting, music, drama, dance and mime can provide alternative ways of expressing and understanding anger in contained situations. Novaco (1975) used *stress inoculation* techniques to help people to control their anger by imagining provoking situations and working mentally through the scenarios, starting with the least and ending with the most annoying.

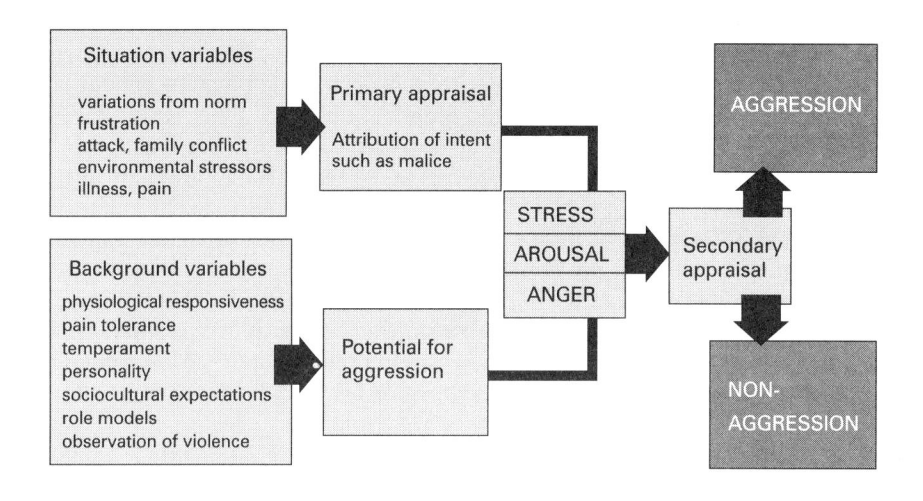

Figure 1.1 Model of variables and processes in affective aggression (*modified from Geen, 1990*)

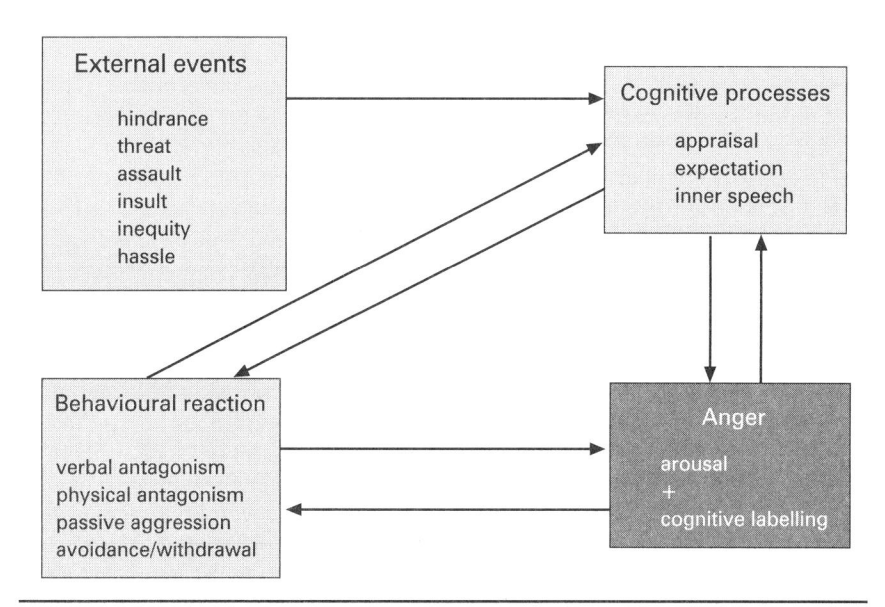

Figure 1.2 Determinants of anger arousal (*adapted from Hollin and Howells, 1989, from material by Novaco, 1978*)

A behavioural systems approach to therapy with couples for those who engage in frequent rows may include paradoxical techniques such as 'timetabled arguments' (see for example, Crowe and Ridley, 1990), in which the couple are instructed to have deliberate arguments or rows to order at set times of the day. The hope is that through confronting the rows and deliberating simulating them, greater understanding will be reached. There is also the possibility for comedy in this approach, which may be helpful.

Another comic technique for discordant couples involves a ritual stamping on crunchy cereal and calling out of frustrations preferably while holding hands. This is thought to be cathartic (see *catharsis*) and may introduce an element of humour. It does not appear to be supported by empirical research and is said to be most effective when the couple own a dog that will subsequently clear up the mess! As discussed in *expression of emotion* (see Chapter 6), it is not possible to predict whether this simulated emotion will reduce or increase the number of rows in the long term as this will depend on whether it resolves the difficulties or reinforces the habit. All techniques need to be used with care and be supported by other forms of counselling (Suinn, 1990). See also Chapters 4, 6, 8, 17 and 20.

Anxiety: in a situation where self-esteem or security is threatened, unconscious anxiety may arise. In order to avoid experiencing this anxiety, the feelings may be displaced as anger and expressed aggressively. See Chapters 2 and 17.

Appeasement gesture: a term used in ethological approaches for an instinctive act by a victim that inhibits the victor's aggression and thus prevents a dominant animal from killing the victim. Humans may adopt appeasement or conciliatory behaviours by making concessions in conflict situations, for example giving in or admitting defeat to avoid further conflict.

Argument: verbal fighting that may involve emotional arousal. Within families or between friends, arguments may be seen as unpleasant or upsetting and can lead to major rows or serious quarrels. These may have a cathartic effect or may lead to a deteriorating situation if unresolved.

In contrast, academic arguments are ideally not usually associated with emotional disturbance but are carefully structured logical debates that compare and contrast beliefs and empirical evidence, usually leading to a conclusion that may or may not be passionately believed in.

Arguments and family therapy: for a family or couple presenting with arguments as the problem, the goal of therapy may be to facilitate more effective communication, introduce more flexible behaviour or alter perceptions of the arguments towards seeing them as sometimes good and constructive rather than dangerous. An inhibited couple who are, perhaps, unable to express mutual frustration and aggressive feelings may benefit from having an unaccustomed argument or heated discussion (Crowe and Ridley, 1990).

Assault: hostile, personal attack that may be physical or verbal in nature.

Assault cycle: Kaplan and Wheeler (1983) propose that an assault follows a sequence of phases in an 'assault cycle' that will be experienced by both the assailant and the victim, and show how recognition of these phases can help in the development of skills in dealing with violent clients. These phases are:

- triggering
- escalation
- crisis
- recovery
- post-crisis depression.

Assaulter: in general hospitals, patients suffering from high levels of pain and patients in intensive care units and accident and emergency departments are often the most assaultive. In psychiatric units, people with schizophrenia, personality disorders, alcohol and drug abuse problems, and organic disorders such as dementia and epilepsy or following a cerebrovascular accident show an increased tendency to be aggressive. With diabetes, the electrolyte imbalance in the hypoglycaemic state can create a confusional state in elderly patients that may result in aggressiveness.

Assertiveness: putting forward one's point of view in order to achieve desired goals; behaving positively and in a forthright manner without being combative or causing harm. Assertiveness and aggression are frequently used synonymously, but assertiveness is associated with self-confidence and tact, speaking out in a spirit of co-operation, negotiation and compromise rather than competition or hostility. See also *traps*.

Assertiveness training: short courses or workshops designed to enable people to learn to put forward their point of view or defend themselves in a non-aggressive way. Most focus on verbal and non-verbal communication skills and are based on the need to avoid being hurt or injured by an aggressor or caught up in a state of conflict. This may range from being in a state of readiness and overcoming timidity to controlling aggressive reactions to provocation. In some contexts, a course may also include physical self-defence (mainly for women wanting to know how to deal with attempted rape or mugging), but this is likely to include some aggressive behaviour.

Bullying at work: see adult bullying.

Catharsis hypothesis: Berkowitz (1962, 1993) describes an early model of motivation proposing that aggression is spontaneously generated energy and that any aggressive action temporarily reduces the inclination to be aggressive, (see also Chapter 17). There is insufficient empirical support for this approach and it can be argued that if aggression is a learned response that is reinforced, the expression of aggression may result in an increased incidence of aggressive behaviour.

Classification of aggression: Buss (1961) suggests that any incidence of aggression may be a combination of the following:

- physical/verbal
- direct/indirect
- passive/active.

For example, spreading malicious gossip about someone would involve verbal, active and indirect aggression.

Moyer (1976), in his ethological approach, identifies several categories of aggression that promote survival chances by helping the animal to find food, emphasise its place in the hierarchy, compete for a mate and reproduce (survival of the fittest), and defend its territory (Table 1.1).

Table 1.1 Ethological classification of aggression
(adapted from Moyer, 1976; Berkowitz, 1993)

Type	Stimulus	Biochemical process or mechanism	Form
predatory	natural prey	lateral hypothalamus amygdala hippocampus	instrumental
intermale territorial defence sex related	male of species	septum anterior hypothalamus	ritualised responses
fear induced	threat	amygdala hypothalamus	automatic reactions defensive behaviours
irritable	frustration	hypothalamus reticular activating system	diffuse reaction
maternal	threat to young	pregnancy parturition lactation	attempts to avoid conflict

Ticklenberg and Ochberg (1981) classified criminal violence according to five types:

- instrumental
- emotional, impulsive in anger or fear
- felonious, in the course of another crime
- bizarre, insane
- dyssocial – violent acts upheld by a peer or reference group.

Feshbach (1964) and Manning *et al.* (1978) used four categories of aggression in children:

- specific or instrumental
- teasing or hostile
- games
- defensive.

Coercion: aggression may be used in an attempt to influence another person's behaviour by trying to get them to do what the aggressor wants. Threats of suicide are sometimes seen as coercive acts (see also Chapter 7).

Cognitive appraisal: sorting out the beliefs, knowledge and understanding a person may have about the situation, the aggression experienced, the value placed on the experience and expectations. See also Chapter 6.

Cognitive labelling: beliefs formed by an aroused person about the cause and nature of bodily sensations, which changes these sensations from 'an undifferentiated arousal state into the specific emotional experience' (Berkowitz 1993: 90). See Chapter 6.

Crowding: Welch and Booth (1975) studied aggression within the family and its relationship to the amount of space in which families lived. They found that density, objectively measured, was unrelated to family aggression. However, subjective perceptions of being crowded were related to family fighting. The families which reported feeling crowded showed more aggression that those which did not. See also *personal space*.

Cycle of violence (intergenerational transmission of aggression): Berkowitz (1983) argues that aggression is transmitted between generations so that people who are exposed to violence when young develop an aggressive tendency themselves.

Depression: if a person is suffering depression as a result of repressed aggression or anger, the task of therapy is usually to encourage greater *assertiveness* rather than an outward show of hostility.

Desensitisation: the more a person is exposed to aggressive behaviour, the less likely he or she is to be disturbed by it. This has been discussed in relation to television violence. It is argued (for example, Drabman and Thomas, 1974) that repeated exposure to violent programmes reduces emotional impact, and greater violence is then needed to produce an emotional reaction.

Displacement: destructive feelings that are held towards someone or something but which cannot be expressed may be redirected on to someone or something else. Patients who have unresolved or unexpressed feelings of anxiety about their health problems may develop feelings of aggression, which they then direct towards health care workers. See Chapter 17.

Distraction: a technique used to deal with aggression, which involves diverting the aggressor's attention away from the target, for example by changing the subject of conversation or moving away from the situation. Diversionary strategies can be used in health-care settings to distract patients' attention and help to avoid aggression, which may be due to lack of stimulation. For example, magazines, piped music and toys for children may be provided in waiting areas.

Empathy: one of the difficulties for therapists working with aggressive clients is being able to stay with the expression of aggression without being pulled into arguments, taking sides or making judgements. Crowe and Ridley (1990) suggest a programme of training for therapists that includes role-play and a detailed discussion of emotional responses. See also Chapter 8.

Environmental antecedents: adverse environmental stimuli such as heat, noise and crowding have been found to increase aggression by producing high levels of *negative affect* and irritation (see also Chapter 4). Mueller (1983) suggests that environmental stressors produce four effects that have links with *affective aggression*:

- arousal
- stimulus overload
- interference with ongoing behaviour
- negative *affect*.

A carer can attempt to control or reduce aversive environmental stimuli by minimising noise, maintaining adequate temperature and ventilation and respecting personal space.

Expectation: responsibility for harm may be avoided if the aggressive persons can use as an excuse the claim that in the circumstances their behaviour could have been anticipated. For example, an anxious person who is kept waiting to see a doctor and is abusive to the receptionist in the outpatients department may state that the behaviour is typical of people kept waiting.

Frustration: this refers either to an external barrier that prevents an individual from attaining a goal, or to an emotional reaction.

Frustration–aggression hypothesis: Dollard *et al.* (1939) argue that aggression is a learned response to frustration. They suggest that if an individual is unable to achieve his or her goals, the resulting frustration will be expressed in the form of aggression towards the person or object believed to be causing the obstacles. On occasions, this may be the patient him or herself, resulting in self-injurious behaviour. If aggression cannot be directed at the cause of frustration, it may be displaced on to someone or something else – the kick-the-cat syndrome. For example, a patient's behaviour may be restricted as a result of health problems such as an inability to walk, to leave hospital when wanted or to be understood: this can lead to frustration that may be displaced on to an innocent victim such as the nurse. A patient's behaviour may also be restricted by health-care professionals who may need to enforce rules, deny requests, impose delays or use limit-setting. Explanations for such restrictions can help to reduce frustration and prevent an aggressive response. If unable to provide an explanation for any of the rules or restrictions, the health-care professional should question the necessity for them.

Heat: high temperatures have been shown to produce increases in aggressive motive and tendencies. Rule *et al.* (1987) showed that heat increases the probability that participants will have aggressive thoughts when aggression-related stimuli are present, and proposed that heat primes aggressive thoughts. Carlsmith and Anderson (1979) studied the incidence of urban riots in several American cities between 1967 an 1971 in relation to average daily temperatures and found a direct correlation: the higher the temperature, the greater the incidence of aggression. Anderson (1987) showed that temperature has a direct effect on the incidence of violent crimes. These findings suggest that, in hospital settings, high temperatures may lead to an increase in aggression.

Hormones: increased blood levels of testosterone correlate with increased aggressiveness (Archer, 1991). Premenstrual decreases in blood levels of progesterone may result in irritability and increases in hostility.

Hospitalisation: insecurity and anxiety on admission to hospital, or during a longer stay when progress is not as expected, can lead to aggressive behaviour, either active or *passive*. It may reflect a more general impatience with procedures that are not understood, and can involve relatives. A case example is given for discussion (Figure 1.3).

Hostile aggression: see *affective aggression*.

> I had just arrived on the ward for a late shift and hadn't had a handover, when Mrs K, the daughter of one of our patients, asked to see me. She started complaining about the care her mother was getting. I tried to explain to her that I had just returned from my two days off and she might be better off speaking to one of the other nurses. Ignoring me, she repeated her complaints. She started raising her voice and was clearly annoyed, as she began emphasising her words in a menacing way. She told me she was fed up with excuses from staff and that nobody seemed to want to accept responsibility for the deterioration in her mother's health. I tried to calm the situation down by saying that I was sorry she was upset.
>
> 'Upset!', she shouted, 'You'd be bloody upset if your mother was in this state!'
>
> I suggested that we went to see her mum so I could see for myself what the problem was, but she demanded to see the ward manager. I told her I was the most senior member of staff on duty that afternoon, but she kept screaming that she wanted to see the manager.
>
> At that moment, Cathy, one of the other staff nurses, rushed up and said that handover was about to start. I tried to explain to Mrs K that I needed to find out what had been happening to all the patients since I was last on duty and that I would return to speak to her when the handover was finished in about 20 minutes.
>
> I was about to ask her if she would like to talk to one of my colleagues from the early shift when she swung her fist at me and started yelling abuse…

Figure 1.3 Aggression in hospital: a case example for discussion

Humour: a light touch and a sense of humour may be beneficial in defusing an aggressive situation. In therapy, where a couple are too embarrassed to discuss an unusually emotional argument, the therapist may be able to help the couple in viewing their behaviour as amusing by smiling and saying something like, 'So you had something of a screaming match' (Crowe and Ridley, 1990: 78). This may help the couple to see their behaviour in a new perspective and give greater freedom for discussion.

Conversely, humour may be destructive if jokes or teasing indicate that one person is not taking the other seriously. This may happen unintentionally when one person thinks he or she knows the other well enough and believes the teasing is enjoyed but neglects to check whether this is so. It may of course be intentional *bullying*.

Indirect expression: psychodynamic approaches argue that when direct expression of aggression is blocked, either by circumstances or because the individual has been socialised into not showing violent behaviour, aggression may be turned inwards towards the self, resulting in deliberate self-harm or *suicide*, or be displaced towards another person. See also Chapters 7 and 17.

Inducement of arguments: a technique used in behavioural systems approaches to couple therapy in which couples who complain of arguing are encouraged to argue either continuously or to a timetable. See *paradoxical prescriptions*.

Instrumental: a term used to denote behaviour that is goal directed, that is intended to achieve something which is desired. For example, a person may inflict self-injury to try to sustain a relationship that is floundering. Threatening another person may bring feelings of power. See also Chapter 4.

Instrumental aggression: the least common but most frightening type of aggression in which the usual inhibitors such as guilt, anxiety and pity are absent. It is characterised by a cold, calculated determination to obtain a specific goal rather than the victim's suffering.

Insult: see *verbal aggression*.

Intent: purpose in behaving aggressively.

Intergenerational transmission of aggression: see *cycle of violence*.

Intractable arguments: arguing can sometimes become part of repetitive, 'symmetrical' or ritualistic sequences, continuously going over old ground without resolving anything. Behavioural therapy for couples would take the form of setting tasks that break the pattern, such as prescribing that the couple 'must not go over old topics' (Crowe and Ridley 1990: 228), even if this means sitting in silence for some time. Alternative behavioural techniques may involve planning *timetabled arguments* or a *paradoxical prescription* for continual arguments. See also *traps*.

Jealousy: therapy may reveal that one of the underlying causes of aggression and arguments in families or couples may be jealousy, which may in turn result from low self-esteem concerning whether one individual feels attractive to the other or feels needed. As with *intractable arguments*, jealousy in couples may respond well to *paradoxical* behavioural techniques.

Malice: the intention to do evil or desire to tease, especially cruelly. In law, wrongful intention.

Negative affect: aversive unpleasant feelings or mood such as disgust or fear, which may serve as a stimulus for aggression. See also Chapter 6.

Noise: noise reduces an individual's ability to withstand and tolerate frustration and intensifies the expression of aggression. Glass and Singer (1972) found that controllability and predictability are important variables in reducing the stress potential of noise. See also Chapter 20.

Pain: Berkowitz (1983) found that pain is a strong source of *negative affect* and aggression.

Paradoxical prescription: a behavioural systems approach to therapy with couples, particularly those complaining of *intractable arguments* and jealousy, in which the couple are encouraged to display the problematic behaviour either continuously or to a timetable. This approach is, of course, not recommended where the behaviour is dangerous.

Passive aggression: withdrawal from a situation or refusal to co-operate, with the intention of annoying someone producing an outcome undesirable or harmful to the other person (Buss, 1961). This can be in the form of refusing to attend planning meetings, not offering help or deliberately 'forgetting' to do something. In relationships, there may be sulky silences and unspoken resentments. See also *silence*, Chapter 9.

Personal space: Worchel and Teddle (1976) found an association between violation of personal space and state of arousal resulting in aggression. If health-care professionals have to invade a patient's personal space, for example to carry out a procedure, an explanation should be given and permission sought. Kinzel (1970) found that inmates in a prison who were regarded as violent needed to maintain large areas of personal space around themselves. See also Chapter 9.

Power struggle: aggression, particularly *passive aggression*, may be the outward expression of a struggle for dominance within a relationship. For example:

> Sexual refusal by one partner may be part of a power struggle in which one partner dominates in their non-sexual interaction and the other dominates in their sexual interaction (Crowe and Ridley, 1990: 162).

Primary appraisal: the judgements and interpretations that are made by a person about situational factors and which have the potential to influence the physiological and emotional state. If the situation is thought to arise from malicious or intentional actions, arousal and anger or fear are likely.

Reciprocity negotiation: a therapeutic technique for helping couples with management of relationship problems. It is particularly helpful with problems involving arguments, fights, bilateral complaints, nagging and threats of violence, in which neither partner is labelled as 'patient', but both are seeking guidance (Crowe and Ridley, 1990). The method involves identifying a number of issues of complaint for which it is feasible for each partner to agree to a change of behaviour. The picture is not simple, but in some instances useful effects can be achieved (Figure 1.4).

To take a typical example where reciprocity negotiation was useful, a couple in their fifties were referred by their general practitioner with a complaint that the husband had become rather withdrawn and silent, while the wife was described as hostile and aggressive. The couple were thinking of separation, and the husband had also become sexually uninterested in his wife, a fact which tended if anything to increase her hostility. In the first session some tasks were worked out which they both agreed would be practicable and which each had requested of the other. The husband was to try to be home within 20 minutes of the time he had predicted, and if he was delayed he would telephone his wife to let her know. The wife was to spend the first 10 minutes after his arrival home listening to his news of the day, not interrupting, and giving him a 'soft answer' rather than challenging or criticising what he said.

As a result of these initial tasks the couple greatly improved their interaction and the husband found, to his surprise, that he was finding his wife much more attractive in her new approach, so much so that the couple had sexual relations for the first time in several months.

Figure 1.4 Reciprocity negotiation (*Crowe and Ridley 1990: 64*)

Secondary appraisal: an individual's assessment of potential to cope with stress in ways other than with aggression.

Stimulus overload: if the environment becomes too exciting or irritating, a person's ability to process environmental information may be impaired. This impairment can cause annoyance and frustration and may result in aggression.

Suicide and aggression: Retterstol (1990: 75) suggests that 'women, more than men, use the act of suicide as an aggressive weapon, as a defensive weapon or as a means with which to manipulate their environment'. It appears that if women are socialised into acting in a restrained way and not showing violence, they are likely to retain this behaviour even when desperate and take out their aggression on themselves. Hendin (1964) has argued that aggressive antisocial behaviour, when accompanied by puritanical and pious attitudes, may lead to a moral form of suicide. Suicide and deliberate self-harm can also take the form of martyrdom or instrumental self-harm, such as in protesters who starve or burn themselves to death in order to bring about social reform.

Suicide risk and aggression: aggression is listed by Ringel (1953, cited by Retterstol, 1990) as the second of three phases (with narrowing/isolation and flight from reality) that precede suicide: the presuicidal syndrome. Retterstol (1990) identifies the three As – aggression, appeal and ambivalence – as key identifying behaviours in the study of suicide. See also Chapter 7.

Territoriality: see Chapter 9.

Tolerable aggression: aggression which Breakwell (1989) suggests is regarded by an individual as expected behaviour. It is influenced by the values held by health-care professionals who accept that a certain amount of aggression is to be accepted from those in their care.

Traps: Ryle and Cowmeadow (1992: 105) define traps as:

> things we cannot escape from. Certain kinds of thinking and acting which result in a 'vicious circle' when, however hard we try, things seem to get worse instead of better. Trying to deal with feeling bad about ourselves, we think and act in ways that tend to confirm our badness.

They argue that people often get trapped because they confuse *aggression* with *assertiveness*. Believing that aggression is wrong, many people bottle up aggression or anger until they cannot help letting it out in a burst of childish behaviour. Seeing themselves acting childishly or causing harm confirms their belief that the aggression is wrong, and they do not easily see that being assertive and asking for their rights is acceptable.

Trauma: Hohmann (1966, 1975) suggests that aggression is one of the normal stages of reaction to the trauma of a major disabling incident. He distinguishes between depression, which he sees as withdrawal and internalised hostility, and aggression or externalised hostility. Evidence for 'stages' is not reliable. See also *indirect expression* and Chapters 7 and 10.

Verbal aggression: this can take the form of insults, threats, sarcasm, gossip, graffiti or any other spoken or written activity that is intended to cause harm.

Weapons effect: the realisation (for example, Dixon 1987) that the mere presence of weapons can lead to violent behaviour.

2 ANXIETY AND DEPRESSION

Anxiety is usually listed as one of the basic emotions (see Chapter 6). It can range from mild to severe, is generally unpleasant and is usually accompanied by heightened autonomic arousal and sometimes by a characteristic facial expression. Anxiety may constitute a warning and can be seen as useful in helping a person to cope with threatening situations, but in excess it may interfere with coping.

Distress or sadness is also considered to be a basic emotion. However, depression, as the word is used clinically, is not mere 'sadness' or a temporary mood of feeling 'low'. It involves a feeling of deep emptiness, of thinking nothing is worthwhile, a wishing to withdraw, feelings of being to blame, of being unloved and unlovable, and of being weak and useless, based on assumptions about the self, the world and the future.

Definitions

Spielberger et al. (1968)	Anxiety is... a palpable but transitory emotional state or condition characterised by feelings of tension and apprehension and heightened autonomic nervous system arousal.
Stratton and Hayes (1993)	Anxiety is... a stressful state resulting from the anticipation of danger. Anxiety has a physiological component (the alarm reaction or fight or flight reaction), cognitive aspects, particularly in narrowing attention, and a subjective experience of discomfort. Each of these components may help the person deal effectively with clearly recognised, real and immediate dangers, but can be damaging both psychologically and physically when the anxiety persists, as in occupational stress or unresolved unconscious conflicts.
Rowe (1983)	Depression is the greatest isolation that we can experience. When we are simply unhappy we can seek comfort from others and we can

Definitions (cont'd)	
	comfort ourselves. But in depression we can neither give nor receive comfort, for we are alone in a prison, and that prison is filled with fear, anger, guilt and despair.
Twaddle and Scott (1991)	The central features of the syndrome of depression are depressed mood, pessimistic thinking, loss of interest and reduced energy level. The abnormality of mood is the most consistent and prominent feature. It is differentiated from sadness because it is more persistent, perhaps exaggerated in response to the provoking stress and varies qualitatively from previous experiences of unhappiness.
Montgomery (1990)	Anxiety and depression are inextricably linked. The traditional separation into many different disorders has been difficult to apply to the majority of those suffering from mixtures of anxiety and depression.

Approaches, Arguments and Applications

Montgomery (1990) argues that it is not helpful to regard depression and extreme anxiety as separate syndromes since the two states are most often seen together, and anxiety and depression inventories both include measures of depression and anxiety. The ICD-10 classification (World Health Organisation, 1992) now recognises the mixed anxiety depression syndrome, whereas the DSM IV (American Psychiatric Association, 1994) proposes separate syndromes. This has significant implications for drug therapy since the main drugs treat separate states.

All types of depression and anxiety can be treated by drug therapy, talking therapies (cognitive, cognitive-behavioural, psychodynamic or person centred), expressive therapies using the creative arts or a mixture of these. Difficulties lie in deciding on diagnosis and the best form of management to take.

Biopsychological approaches: these relate the psychological experience of anxiety to physiological functions and changes. Drug therapy, informed by medical practice, seeks to intervene with the *adreno-SNS* arousal and other physiological processes related to mood or emotional state. Depression is linked to neurotransmitter disturbances.

Behavioural approaches: these describe processes of conditioning by which a person learns certain anxiety responses to situations either by association or reinforcement. Anxiety may be learned by classical conditioning, when adreno-SNS arousal becomes associated with certain situations. This may be specific at first, but can generalise. The anxiety may then be maintained by operant conditioning if behaviour is reinforced. There are several types of behaviour therapy, for example behaviour modification and progressive desensitisation, which seek to develop new learned responses and in which a goal is reached via small manageable steps.

Social learning theory approaches: these propose that anxious responses are learned in a social context through observation and imitation. The family, peer group and culture determine what situations will be viewed as anxiety-provoking and what behaviour is appropriate. For example, children brought up in a household where electrical storms are regarded as frightening are more likely to display anxiety during storms. The situation with depression is less clear. Family or group therapy focuses on the sharing of experiences and learning or relearning of constructive coping strategies.

Cognitive approaches: these assume that all emotions are controlled by cognitive processes. Understanding and perception, whether conscious or unconscious, of a situation will determine whether a person becomes aroused or experiences a drop in arousal and how the level of arousal is interpreted. Cognitive therapy focuses on beliefs, knowledge and understanding with a view to cognitive restructuring and hence reduction of anxiety or depression. This approach may be used with behavioural techniques to treat phobias or obsessive-compulsive disorder and can be used with moderate anxiety or depression related to lack of self-confidence or learned helplessness. See Chapter 6.

Psychodynamic approaches: these theories emphasise the unconscious processes by which anxiety and depression can arise from unresolved tensions, particularly those developed during childhood. Therapies seek to intervene by helping the client to acknowledge conflicts and address them.

Humanistic and integrative approaches: these focus on the autonomy of the patient or client and individual qualities and needs. Therapy seeks to help in exploring whatever the individual feels is necessary or desirable. Any intervention that breaks an unhelpful cycle of behaviour and emotional distress may enable a person to develop new ways of coping. Some complementary interventions may also modify physiological processes. Examples include biofeedback, hypnosis, exercise, relaxation and meditation.

Key Terms and Concepts

Abnormal anxiety: there is no single clinical definition of abnormal levels of anxiety. People may be considered to have abnormal anxiety if their anxiety falls into one or more of the following four groups, being:

- unusual, either higher or lower than the normal
- socially unacceptable
- a medical diagnosis
- so personally distressing that it interferes with the sufferer's daily living (see anxiety disorders).

Aggression: when people are anxious, they may become aggressive. For example, when entering the strange environment of the hospital, patients or relatives may act aggressively towards health-care professionals. See Chapter 1.

Agitation: a state of unrest, disturbance or excitement, often associated with anxiety, the cause of which may or may not be recognised. Patients presenting with an agitated form of anxiety or depression may be treated with antipsychotic drugs such as haloperidol rather than benzodiazapines. When associated with signs other than behavioural ones, for example euphoric mood punctuated by irritability, grandiosity or distractability, agitation may be diagnosed as mania (see bipolar disorders).

Agoraphobia: the word is derived from the Greek *agora* meaning market place and literally means a fear of public spaces. It is usually associated with fear of going out of doors and may be characterised by a fear of social interaction. Agoraphobia restricts sufferers' daily living if they cannot enter any crowded area and become unable to leave home. Psychodynamic approaches indicate that this phobia may be a defence mechanism enabling the sufferer to avoid tackling some other source of anxiety. However, psychodynamic therapies are not often found to be effective in treating agoraphobia, behavioural approaches usually being preferred. Behavioural approaches attempt to reduce the symptoms of the phobia by such techniques as *exposure*. See also *phobia*.

Antidepressants: noradrenaline and serotonin levels are involved in some, if not all, forms of depression. General dissatisfaction with older tricyclic antidepressants (TCADs or TCAs) led to the introduction of a number of new antidepressant drugs, such as newer TCAs, tetracyclic antidepressants (for example, mianserin), monoamine oxidase inhibitors, lithium salts and 5HT uptake inhibitors (for example, Prozac).

TCAs affect the reuptake of noradrenaline, serotonin and other neurotransmitters into the neurones, prolonging the effects of these transmitters and, in some cases, producing a sedative effect. Tetracyclic antidepressants also seem to affect noradrenaline and serotonin levels, although their action is not well understood.

Examples of 5HT inhibitors are fluoxetine, fluoxamine and citalopram. Prozac is fluoxetine hydrochloride. 5HT inhibitors block the reuptake of 5HT (serotonin only), producing an increase in the amount of this neurotransmitter at central synapses. They appear to have little or no effect on the reuptake of other central neurotransmitters. They are effective over a broad range of depressive symptoms with the same efficiency as TCAs but have little sedative action and fewer undesirable effects. 5HT Inhibitors are thought to be particularly useful for obsessive-compulsive disorder and possibly for suicidal patients, but less so for agitated depression.

Anxiety disorders: a medical term used for severe psychological disorders in which abnormal or chronic anxiety interferes with daily living. There are three main diagnostic categories in common usage: panic attacks, phobias and obsessive-compulsive disorder. DSM IV (American Psychiatric Association, 1994) splits anxiety into sub-groups:

- panic disorder without agoraphobia
- panic disorder with agoraphobia

- agoraphobia without history of panic disorder
- specific phobia
- social phobia
- obsessive-compulsive disorder
- post-traumatic stress disorder
- acute stress disorder
- generalised anxiety disorder
- anxiety disorder (related to general medical or substance-induced condition)
- anxiety disorder (not otherwise specified).

Anxiety hierarchy: a series of goals to be achieved by the client during therapy (Milne, 1993: 122). See also Chapter 4.

Anxiety management: techniques for controlling anxiety can be taught individually or within a group setting where members can offer support to each other. Anxiety management training is usually offered as a course comprising a number of sessions which may include:

- explanations of anxiety
- relaxation therapy
- breathing control
- thought-challenging/cognitive restructuring
- assertiveness training.

The client is encouraged to practise skills as 'homework'. Where the anxiety is associated with a specific phobia, exposure to the feared object or situation is included in the programme.

Anxiety neurosis: a vague term used by some people to describe undesirable or socially unacceptable anxiety. It is not normally used as a medical term.

Anxiolytics: drugs that have an anxiety-reducing effect. These include *benzodiazepines*, barbiturates, beta-blockers and some of the *antipsychotic* drugs. See also Chapters 5 and 12.

Apprehension: a word derived from understanding or grasping of ideas, commonly used instead of 'apprehensive' to signify a feeling of unease or dread concerning some future event.

Arousal: the physiological arousal experienced in anxiety is not distinguished from arousal felt in any stressful or painful situation, but can be distinguished from anger or other *basic emotions*. See Chapters 6 and 20.

Assessment of anxiety and depression: assessment may be objective or subjective, using tools such as an adjective checklist, a linear scale (from no anxiety to worst possible anxiety) or a questionnaire. Examples of questionnaires include the Self-Evaluation Questionnaire for State and Trait Anxiety (Spielberger *et al.*,1968), the Hamilton Depression Rating Scale, the Hamilton Anxiety Scale and the Montgomery and Asber Depression Rating Scale (cited in Montgomery, 1990). Any of these assessment tools may be used in one or more of the following categories:

- **observation** (physical, verbal and non-verbal signs): sweating, raised pulse rate, raised blood pressure and other physical signs; expression of

anger, aggression, agitation or impatience; facial expressions, posture, mannerisms, excessive talking, withdrawal, indication of cognitive impairment or regression
- **self-report** (physical, cognitive, emotional and behavioural symptoms) physical symptoms may include 'butterflies', headache, nausea, bowel movement disturbances and generalised aches and pains. Emotional symptoms may include mood fluctuations, lack of confidence, or worry and fear. Alterations to thinking and behaviour may include feelings of confusion and an inability to think straight, increased clumsiness, forgetfulness, preoccupation and a lack of concentration.

Benzodiazapines: hypnotic and anxiolytic drugs which are thought to act by facilitating an inhibitory transmitter (GABA) that dampens neuronal activity in the brain. Different preparations may work in slightly different ways to achieve some or all of the desired effects and may bring different undesired (side-) effects:

Desired effects
- muscle-relaxant
- anticonvulsant
- hypnotic (sleep-inducing)
- sedation (calming)
- reduce anxiety.

Undesired effects
- incompatibility with alcohol
- tolerance
- drowsiness
- 'rebound' insomnia
- dependency
- impaired psychomotor performance
- dizziness
- dry mouth
- involuntary motor activity at high dose.

Benzodiazapines can be divided into two groups:

- Intermediate-acting compounds act for 6–10 hours and carry a greater risk of withdrawal symptoms but less risk of excessive accumulation
- Long-acting compounds, lasting up to 24 hours, have less risk of withdrawal problems but repeated doses may lead to the accumulation of drug metabolites, with their undesirable effects.

Although benzodiazapines used to be thought to be harmless, it is now recognised that their continued use carries significant risks. Treatment is recommended to be restricted to 2–4 weeks for the relief of severe anxiety only. The elderly and those with hepatic or renal difficulties are likely to be particularly susceptible to the adverse effects.

When long-term use of any drugs is not advisable, some form of psychological intervention is preferable. Benzodiazepines are not recommended for phobic or obsessional states.

Bipolar disorders: the term 'bipolar disorder' may be used to encompass a range of possible mood disturbances that are experienced over time. The term comes from the recognition that a few people with a bipolar disorder may experience two opposite extremes, swinging between periods of depression and excitement (mania). People suffering this condition used to be known as manic-depressives, but this label has unhelpful connotations and, as with all names that label the person rather than the condition, is best not used. The diagnosis of bipolar disorder may be used wherever a person experiences episodes of overexcitement or mania, or a more moderate hypomania, with or without periods of depression, in a pattern that does not necessarily alternate.

Compulsions: actions, often linked to obsessions (thoughts), that a person has an irresistible urge to carry out. These are irrational and may occur with or without some understanding of what drives them. Attempting to resist the compulsions may create anxiety, so the actions tend to be repetitive in order to avoid this. Compulsions are often associated with ritualistic behaviours involving adherence to a specific sequence of activities. Common compulsions include cleaning, checking, counting and hoarding. See also obsessions and obsessive-compulsive disorder.

Conditioned anxiety: the behaviourist approach suggests that anxiety may be learned by *classical conditioning*, when adreno-SNS arousal becomes associated with certain situations. This may be specific at first but can generalise. The anxiety may then be maintained by *operant conditioning* if the behaviour is reinforced. Behavioural approaches attempt to reduce the anxiety by such techniques as *systematic desensitisation*. See Chapter 4.

Defence mechanisms: psychodynamic approaches suggest that many of the symptoms of anxiety disorders such as phobias are defence mechanisms that enable the sufferer to avoid tackling other emotional issues. See Chapter 17.

Depression: a diagnosis of depression or depressive illness is made where a person has a persistent or pervasive condition characterised by low mood, pessimism, feelings of low self-worth and reduced energy level. The condition may be mild or severe. Depression appears to be the most common formal psychiatric disorder. The incidence of either depression or anxiety is thought to be about 15 per cent of the general population over a period of a year. Estimates vary according to the population studied and the diagnostic criteria used. Significant differences are found in the literature between diagnoses for males and females, and for different age, socioeconomic and ethnic groups.

The word 'depression' is often used loosely in lay terms to refer to a low mood or sadness, and this needs to be distinguished from the clinical use of the term. If a piece of research suggests, for example, that the diagnosis of some spinal cord injuries is not generally associated with depression, it is not being suggested that the patients are not profoundly upset and sad but that they are not outside normal limits of feelings of self-worth. There is a common assumption that such patients will, and should be, depressed. This may lead to depression, when it does occur, being taken for granted instead of being recognised as abnormal and serious. It is therefore likely to be left untreated.

All people experience periods of despondency and despair, as well as feelings of extreme well-being. One view is that depression and bipolar disorders are simply extremes of otherwise normal emotional swings. However, the biology of mood or *affective* disorders suggests that these illnesses represent major alterations in normal brain function (Wingard *et al.*, 1991). This debate has implications for interventions. If the illnesses are merely extreme forms of normal behaviour, this might suggest that they are amenable to talking therapies (for example, Rowe, 1983). If, on the other hand, there is significant alteration in brain function, drug therapy might be an important part of treatment. There is ongoing debate about which approach is preferable, with strong feelings on both sides.

According to Montgomery (1990), classifications tend to depend on symptoms. Traditionally, the clinical diagnosis of depression has identified two main types: exogenous (reactive) and endogenous. If the depression seems to have been brought on by events and the causes can be identified, the depression is labelled 'reactive', that is, reacting to the environment. If there is no known cause and the person just seems to be depressed for no reason, or it seems part of his or her personality, the depression is labelled 'endogenous' or within the person. There is no clear distinction between reactive depression and the kind of depression that would be seen as part of post-traumatic stress disorder. In many cases, there may be a mild underlying endogenous depression or potential for depression that is brought to the fore by distressing events. Diagnosis into these two categories is difficult and can be misleading.

Other diagnoses of depression include retarded depression and agitated depression. Retarded depression means psychomotor retardation or slowing down. The condition responds to some antidepressants and the label can avoid the stigma associated with clinical depression. Agitated depression is characterised by moderate-to-high levels of anxiety. The accompanying continuous physical restlessness is referred to as psychomotor agitation and may be observed in pacing or fidgeting behaviours. It may also be seen as restlessness combined with slowing down. It used to be treated with sedatives but this practice is now questioned.

The current classification of depression depends on:

- origins:
    exogenous (reactive)
    endogenous
- pattern:
    unipolar
    bipolar
    seasonal affective disorder
    postnatal
    cyclothymic disorder

ANXIETY AND DEPRESSION   23

- features:
    psychomotor agitation
    psychomotor retardation
    presence or absence of perceptual distortions.

Desensitisation: in this context, a behavioural technique used to treat anxiety disorders. See also Chapters 1 and 4.

Dimensions of anxiety: there are a number of ways of classifying anxiety, including:

- duration – transitory or enduring
- strength – mild or severe
- context – localised, generalised or free-floating
- state or trait.

Endogenous depression: see *depression*.

Fear: the words 'fear' and 'anxiety' are often used interchangeably. However, it is sometimes useful to make a distinction and there are various ways of doing this. Some people use the word 'fear' when the object of the emotion is known, and 'anxiety' when the object is unknown. To some, fear represents a stronger emotion than anxiety, linked with a greater perceived threat. Others use anxiety for the state of emotional arousal, and fear for the belief or cognitive component – such that when we *know* we are frightened we may *experience* symptoms of anxiety. See also Chapter 6.

Free-floating anxiety: a term used for trait anxiety where a person has a tendency to be anxious all the time about many things that are not related to specific situations.

Generalised anxiety: when someone has developed a localised anxiety, this may generalise to associated items. For example, anxiety associated with going to a dentist who wears a white coat may generalise to all people in white coats.

Hospitalisation: anxiety may be one of the outcomes of stress or uncertainty precipitated by hospitalisation. Wattley and Muller (1984) referred to the work of Volicier and Bohannon (1975) and compared nurses' and patients' expectations of what was most likely to create anxiety. They found that patients were less anxious than nurses thought they would be about thinking that they might have pain after surgery or might have their appearance altered. Patients were unexpectedly worried about having nurses be in too much of a hurry or by not having the call light answered. Important on all lists was anxiety about not being told the diagnosis, the results of tests or the reasons for treatment.

Localised anxiety: a term used to describe anxiety that occurs in response to a particular object or event such as going to the dentist or having an injection. This is also referred to as situation-specific anxiety. In many cases, the word 'phobia' is popularly used for this kind of anxiety. However, it is usually better to reserve 'phobia' for where the anxiety is extreme and interferes with all normal daily living activities.

Neurosis: excessive anxiety or worry that has become an unhealthy, overly distressing or destructive part of an individual's personality or lifestyle.

Traditionally, mental illnesses have been classified as either neurotic or psychotic, with the implication that 'neurotics' are aware of their disabilities and 'psychotics' are out of touch with reality and thus not aware. However, this approach to mental health and this kind of labelling of people is considered controversial and not a useful part of person-centred approaches.

Neurotic: sometimes used as a lay term to describe excess worry or anxiety; it can be distinguished from 'neurosis' as used in classifications of mental health disorders.

Normal anxiety: in everyday life, a certain level of anxiety is normal and may help to prepare us physiologically for coping with demands. It is accepted as normal if it is appropriate to the circumstances, improves (or at least does not impair) performance and does not interfere unduly with daily living. Views of what is appropriate may vary with social grouping and circumstances. See also Chapter 3.

Obsessions: recurrent and persistent intrusive thoughts and beliefs over which the individual has no apparent conscious control, often resulting in compulsive behaviour. In the medical sense, obsessions are seen as disorders. Treatment may be needed where the individual is badly affected by obsessions and cannot continue with the desired lifestyle. Cognitive and behavioural treatment involves helping people to recognise that the thoughts are generated by them; it may focus on *thought-stopping*. See Chapters 4 and 6.

Obsessive-compulsive disorder: a medical diagnosis of a disorder in which an individual suffers recurrent, persistent intrusive thoughts that compel him or her to carry out specific actions interfering with daily living. If the person is prevented from carrying out these actions, severe anxiety is experienced. Psychodynamic approaches (see Chapter 17) suggest that the disorder arises as a *defence mechanism*, which, through displacement, is shielding the individual from having to deal with some other emotional issue. In practice, psychodynamic therapies that address hidden emotions are not often successful in treating this disorder, and cognitive and behavioural approaches are more often used. However, psychodynamic therapists sometimes argue that behavioural techniques result only in short-term benefits.

Obsessive-compulsive personality: this label may be applied to a person whose behaviour patterns are inflexible and governed by a desire for perfection. Such people do not recognise the senselessness of their behaviour and differ from those with an obsessive-compulsive disorder, who recognise that their behaviour is irrational or absurd. The term implies that if particular obsessions or compulsions are eliminated through behavioural techniques without addressing underlying emotional components, the individual may later develop other obsessions and compulsions.

Outcomes of anxiety: anxiety may have consequences for health status and precipitate conditions such as:

- migraine
- angina
- aggravation of psoriasis, asthma, eczema and other disorders

- disturbances of bowel movement resulting in constipation, diarrhoea or irritable bowel syndrome
- unstable maintenance of diabetes
- vulnerability to hospital-acquired (nosocomial) infections
- cognitive impairment, which has implications for patient teaching and self-care
- altered appetite and eating habits, which affect nutritional state
- insomnia and restlessness, perhaps leading to reduced healing
- lethargy, which may lead to low motivation and rejection of help
- a lowered pain threshold.

Panic: an intense, sudden, overwhelming, uncontrollable feeling that is interpreted as terror and accompanied by immediate physiological changes that may result in immobility or senseless 'hysterical' behaviour.

Panic attacks: sudden discrete episodes of intense fear. Attacks can be initially unexpected, as in panic disorder or post-traumatic stress disorder, or they may occur as a reaction to a feared object or situation as part of a phobic disorder. The DSM IV (American Psychiatric Association, 1994) states that for a panic attack to be diagnosed as such, four of the following somatic or cognitive symptoms must be experienced and that these must reach a peak within 10 minutes:

- palpitations
- sweating
- trembling or shaking
- sensations of shortness of breath or smothering
- feelings of choking
- chest pain or discomfort
- nausea
- feeling dizzy, unsteady, lightheaded or faint
- derealisation or depersonalisation
- fear of losing control or going mad
- fear of dying
- paraesthesia
- chills or hot flushes.

Montgomery (1990) argues that panic attacks cannot be considered as a separate anxiety disorder and that they occur in many patients diagnosed as suffering from major depression.

Panic disorder: a relatively recently developed construct used to label the recurrence of panic attacks where there is no apparent precipitating factor. The DSM IV criteria are that the attacks are recent and unexpected, and that at least one of the attacks has been followed by persistent worry about having further attacks, concerns about the implications or consequences of the attack or a change in behaviour related to the attacks. These are distinguished from phobias, in which the symptoms may be similar. However, the distinction is sometimes blurred if the person believes that attacks are more likely in certain contexts. Avoidance of situations where panic attacks have been experienced may lead to a restricted lifestyle, and in severe cases the sufferer may become completely housebound, as in some forms of agoraphobia.

Phobia: an abnormal or morbid fear or aversion that is inconsistent or incompatible with the threat posed by the feared object or situation (Greek *phobia* = fear). This may be accompanied by panic attacks. Individuals may have one specific phobia (monophobia), several phobias that may be linked (polyphobia) or a generalised diffuse phobic disposition. Onset may be sudden, following one disturbing incident, or gradual with no apparent triggering event.

Psychodynamic explanations view phobias as resulting from the repression of memories of traumatic events. Behavioural and social learning approaches describe phobias as learned through conditioning and copying the behaviour of others. It is argued that phobias are reinforced and maintained by increased attention from others and the avoidance of unwanted activities.

If a precipitating incident is recognised and resolved, through either psychodynamic, cognitive or person-centred counselling, the phobia may lesson or even disappear. However, in many cases it is not possible to discover any original event, or if one is known, its recognition alone does not lead to a reduction of symptoms. In practice, the behavioural approach of progressive desensitisation is found to be most successful in reducing symptoms (see Chapter 4). However, if there is an underlying unresolved problem, different symptoms may emerge at a later date.

One feature of phobias is that people report seeing a great many examples of the feared object. When they are better, far fewer are noticed. For example, a patient may report that there are now fewer cats in her neighbourhood since she has been cured of her phobia of cats.

Post-traumatic stress disorder (PTSD): a maladaptive response to major trauma: either a single dramatic trauma such as a natural disaster or injury, or extreme enduring circumstances such as persistent harassment at work. Features are intrusive imagery, avoidance of anything reminiscent of the trauma and uncharacteristic irritability. See also Chapter 20.

Reactive depression: see *depression*.

Retarded depression: see *depression*.

Seasonal affective disorder (SAD): this is best translated as seasonal mood disorder (see also Chapter 6) and is the name given to a recently identified syndrome in which people are seen to become much lower or negative in mood, some tending towards depression, in the winter months. It has been suggested that the condition may be related to a change in serotonin levels due to lack of light stimulation perhaps of the pineal gland, and some treatments involve exposure to light (for example, Dalgleish and Rosen, 1996).

State and trait effects: it is suggested that there is a significant difference between conditions that are inherent in an individual as personality or temperament traits and those which are the outcome of specific events. There are measurable differences, but if only the 'state' scores are known, it may not be possible to distinguish between different precipitating factors.

Spielberger *et al.* (1968) distinguish between state and trait anxiety:

Dimension	**State anxiety**	**Trait anxiety**
duration	transitory	enduring
context	situation specific	free-floating or generalised
emotion	fear and tension	apprehension
explanation	cognitive appraisal linked to adreno-SNS arousal	personality characteristic or disposition

In relation to depression, Williams *et al.* (1988) use research in human *information processing* to work towards a distinction between cognitive disturbance that is a response to particular events (state) and that which arises from a particular cognitive style or trait disposition (trait). This can be compared with the medical diagnoses of reactive and endogenous depression.

3 ATTITUDES, ATTITUDE CHANGE AND PERSUASION

Attitudes are settled or fixed ways of responding to people and objects in the environment. They involve what people know or believe and what they feel, as well as what they say and do. Attitudes can be stuck in a rut or can change in response to new experiences or persuasion. Psychological study is concerned with how attitudes are expressed and how they develop and change throughout the lifespan.

Definitions	
Allport (1937)	An attitude is a mental and neural state of readiness, organized through experience, exerting a directive or dynamic influence upon the individual's response to all objects and situations with which it is related.
Thurstone (1948)	An enduring, learned predisposition to behave in a consistent way toward a given class of objects, or the persistent mental and/or neural readiness to react to objects, not as they are, but as they are conceived to be.
Rokeach (1960, 1968)	A learned orientation, or disposition, toward an object or situation, which provides a tendency to respond favourably or unfavourably to the object or situation.
Triandis (1971)	A person can be said to have an 'attitude' towards an object, person or situation if his or her emotional reaction, thoughts or behaviour towards that object, person or situation is similar on various different occasions.
Bem (1970)	Attitudes are likes and dislikes.
Tajfel and Fraser (1978)	An attitude can be compared with 'set' or fixity in problem-solving, and is a mental organisation that intervenes between basic psychological processes like 'needs' and 'motives' and the action that is caused by them.

Approaches, Arguments and Applications

Triandis (1971) gives the following reasons for holding settled attitudes. They:

- help us understand the world around us, by organising and simplifying a very complex input from our environment
- protect our self-esteem by making it possible for us to avoid unpleasant truths about ourselves
- help us to adjust in a complex world by making it more likely that we will react so as to maximise our rewards from the environment
- allow us to express our fundamental values.

Attitudes help us to function with least effort. Once we have established a pattern of reactions to a given category of attitude objects, we are saved from having to decide again, starting from first principles, what our reaction should be. Our previous experience is a guide. Moreover, we can adjust socially by making it easier to get along with people who have similar attitudes (Newcomb, 1953).

Much psychological research into attitudes explores the relationship between three basic components, or psychological domains – cognitive, affective and behavioural – looking at the consistency or inconsistency between beliefs, feelings and actions. Some standpoints focus only on the emotional aspects of the attitude or on one aspect at a time.

A significant theoretical approach is the *three-component model* (from Rosenberg and Hovland, 1960). This is based on behavioural principles and considers the expression of all three domains to be the behavioural outcomes of an attitude, with equal emphasis on each component. Observation of all outcomes leads to inferences about the attitude. The attitude itself is defined as an 'intervening variable' or abstract concept that cannot be measured directly (Figure 3.1).

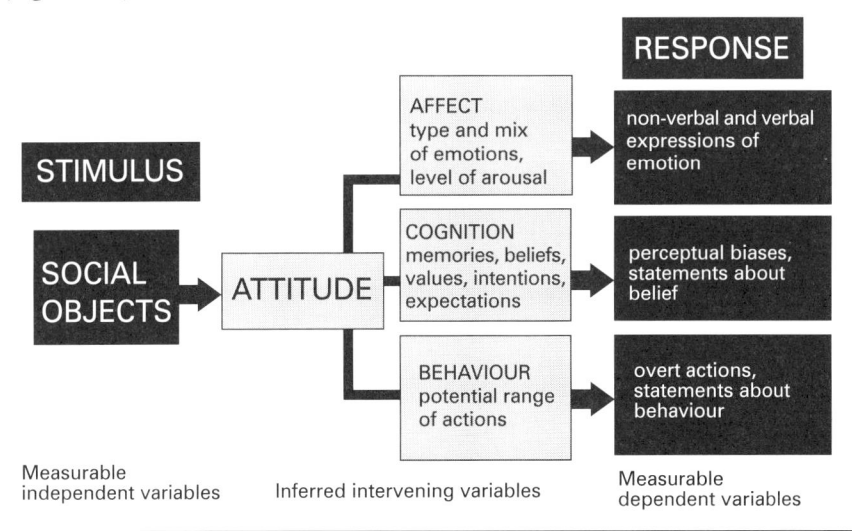

Figure 3.1 Three-component model of attitude (*after Rosenberg and Hovland, 1960*)

In most common usage, an attitude is regarded as having mainly cognitive and emotional components, which then lead to behaviour. From this point of view, questioning a person about beliefs and feelings is thought to give direct information about the attitude. The main debate is whether attitudes can be measured directly by questionnaire or only indirectly, by observing all responses.

Current trends towards the integration of cognition and affect (see Chapter 6) and away from viewing these as separate domains may gradually lead to a new way of assessing attitudes.

Key Terms and Concepts

Affective domain: one of the traditional domains of psychology (after Kant), which is viewed as a component of attitudes, involving the emotional aspects.

Ambivalence: having two opposite emotions, attitudes or motivations towards an object, for example love–hate. The prefix 'ambi' means on both sides, and the word ambivalence comes from the idea of being equally powerful on both sides. An ambivalent attitude to smoking might involve wanting a cigarette at the same time as wanting to give up smoking. It is believed that the two opposites develop quite separately so that the person finds it impossible to integrate them and either hesitates or alternates between the two extremes or represses one of them until a choice can be made. In casual usage, the word 'ambivalent' is often used simply to mean hesitancy.

Attitude change: a change in cognitions, emotions or actions in relation to an attitude object that can come about either because it is intrinsically desired by the person concerned or as a result of the deliberate persuasion by others. See persuasion.

Attitude object: almost anything can serve as an attitude object, and what seems trivial to one person may evoke strong reactions in another, such as which end of a boiled egg to crack open, a theme explored satirically by Jonathan Swift in *Gulliver's Travels*. Stroebe and Stroebe (1995: 14) define an attitude object as 'any discriminable aspect of the physical or social environment, such as things (cars, drugs), people (doctors, the British), behaviour (jogging, drinking alcohol) or even abstract ideas (religion, health)'.

Attitude questionnaires: the simplest way of directly measuring attitudes is through questionnaires. These usually consist of a set of questions or statements to each of which the respondent assigns a score on a Likert-type scale (see Chapter 18). Designing an attitude questionnaire usually involves the following steps:

- Define the topic, attitude object and participants
- Sort out the aspects – cognitive, affective, behavioural
- Choose the *dimension,* such as favourability/unfavourability
- Select the statements and test them for validity
- Construct a *Likert scale.*

See Chapter 18 for details of constructing questionnaires.

Cognitive dissonance: Festinger (1957) developed cognitive dissonance theory based on the proposal that there is a basic need or drive for consistency of beliefs. If a person holds two ideas that are inconsistent, this is likely to result in discomfort, so the person is motivated to remove the inconsistency. This may be done by changing one of the ideas or by ignoring or repressing one of them. An example of cognitive dissonance can be seen when a person holds humanistic beliefs that every individual has the right to be self-determining that conflict with religious beliefs that certain actions such as euthanasia, suicide and abortion are morally wrong. The concept of dissonance is also often used to refer to inconsistency between beliefs and behaviour. Where behaviour is inconsistent with a belief, either the behaviour or the belief may be changed to reduce the dissonance. In practice, it is found that most people are more likely to change their beliefs than their behaviour. For example, someone who 'knows' that increased exercise would promote health but does not want to exercise may justify the lack of exercise by finding reasons to suggest that exercise can be harmful.

Development of attitudes: Niven (1994) identifies three main ways in which attitudes are formed: *operant* (or *instrumental*) *conditioning*, *modelling* and direct experience. The principles of operant conditioning (see Chapter 4) are based on the reinforcement of responses to stimuli. A child's parents, teachers and friends will often provide reinforcement for expressing the 'right' attitude and criticise the 'wrong' one. When the child is rewarded for saying or doing something, he or she is more likely to repeat this action. The reward may be only slight, such as a nod or continued attention. (The outcome of criticism or punishment is not usually predictable; an individual may drop or change an unwelcome attitude or may find ways of avoiding its being noticed.) Modelling refers to copying others who may or may not realise they are being used as 'role-models'. Many attitudes are learned by children acting out in play things they have seen their parents do or have watched on television. Attitudes acquired through direct experience with an attitude object or person tend to be stronger and more vivid that those acquired 'second hand' through conditioning or modelling (for example, Fazio and Zanna, 1978).

Dimensions of attitudes: when measuring attitudes, a number of different dimensions can be considered:

- polarity or sign (+ve or –ve, that is favourable or unfavourable)
- clarity
- specificity
- consistency
- strength
- importance.

The most common of these to be measured, using *attitude questionnaires* with *Likert-type scales*, is polarity or favourability/unfavourability.

Discrimination: the observable behavioural component of prejudice, in which people express or demonstrate unfavourable attitudes towards an individual or group. Allport (1954) proposes five levels or strengths of discrimination:

- antilocution: hostile talk, verbal insults, racial or sexual jokes
- avoidance: keeping a distance without inflicting any harm
- discrimination: exclusion – from housing, civil rights and employment
- physical attack: violence against persons or their property
- extermination: violence against an entire group.

Labelling: referring to individuals in terms of a medical diagnosis or membership of a group, based on a particular feature such as an impairment, disability or age group, for example 'a schizophrenic', 'a diabetic', 'the elderly', 'the disabled', 'the deaf' (Figure 3.2). Some of the disadvantages of such labelling can be summarised as follows. The individual:

- no longer has equal opportunity or rights in 'normal' society but has become part of a minority group and cast in a particular role associated with the group
- is in danger of the labelling becoming a self-fulfilling prophecy of worthlessness, with consequent loss of self-esteem and alienation from society
- experiences less choice about his or her care and treatment because a label brings 'a packet of treatment' instead of an individual approach for that unique person
- is prevented from partaking in an holistic approach to therapy but instead has to submit to the treatment system associated with a particular condition
- is denied control of his or her own life and its health/disease balance, and is placed in a subordinate role as the receiver of care and treatment. Insight is not encouraged so preventive action on the part of the individual is not fostered.

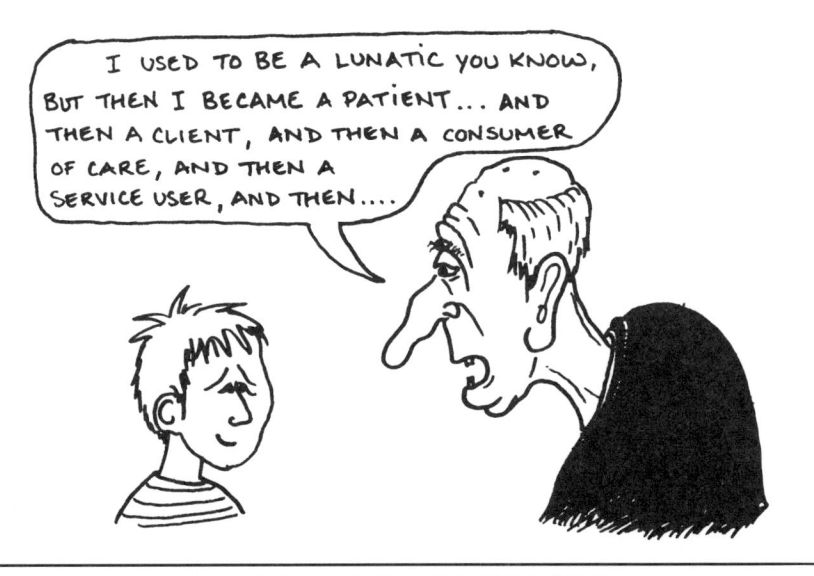

Figure 3.2 Labelling (*Bill O'Neill, 1997*).

Instead of labelling the *person* in terms of a particular attribute, it can be more productive to name only the *attribute*. For example, it might be better to say 'Mrs Smith has diabetes' instead of 'Mrs Smith is a diabetic.' The slight change in wording makes a significant change to the emphasis, such that if we know that Mrs Smith has diabetes, we can work with Mrs Smith to help her manage her lifestyle, but if she is seen primarily as 'a diabetic', the emphasis is more likely to be on the medical condition and a set of common findings or a stereotype associated with it. Compare the instruction 'Nurse, please give an insulin injection immediately to the diabetic in bed 3' with 'Sarah, please could you help Mrs Smith with her insulin injection, which is due now.'

Interestingly, we readily label many people in terms of conditions such as 'diabetics' and 'epileptics' but do not do so to people with multiple sclerosis, cancer or heart disease. It has been pointed out by a colleague that the latter conditions are life-threatening and it may be that we refrain from labelling the person in such situations. See also Chapter 9.

Manipulation: behaving in a way that results in changes in the environment or the behaviour of others, usually to their detriment, with or without conscious awareness. Describing a person in lay terms as manipulative usually implies that the person is deliberately and unfairly controlling other people through emotional blackmail or threats. Within psychodynamic approaches, the label may be used to describe behaviour that is unconsciously determined so that the person does not appreciate, in a normal way, the emotional effects of the behaviour on other people or understand his or her own motives.

Message (*text*) variables: in constructing a persuasive communication, a number of decisions have to be made. For example, should the strongest arguments be saved until the end or given first? Should counterarguments be included? To what extent is it effective to arouse an emotional response?

In a one-sided argument, putting the strongest argument first is an advantage only if the audience is initially uninterested in the topic. If each side is being presented by different people, as in a formal debate, there is no particular advantage in being first. The inclusion of counterarguments is more effective if the audience initially disagrees with the speaker or if the listeners are highly educated. A two-sided argument is also better if the participants are already familiar with the topic. It seems that if participants are likely to counterargue between themselves, the speaker (or writer) is more likely to win them over when he or she recognises the counterargument.

Insko (1967) demonstrated that strong fear is more effective if participants are, at the same time, given some reassuring recommendation as to how the threat can be averted. In particular, it was demonstrated that strong fear can be effective in strengthening the resolve of non-smokers never to smoke, but low or moderate fear is better in changing the opinion of smokers against smoking.

It also makes a difference whether information is spoken, written or developed through role-playing or other interactive techniques. See Figure 3.3 and also receiver (*consumer*), sender (*producer*) variables and Chapter 9.

Producer	Text	Consumer
prestige intention success bias self-interest similarity	order counterarguments emotional appeal involvement role-playing	personality gender previous experience reference group reasons for attitude stage of formation

independent variables

→ **dependent variables: ATTITUDE CHANGE**

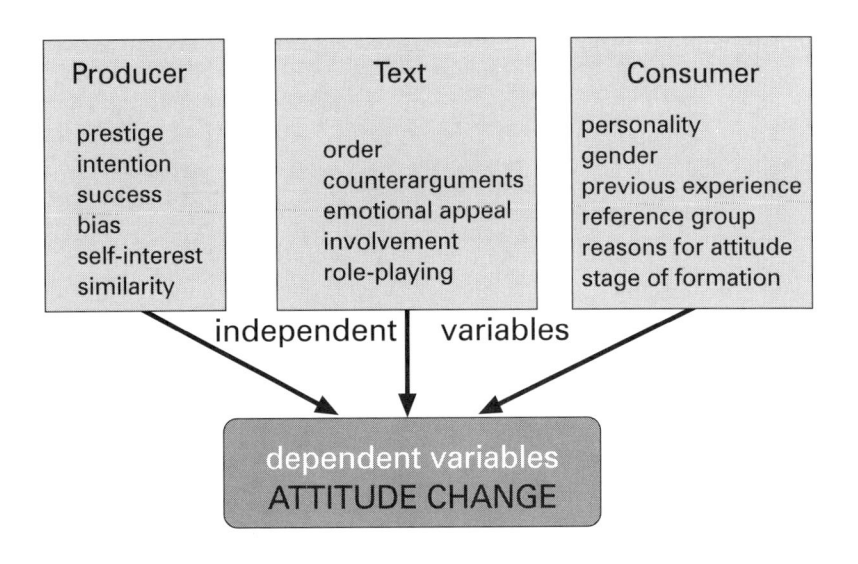

Figure 3.3 Communication variables

Opinion: a *verbal* statement of an attitude or of what a person believes or values. In common usage, the words 'opinion' and 'attitude' can be used interchangeably. However, it is generally understood that an opinion is something explicitly stated, whereas an attitude need not be. It is found that people's statements of their opinions, or what they think is their attitude, can differ widely from what is observed in their behaviour (for example, La Piere, 1934). It is this kind of finding that has fostered the development of the *three-component* approach to attitudes, since the integration of information concerning beliefs, emotions and actions, separately gathered, gives a more reliable picture than does simply asking people to state an opinion or attitude.

Persuasion: a deliberate attempt by an individual or an organisation to bring about a change of attitude, opinion, belief, value, feelings or actions in another individual or group (Figure 3.4).

Most persuasion aims to get people to do things that they would not otherwise have done. People will not normally act before they see that it is in some way to their advantage to do so. Persuasion helps them to make up or change their minds. From the point of view of the person being persuaded, the process may entail a certain degree of emotional pressure. The word 'persuasion' may be used with or without the implication of emotional pressure.

A scale can be drawn with influence at one end and coercion at the other, persuasion lying somewhere in between (Gill and Adams, 1992). In this model, the word persuasion is taken to imply some emotional pressure:

Influence ← .... persuasion .... → coercion

(rational argument) .... (reason + emotion) .... (threat)

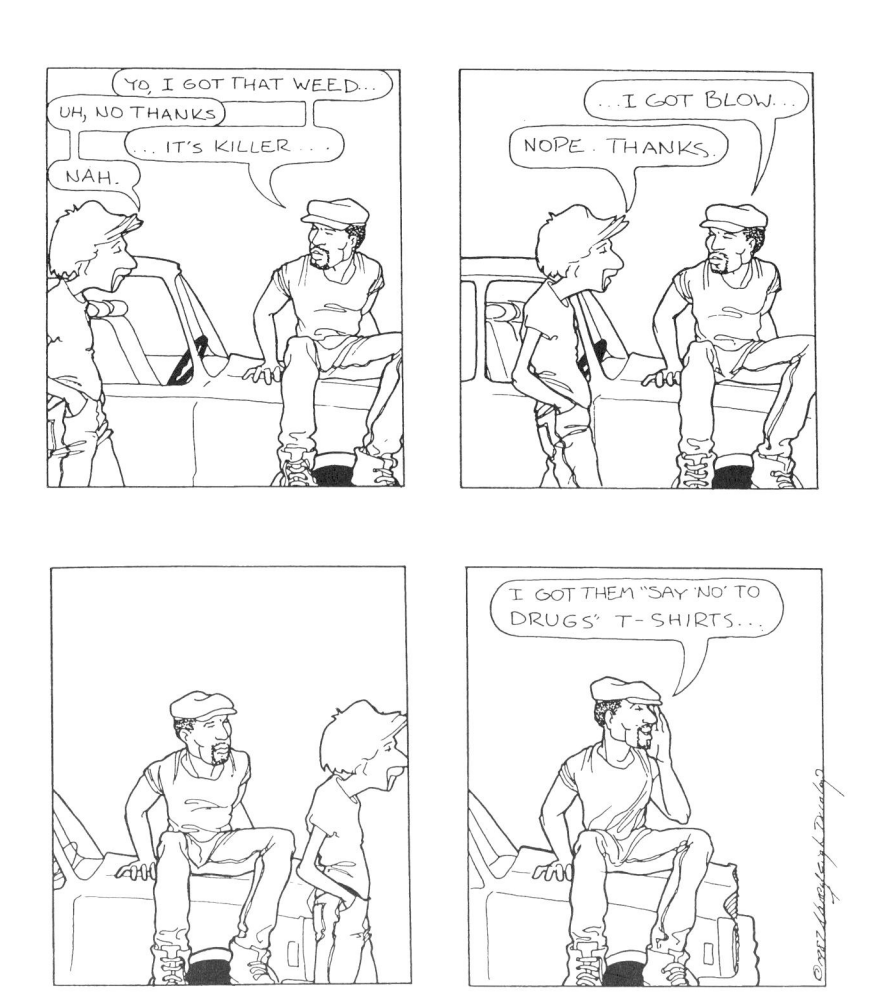

Figure 3.4   Persuasion (*N. Leigh Dunlop, 1987*)

The term 'influence' can refer to the way in which a person may be responding simply to information, education and rational argument, free to make up his or her own mind without emotional pressure. At the other extreme, the pressure is a threat of punishment that coerces or makes someone do something against their will. Brown (1988) suggests that, historically, it is the development of speech that has provided the possibility of changing people's attitudes or opinions without the use of force. Freedom to resist persuasion dwindles the more that coercion, or techniques appealing to emotions of which the recipient is not fully aware, is used.

For effective persuasion, it is first necessary to decide what one desires to change. Research in this area was prominent in the first half of the twentieth century, mostly in connection with propaganda and persuasive communication. For example, Lasswell (1948, cited in Gill and Adams, 1992) developed a political propaganda model of communication 'Who, says what, in which channel, to whom, with what effect?' This early work was based on process models of communication identifying the three key elements of the process as *sender*, *message* and *receiver*. These may be renamed *producer*, *text* and *consumer* (see Chapter 9).

To bring about an attitude change, it is possible to examine and manipulate variables of all three elements. In any experiment, one or more of these is varied systematically and the remainder held constant or randomised. See Figure 3.3, and separate entries for *sender* (*producer*), *message* (*text*) and *receiver* (*consumer*) variables.

This separation of variables can be directly compared with a behavioural model of effective communication devised by Berlo (1960), who identified the characteristics of sender, message and receiver in terms of individual attributes and the sensory channels available. See also Gill and Adams (1992).

Prejudice: the word 'prejudice' literally means prejudgement and is used when someone has formed an attitude about an individual person or object without taking into account any knowledge about the individual. Such prejudgements are usually based on assumptions about a *group* of which the individual is perceived to be a member (see also Chapter 19). In the widest sense, a prejudgement could be favourable or unfavourable; Atkinson *et al.* (1996) suggest, for example, that a person could be strongly prejudiced in favour of eating oranges. However, in common usage, the term is usually reserved for negative or demeaning attitudes towards people. Allport (1954) defines prejudice as:

an antipathy based on a faulty and inflexible generalisation directed towards a group as a whole or towards an individual because he is a member of that group. It may be felt or expressed.

There are a number of theoretical approaches that attempt to identify the main causes of prejudice, for example:

- authoritarian personality
- social norms
- intergroup conflict
- scapegoating.

People with the cluster of traits viewed as the authoritarian personality (see Chapter 15) are those who are submissive and obedient to authority, emphasise discipline and conventionalism, tend to see everything in terms of 'black and white', reject groups other than their own and like to ally themselves with an authority figure. This does not, however, explain all prejudice. It can be observed that many people hold specific prejudices in relation to a target group rather than being prejudiced against all those who do not belong to their own group. Personality scores fail to distinguish between high and low prejudice. However, endorsement of social norms by those in positions of authority is significant, and prejudice can be readily created. This was demonstrated by Jane Elliott in her 'blue eyes – brown eyes' exercises (Aronson and Osherow, 1980 and shown on Channel 4 TV in *The Class Divided*). She showed how young children and adults very quickly adopt unpleasant behaviour towards each other when a group is divided according to eye colour and the participants are told that blue-eyed people are better than brown-eyed or vice versa.

People can be shown to demonstrate different prejudices in different social groups, and it appears that many prejudices, like attitudes in general, are learned by processes of conditioning and modelling. As with all attitudes, prejudices can be seen to have cognitive, affective and behavioural components. The behavioural component is observable as *discrimination*.

Receiver (*consumer*) variables: there are two main questions here:

- Are some personalities or types more susceptible to persuasion?
- Are different activities likely to affect attitude change?

Variables include gender, age or other 'reference group', personality and previous experience with the attitude object.

There is some suggestion that suggestibility or persuasability is greater in females (Whittaker and Meade, 1967), declines between the ages of 14 and 32, and is in men related to self-esteem. Cox and Bauer (1964) found an inverted U-curve (curvilinear) relationship between self-esteem and persuasability. Men with medium self-esteem were most susceptible; those with low self-esteem tended to react against the communication and shift their opinions further away, whereas those with high self-esteem were not affected at all. Suggestibility is also found to increase in situations where people have reduced sensory input (Heron, 1957). All this has implications for the care of older people with sensory loss, average self-esteem or a lifestyle lacking in variety or challenge, who may be overly susceptible to attempts to persuade them to adopt a particular course of action such as giving up their home.

Counterattitudinal role-playing is a potent determinant of change. In a study by Janis and King (1954), participants were required to play the part of 'sender'. They were given an outline of the argument, which advocated a position discordant with their own, and were then asked to present this argument to others. Their attitudes changed significantly more than did those of the control participants who listened passively. Improvising a communication was found to be more effective than reading it aloud or silently. Janis and Mann (1965) required participants to play the role of patients who had just been told they had lung cancer. Not only were their opinions of smoking modified to a greater extent, but they also changed their actual smoking habits more than did participants who had simply heard the procedure recorded on tape. See also Figure 3.3 above.

Rhetoric: the art of using language in order to influence or persuade others. In practice, rhetoric often consists of familiar or regularly used one-sided arguments, employed on the grounds that many people will be persuaded to believe something that they hear repeatedly.

Sender (*producer*) variables: the success of a persuasive communication depends on how the source of the communication is perceived and evaluated.

Hovland and Weiss (1951) gave two groups of participants the same four items of persuasive information on different medical topics. For one group, the source was presented as highly credible, for example a prominent doctor or a journal of biology. The other group were told it came from a glossy magazine or newspaper. The participants, who were university students, were more likely to have a greater opinion change for the highly credible source.

In 1942, Ewing examined the effects of the communicator declaring a bias. Having ascertained that the participants had a generally favourable attitude towards Henry Ford, Ewing gave them a communication recommending a less favourable attitude. Under one condition, the communicator announced that he was biased towards Henry Ford, in the other that he was biased against him. Participants' opinions altered more in the first case. One suggestion made at the time was that it is important that listeners do not notice the discrepancy between the declared bias and the actual communication.

Walster *et al.* (1966) found that a communication is more effective if it is seen as running counter to the self-interest of the communicator. They gave participants communications that advocated either more or less power to the courts and which purported to come from either a criminal or a prosecuting lawyer. The criminal was less effective than the prosecutor when advocating less power for the courts but more effective when advocating more power.

On the other hand, when the communicator is seen as trying to be persuasive, counterarguments are provoked more in the listeners. The more the listeners engage in counterarguments that have not been addressed by the speaker, the less effective the communication. Allyn and Festinger (1961) tested this by comparing groups who had, or had not, been forewarned. In one group, participants were informed beforehand that the speaker was going to try to convince them of a point of view that ran counter to their strongly held beliefs. In the second group, participants were not forewarned and were distracted from thinking of counterarguments by being asked to assess the speaker's personality while listening. Opinion change was much greater in the second condition.

It is also found that 'overheard' communication is often more effective than something explicitly directed to an audience, at least when the listeners are initially somewhat favourably disposed towards the position advocated (Walster and Festinger, 1962). Responses are also greater when the audience perceive themselves to be in some way similar to the speaker.

In summary, the persuasive effect will vary according to whether the person is regarded as being credible, as having good intentions or those related to the needs of the recipient, as being similar in some way to the recipient and as being unbiased or impartial. See also Figure 3.3 above.

Stereotypes: these can be seen as fixed attitudes towards groups. The word means something fixed or constantly repeated and in technology refers to the type-metal used for printing. The term was first used in the social sciences by Lippman in 1922, who saw stereotypes as 'pictures in our heads' that cast or mould attitudes. They constitute part of a person's *implicit personality theory* or system for categorising others. Stereotyping refers principally to obvious characteristics related to appearance, such as sex, age and apparent ethnic group, but can be extended to any group identity, for example that of doctors, nurses or social workers. A few, usually negative, aspects of group or role-related behaviour may be used to characterise the whole group. This may lead to faulty interpersonal perception or to prejudice and discrimination. Stereotypes may be confused with archetypes, which are intended to refer to ideal characteristics (see Chapter 17).

Value: an abstract idea of what is desirable. See also Chapter 6.

4 BEHAVIOURISM AND BEHAVIOUR THERAPIES

Behaviourism proposes an objective approach to the study of human behaviour and aims to explain, predict and control behaviour by exploring the extent to which environment determines behaviour. This school of thought, or perspective, regards mental processes and the mind as unknown and unknowable (a black box) and considers only observable, measurable phenomena.

Definitions	
Bandura (1969)	Behaviour that is harmful to the individual or departs widely from accepted social and ethical norms is viewed not as symptomatic of some kind of disease but as a way that the individual has learned to cope with environmental and self-imposed demands. Treatment then becomes mainly a problem in social learning rather than one in the medical domain.
Hirschorn (1979)	Behaviourism [is] an approach which focuses on how the developing human organism is shaped through its constant interactions with the environment. You enter the world with a genetic potential that contributes to your ultimate patterns of adjustment. But learning and experience also determine the kind of person you become.
Marks (1986)	Behavioural psychotherapy comprises a variety of therapeutic methods that aim to change abnormal behaviour directly rather than by analysing hypothesised conflicts. The problem may be a behavioural deficit... or excess...

Approaches, Arguments and Applications

A key assumption of the school of behaviourism is that learning takes place by conditioning and that this learned behaviour can be described in terms of stimulus–response units (S–R units). That is, learning can be seen to have taken place whenever a particular response predictably follows a particular stimulus without the need for conscious effort or will. There are two types of conditioning, one which just happens passively through repeated exposure to associated stimuli (classical conditioning), the other in which actions are reinforced (operant or instrumental conditioning). Both of these can also be thought of as 'trial and error' learning. Behaviourism also covers other aspects of animal behaviour such as instincts and imprinting.

Behaviourism developed in the 1920s as a reaction to other early types of psychology, such as introspection, and reached its heyday in the 1960s. Psychology, particularly in the USA, is sometimes referred to as behavioural science, notably where behaviourism forms the dominant perspective of the psychology being taught in an institution. (This was illustrated in the film *The Silence of the Lambs*.)

Various interesting results emerged from the early studies with animals. For example, behaviour learned in connection with intermittent reinforcement takes much longer to extinguish than does behaviour that has been conditioned by regular reinforcement. Punishment, which is often naively assumed to be a deterrent, does not necessarily lead to the extinction of previously learned actions and may be found to reinforce unwanted behaviour.

If we extend these findings to people, we might say that when 'socialising' children, it is likely that predictable *rewards* such as sweets or regular praise for good behaviour (or good school results) will be less effective in reinforcing that behaviour than an irregular and unpredictable assortment of attention, treats and the child's own evident pleasure in the activity. Reinforcement is more successful if it meets intrinsic rather than superficial or extrinsic needs and interests. If sweets come to be expected, good behaviour may not be forthcoming without them. Regular praise can sound empty and patronising and, if too predictable, may not leave anything to strive for. Genuine pleasure that erupts occasionally and spontaneously in response to new actions may be a better reinforcer. Ignoring mildly naughty behaviour and diverting the child to desirable activities and giving added attention is likely to be more effective than punishment. Frequent predictable punishment, even if painful, frustrating or humiliating, may well provide much-needed attention and act as a reinforcer.

One of the main problems with applying many of the behavioural principles to human behaviour lies in the difficulty of identifying what needs are likely to be met by the available reinforcers. It can be helpful to refer to *Maslow's* (1962) *hierarchy of needs* (see Chapter 7) to see that an extensive range of psychological needs exists beyond the basic needs for food and freedom investigated by Skinner and Thorndike.

Pure behaviourism was not concerned with beliefs, intentions, social influences, expectations, emotions and evaluations. It emphasised measurement of a known need state, observation of behaviour and the counting of trials.

Opposition to behaviourism comes from cognitive, social, humanistic and psychodynamic perspectives, in all of which it is argued that most learning does not occur in isolation from social interaction, emotional and cognitive processes. Today, where behavioural principles are applied in therapy, they are nearly always used in a way that acknowledges the clients' cognitions, emotions and lifestyle. Behavioural programmes are often combined with cognitive therapy. Moreover, since conditioning is seen as being beyond conscious control, the principles of behaviourism offend anyone who holds that humans, if not other animals, can exercise free will and are not just automata responding mindlessly to the reinforcement of basic needs. It does not leave any room for notions of freedom or free will and cannot adequately explain artistic practice.

Key Terms and Concepts

Acquisition: the strengthening of a response during the process of conditioning.

Aversion therapy: stimuli that trigger undesirable responses are deliberately arranged so that unpleasant events follow. The intention is that if the sequence is repeated frequently, the undesirable response will fade through avoidance learning.

Early in the twentieth century, aversion therapy was associated with eradicating whatever was then thought to be socially undesirable behaviour, such as male homosexuality. The client seeking therapy was shown a series of photographs or slides. The aversion event, such as a painful electric shock, was administered by the therapist whenever the client paid too much attention or exhibited an arousal response to a relevant stimulus, such as a photograph of a man in a sexually provocative pose. Therapy was based on the assumption that homosexual arousal was not natural, that it was a learned behaviour (due to some sort of faulty upbringing) and that it could be unlearned. Usually, both client and therapist shared these assumptions, which were prevalent at the time. Evidence concerning the success of these techniques is conflicting. More recently, less aggressive aversion techniques have been linked to cognitive approaches towards reducing the incidence of unwanted thoughts. For example, someone wanting to reduce or prevent thoughts that induce anxiety can self-administer a small, sharp, mildly unpleasant stimulus such as snapping an elastic band on the wrist whenever the thoughts begin. If an alternative behaviour, rather than an unpleasant stimulus, is introduced in order to reduce unwanted behaviour, the process of relearning may be known as *response prevention*.

Aversive stimulus: a stimulus is described as aversive if it is associated with something unpleasant and leads to avoidance behaviour.

Avoidance learning: a process by which behaviour is learned in response to an aversive stimulus and which results in a possible unpleasant event failing to take place. The removal of an unpleasant or unwanted consequence that increases the likelihood of repetition of a certain behaviour is known as negative reinforcement. For example, a person may learn not to attempt tricky or precise work when tired. Avoidance learning can be more resistant to extinction than other forms of learning. Harm avoidance and pain avoidance are good examples of this, a person or animal learning to engage in behaviour that will prevent harm or pain. For example, a patient with a chronic condition may learn by trial and error that it is better to take analgesics regularly before the pain occurs rather than waiting until the pain is felt. As with most human behaviour, it is difficult in this example to separate any behavioural principles of reinforcement from concomitant cognitive awareness, deliberate planning or perception of motivation. To be purely behavioural, the learning would have to take place without conscious awareness, effort or will.

Behaviour: observable activities, such as speech, which can be measured. Behaviourism does not take account of accompanying thoughts or activities, whose presence can only be inferred. Internal processes, such as those of the brain and nervous system, may or may not be considered to be behaviour, depending on whether they are measurable.

Behavioural analysis: a method of gaining information about a client's experiences when a behavioural problem is manifested (Richards and McDonald, 1990). The analysis contains three parts focusing on:

- antecedents: A
- behaviour: B
- consequences: C.

Antecedents (the stimuli) come before the behaviour and are thought to be associated with it. Consequences (the reinforcers) are events and experiences that follow and are believed to be associated with the behaviour. The antecedents and consequences of a behaviour will influence the likelihood of that behaviour being repeated when faced with similar antecedents.

Analysis of the behaviour itself involves an exploration of how the client acted. This approach is an extension of pure behaviourism, related to *social learning theory*. The antecedents and consequences of the behaviour may be considered in physical, cognitive, emotional, behavioural and social terms. The practical application of this kind of analysis is most often used with problematic or undesirable behaviours.

Behavioural approach: a psychological approach based on the principles of behaviourism. In principle, only observable behaviour is taken into consideration. In practice, however, most so-called behavioural programmes involve cognitive, affective and social elements.

Behavioural contract: an explicit agreement between client and therapist specifying expectations, plans and/or contingencies for behaviour(s) to be changed. The contract may be written or oral.

Behaviour modification therapy (behaviour modification): the therapeutic application of behaviour shaping through operant (instrumental) conditioning. The key ingredients are:

- baseline measurement
- goal-setting

- small, manageable steps
- reinforcement.

In order for the client and therapist to evaluate the success of the behaviour modification programme, baseline measurements of behaviour must be made at the start. An end goal is also established at the outset so that progress towards the goal can be monitored and the remaining work clearly identified. This avoids any tendency to 'shift the goalposts'. It is normally most effective if negotiation between client and therapist occurs at all stages of the programme; this can be formalised through the use of a *behavioural contract*.

It is important that the steps are small and achievable. The client needs to experience success and not be allowed to fail. Achievement serves as its own reinforcer and is likely to promote further attempts.

Humour is very useful, and if the steps can be made into a game, without being patronising, this often works very well. A case example, taken from Davies (1983), is included for discussion in Figure 4.1. Readers might like to design a suitable behaviour modification programme and then compare it with the actual programme that was used.

Miss Offord had moderately good recovery of motor power following a stroke but had residual left sided paresis with neglect of the left side and hemianopia. She could move her left arm and foot but was very unsteady and walked very poorly even with two helpers, her right foot overlapping her left. Miss Offord appeared very frightened. She would not cooperate with physiotherapy or occupational therapy and, at her worst, refused even to turn in bed.

There was no physical reason why Miss Offord should not start walking training, although she experienced panic when attempts were made. Miss Offord was alert and lucid most of the time but was occasionally confused and forgetful.

Figure 4.1 Behaviour modification programme: a case example for discussion (*from Davies, 1983*)

Although the technique is ostensibly concerned with behaviour, if the patient is fully conversant with what is happening and involves notions of reward and punishment, it then ceases to be purely behavioural but invokes a range of cognitive, affective and social influences to do with motivation and compliance.

Behaviour-shaping: the alteration of behaviour or the production of new behaviour through the systematic use of reinforcement, based on the principles of operant (instrumental) conditioning. Although the terms 'behaviour-shaping' and 'behaviour modification therapy' are often used interchangeably, behaviour-shaping is sometimes reserved for a 'purer' form of therapeutic programme in which the success of the programme does not rely on the participant having cognitive awareness of the aims of the programme, so the use of a *behavioural contract* is not applicable.

The term 'behaviour-shaping' is also used where there is no therapeutic attempt and to refer to the training of animals to perform complex tasks.

Shaping is linked to trial and error. Animals engage in a range of behaviours, some apparently intentional, some random. When a certain item of behaviour is followed by a desirable outcome (such as food), that item of behaviour is likely to be repeated. The trainer, with an end goal in mind, waits until a bit of behaviour occurs that, with luck and further training, will lead toward the end goal and then gives a reward. When that item of behaviour is established, the trainer withholds reward until new behaviour occurs that is a little closer to the target behaviour. The behaviour gradually becomes closer and closer to the required goal until the goal is finally reached.

In the context of working with people with severe learning disabilities, it may be only the health-care professional who has any notion of the end goal and the intermediary steps. In practice, the steps are themselves determined by trial and error, depending on what behaviour occurs and when and where the professional decides to give reinforcement or withhold it. Behaviour-shaping of this nature may also be used with those who are very anxious and not able to see the programme as a whole from the outset.

Behaviour therapies (also known as behavioural psychotherapies): a global term for all treatment approaches that apply classical or operant conditioning techniques or other aspects of learning theory to the analysis of behaviour problems in an attempt to change the problem behaviour. In some texts, the term 'behaviour therapy' is used only for techniques based on classical conditioning (see Gregory, 1987), but the term is used in its widest sense here. There are various types, including:

- behaviour modification or shaping
- avoidance therapy
- response prevention
- aversion therapy
- graded exposure
- progressive desensitisation
- implosion and flooding.

Behavioural techniques may also be combined with cognitive therapy to provide a cognitive-behavioural programme. Once suitability has been assessed, the most appropriate type of therapeutic programme can be designed.

Richards and McDonald (1990) give five criteria by which a person's suitability for behaviour therapy can be assessed:

- The problem can be expressed in behavioural terms
- The problem is current and predictable
- Clear behavioural goals can be agreed
- The client understands and agrees to treatment
- Objections to behavioural treatment cannot be seen.

Black box: a term borrowed from experimental electronic science and used to describe the mind or the internal workings of an organism that are regarded as inaccessible to observation and measurement, as if they take place inside a black box. Behaviourists claim that it is not important to know what goes on in the mind and that only the relationships between inputs (stimuli) and outputs (responses) should be studied.

Chaining: the process of identifying a series of meaningful tasks or steps that will lead to a goal-orientated behaviour. For example, when teaching a client to cook a meal, the interim stages towards achieving the goal are identified and then taught sequentially as distinct entities. Chaining can be forward or backward. In forward chaining, the sequence starts with the first step. In backward chaining, the last stage is taught first, so the learner receives immediate reinforcement from the satisfaction of completing the task. The order of the stages is then taught from last to first.

Classical conditioning (also known as associative, contigual or contiguous conditioning): the first kind of conditioning to be described. This shows how learning takes place when an association is made between two stimuli. After repeated exposure to two stimuli together, a natural response to one stimulus is found to occur also in response to the other stimulus. Pavlov found that if he rang a bell whenever a dog was eating and salivating, after a few times the dog salivated in response to the bell even if no food was given. Pavlov's early work was concerned with measuring how many trials were needed for the salivation response to be conditioned to a new stimulus and how many trials were needed for the conditioned response to be *extinguished* if no food was given.

To establish a conditioned response, it is necessary to start with a natural unconditioned response such as a reflex. Before conditioning, the natural behaviour or reflex is known as the unconditioned response and the stimulus that evokes it is the unconditioned stimulus (UCS). That is, the dog's natural salivation in response to food is the unconditioned response and the food is the UCS. At this stage, it is assumed that no learning has taken place. The UCS is then paired regularly with a new stimulus. After conditioning takes place, and learning can be said to have occurred, the new stimulus is known as the conditioned stimulus (CS). The response that previously occurred only naturally but now occurs to the new stimulus is renamed the conditioned response (CR). In our example, the bell is the CS and the salivation in response to the bell the CR.

Classical conditioning may account for some of a baby's learning of 'rooting' and sucking in response to the appearance, feel and smell of the mother (or other carer). Rooting and sucking are natural in-born reflexes that occur in response to anyone or anything touching the baby's cheek or putting anything in the baby's mouth. The sucking reflex is strongest immediately after birth and may fade considerably within a few hours if the baby is not fed. If fed, these responses, after a few days or weeks, occur more strongly in the presence of the regular feeder than any other adult. Responses to other adults may, however, occur, and it is not unusual for a visiting man, holding a new baby for the first time, to find the baby hunting enthusiastically for the breast. Further associational learning leads to finer discrimination between stimuli, and older babies learn which carers provide food. Similar processes may account for much of what is learned by children and adults, but it is usually difficult to distinguish between classical and operant conditioning and to separate this kind of learning from social and cognitive learning. See also Chapters 7 and 16.

Clinical observations may be interpreted as examples of classical conditioning, such as when a person develops a fear of going outdoors following a mugging attack. An unconditioned response of fear to being mugged can become a conditioned response to going outdoors when this is repeatedly associated with memories of the attack. Counterconditioning methods such as *progressive desensitisation* may be used to reduce fear.

Comparative psychology: that branch of psychology which is concerned with studying animal behaviour with a view to being able to compare what is seen in animals with what is known about human behaviour.

Conditioned response: a behaviour that occurs in response to a conditioned stimulus.

Conditioned stimulus: a stimulus that has been paired with an unconditioned stimulus and evokes a conditioned response.

Counterconditioning: the association of an anxiety-evoking stimulus with a stimulus that produces an incompatible response, usually relaxation, in order to modify the anxious response. The technique is based on the principle that one cannot be anxious and relaxed at the same time and forms the basis of *progressive desensitisation.*

Exposure: any method used for treating phobias in which the client is exposed to the feared situation in either imagination or reality. Examples include graded exposure, systematic or progressive desensitisation, implosion and flooding.

Extinction: the diminishing in strength of a behaviour by withholding reinforcers so that the behaviour eventually ceases. The rate at which extinction occurs depends on the *reinforcement schedule* used when the behaviour was learned.

Flooding: a technique that involves rapid, prolonged exposure of the client in imagination or in reality to the stimulus that evokes most fear. It is based on the principle that panic-level anxiety cannot be sustained and eventually subsides, resulting in tolerance of the stimulus. If the exercise is carried out purely in the imagination, it may be referred to as implosion therapy.

Flooding may be used to treat phobias. The client is exposed to a very intense stimulus of the kind known to induce symptoms of fear. Hopefully, as the client realises that there is no actual harmful effect, the usual stimulus will cease to induce fear. This technique tends to be based on intuitive notions of what might work rather than on sound research evidence and should be used with caution. It is something that may be noticed in everyday situations, when people find they are no longer anxious about certain situations after they have survived a particularly bad time. For example, someone might be mildly anxious of driving down a steep spiral exit from a local car park. Later, after a holiday in Crete and some hair-raising experiences of driving round steep bends on the sides of hills with sheer drops, the car park exit may no longer seem upsetting. Encouraging a person after an accident to go back quickly and engage in the anxiety-provoking activity associated with the accident can be seen as a type of flooding. Such prompt behaviour helps people to cope with the wave of anxiety that is likely to be induced before anticipatory fear escalates and leads to avoidance of the feared situation such that daily living is affected.

Goal identification (setting): see behaviour modification therapy.

Graded exposure: a method used for treating phobias in which the client is gradually exposed to the feared situation. The exposure is graded using a client-constructed hierarchy of anxiety-inducing situations so that a number of stages are used in imagination or reality over a period of time. The client is first exposed to the least anxiety-inducing situation and over time progresses up the hierarchy through preplanned stages of increasing difficulty. Exposure at each stage is prolonged and repeated until the client's anxiety levels drop, after which the next stage of exposure is embarked upon until the most feared situation can be faced. The client must practise as homework any exposure undertaken in the session. A more refined version of graded exposure is progressive desensitisation, in which relaxation techniques are used in conjunction with the exposure. Implosion and flooding are versions of exposure that are not graded.

Hierarchy construction: the client is asked to classify anxiety-evoking stimuli related to a feared situation according to the degree of anxiety evoked. The level of anxiety may be linked to proximity of the feared object or situation or to the number of anxiety-provoking stimuli present. The client uses a numerical scale to rate the degree of distress for each stage of the hierarchy before, during and after each exposure. For example, a car driver involved in a serious road traffic accident who has been unable to get into a car since the accident may construct a hierarchy as follows:

- standing beside a car
- sitting in the passenger seat of a stationary car
- being driven as a passenger to the local shops
- sitting in the driver's seat of a stationary car
- driving while accompanied to the local shops
- driving unaccompanied to the local shops
- being driven as a passenger past the scene of the accident
- driving while accompanied in urban traffic
- driving unaccompanied in urban traffic
- driving while accompanied past the scene of the accident
- driving unaccompanied past the scene of the accident.

Implosion therapy: see flooding.

Intermittent reinforcement: one of the findings of early behavioural research was that behaviour followed by intermittent or irregular reinforcement was very resistant to extinction. This has implications for teaching and parenting as it suggests that occasional recognition may be more effective than regular praise or high marks in maintaining high levels of effort after the reinforcement system ceases. See reinforcement schedules.

Learning theory: an early name for the basic behaviourist description of how learning takes place through a process of conditioning, either classical or operant. As there is now a large number of learning theories, based on different theoretical concepts, the original usage is no longer appropriate. See Chapters 7 and 16 for learning theories.

Modelling: an individual can learn many potential styles of response from observing and copying other people's behaviour (Figure 4.2). The person being copied is the 'model' or 'role-model'. The model need not be aware that copying has occurred. See also vicarious learning and social learning theory.

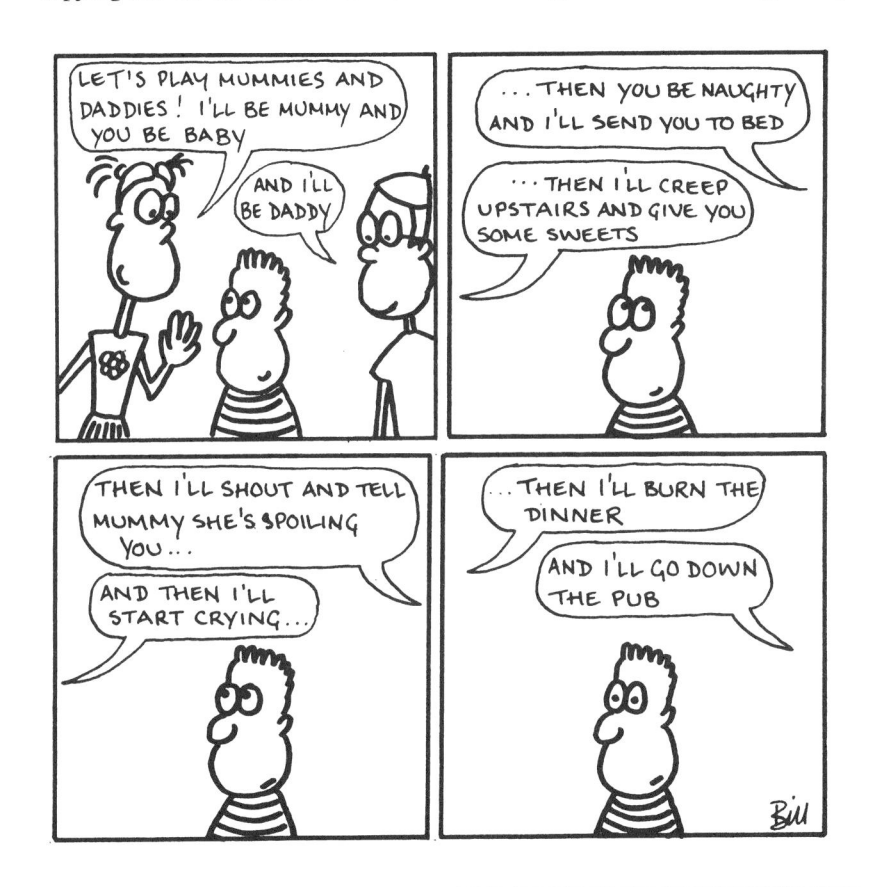

Figure 4.2 Modelling (*Bill O'Neill, 1997*)

Operant (instrumental) conditioning: the terms 'operant' and 'instrumental' are equivalent. Instrumental means doing something in order to gain whatever is wanted. The Latin word *opus* (plural *opera*) means 'work'. In this type of conditioning, some work or action is involved in order to gain something that satisfies a need. Like classical conditioning, the process is seen as happening without conscious effort or will to learn, but unlike classical conditioning, which can be completely passive, operant conditioning is an active process. The term 'operant learning' is sometimes used as an alternative to operant conditioning.

The early researchers (for example, Watson, Thorndike and Skinner) observed that animals have a tendency to repeat actions that have been followed by, for example, food or freedom. Animals were placed in cages having a lever. At first, the animal might happen to hit the lever only by chance, but if the lever opened the door or delivered a piece of food, the animal would, after a few trials, then go straight to the lever and press it. Following on from discoveries within classical conditioning, each associated stimulus and response was identified and linked in stimulus–response (S–R) pairs. For example, the lever would be seen as the conditioned stimulus that evoked the conditioned response of pressing; the food or freedom was seen as the reinforcer. Experiments were concerned with quantifying states of need such as hunger, measuring how many trials were required before the action became conditioned, how many trials were needed to shape behaviour or how many were needed before actions became extinguished.

Progressive desensitisation (systematic desensitisation): a method that involves the systematic lessening of a specific, learned fear through the use of counterconditioning techniques, based on the principles of classical conditioning.

As with *behaviour modification therapy*, three of the essential elements are baseline measurement, goal-setting and small manageable steps. The main difference between the two techniques is that behaviour modification therapy uses operant conditioning principles with reinforcement of actions, while progressive or systematic desensitisation is based on classical conditioning with a focus on the physiological state.

A programme of graded exposure is planned, in which relaxation techniques are used in conjunction with the exposure. The key principle is that a physiological fear arousal state cannot exist at the same time as a relaxed state. Moreover, it is assumed that the exhibited fear response has been learned through a simple process of classical conditioning in earlier life experience and can therefore be unlearned or relearned in a new way.

The exposure is graded using a client-constructed hierarchy of anxiety-inducing situations so that a number of stages are used over a period of time, gradually progressing from the least feared to the most feared situation. The client is first taught relaxation techniques. A least-feared example of the feared object or situation is then introduced. The client practises relaxation until minimal arousal is again achieved. This is repeated until the object does not result in arousal. The next step in the hierarchy is then introduced. Again, the client practises relaxation until there is no arousal associated with the object. This process continues until the client experiences no arousal when faced with the most-feared situation or object. The client should practice as homework any relaxation techniques and exposure undertaken in the session.

This technique is most successful where the feared object or situation is specific and can be clearly identified, such as with phobias of cats, mice or spiders, or some kinds of agoraphobia.

The chief argument against the use of this technique comes from psychodynamics. It is argued that phobias are not always simple conditioned responses but are often symptoms of a more profound underlying anxiety. Even if the behavioural programme eliminates the specific fear response, it does not address the underlying problem, which will manifest itself later in a new way. In practice, progressive desensitisation is found to be extremely helpful to some people in restoring normal daily activities. If the effects are short lived, or other symptoms begin to emerge, clients may be advised to seek other kinds of counselling or therapy. For ongoing problems, integrative, eclectic or multimodal therapeutic approaches may be most appropriate (see Chapter 8).

Punishment: anything perceived as intended to be unpleasant and in recognition of undesired behaviour. This is usually carried out with the explicit intention that it should extinguish the undesired behaviour or decrease the probability of its occurring again on future occasions. However, punishment may also contain elements of retribution or revenge, and since this contains cognitive and social factors, it cannot be explained in terms of behavioural principles alone. The principles of behaviourism would suggest that punishment is ineffective in reducing unwanted behaviour but rather that new behaviours may emerge which circumvent the discomfort (*avoidance learning*). With people, this may involve deceit.

Crucially, a child's perception of punishment will determine whether its behaviour is reinforced or extinguished. For example, if the punishment involves providing more attention, the child may increase the naughty behaviour. Alternatively, a child may avoid punishment by pretending to be good or blaming another child. Hence, punishment sometimes works and sometimes does not.

In behavioural approaches, it is usually recommended that distraction from the undesired behaviour with plenty of attention and reinforcement of desired behaviour should be implemented. The overall level of attention given by parents and carers may be much more important than considerations of punishment or reward. *Time ou*t may be necessary when the undesirable behaviour persists. In general, if consequences are perceived as punitive, or if the person feels punished despite making an effort to comply with a behavioural programme, it may be necessary to review the steps or stages in the programme to ensure that they match the person's ability and that the goals are achievable.

The *threat* of punishment is sometimes effective in preventing unwanted behaviour. However, as this again involves cognitive and social processes, it cannot be explained in terms of behaviourism.

Reinforcement: in operant conditioning, the probability of a response is seen as being altered by its consequences (Figure 4.3). Anything that increases the probability of a response is called reinforcement. In general, reinforcement occurs when the consequences meet a 'need' of the recipient. This does not have to be perceived as pleasant or as a reward but merely has to increase the incidence of the responses to a stimulus. Reinforcement can be either positive or negative.

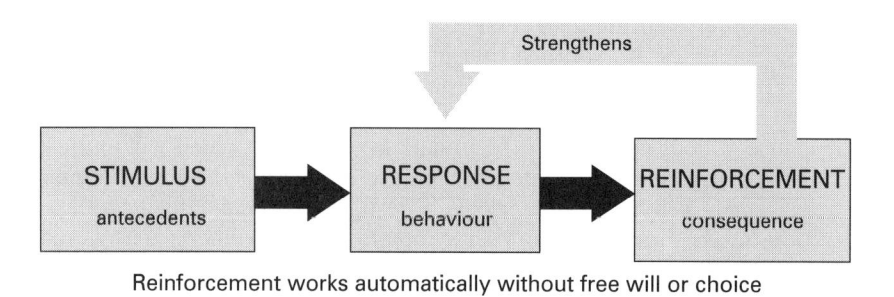

```
                    Strengthens
        ┌─────────────────────────┐
        ▼                         │
┌──────────┐    ┌──────────┐    ┌───────────────┐
│ STIMULUS │ ──▶│ RESPONSE │ ──▶│ REINFORCEMENT │
│antecedents│   │ behaviour│    │  consequence  │
└──────────┘    └──────────┘    └───────────────┘
```

Reinforcement works automatically without free will or choice

Figure 4.3 Operant conditioning: reinforcement of the stimulus–response (S–R) unit

Positive reinforcement involves the addition of something that meets a need, for example giving a child attention.

In negative reinforcement, the removal of something meets a need. For example, privacy can be perceived as a need. When a patient has been 'specialed', that is, nursed under close supervision, because of a tendency to self-harm, the level of supervision can be gradually decreased as a consequence of self-respecting behaviour. This may further reinforce such behaviour, allowing more privacy. This can be regarded as avoidance learning.

Extinction occurs when there is no reinforcement.

Contrary to popular understanding, the theory predicts that where treats and privileges are given as part of a simple positive reinforcement schedule for good behaviour, the absence of these will lead to gradual extinction of the good behaviour. Moreover, the withdrawal of treats, and any associated criticism, may act as a negative reinforcer of avoidance behaviour. That is, the person will try something new in order to avoid the unpleasant consequences. In practice, this does not usually result in good behaviour but in 'escape' attempts. This may be seen in treatment schedules for people with anorexia nervosa who are unwilling participants and sometimes demonstrate 'avoidance learning' such as pretending to eat and filling themselves with water before being weighed in order to avoid criticism and punishment.

Reinforcement schedules: the timing of the association between behaviour and the reinforcement is crucial. Different response rates and extinction rates will be found according to whether the reinforcement is regular and predictable or intermittent and unpredictable. Findings from early work with animals can be roughly compared with different jobs or activities which give financial reward. Simplified assumptions are summarised in Table 4.1. In practice, of course, there are many more needs and interests that are served by these activities, and the real relationship is far from simple.

Response prevention: a method for helping people learn to stop engaging in unwanted behaviours. Therapeutically, this can be applied to behaviours that are detrimental to health. For example, response prevention may be used in helping people with skin disorders not to scratch. As soon as the impulse to scratch is felt, a behaviour linked to this impulse is identified,

Table 4.1 Reinforcement schedules

Schedule	Example	Response rate	Extinction
continuous: every response is reinforced	vending machine	steady, slow	quick
fixed ratio: reinforcement is given for a fixed number of responses	pay for piece work	high, with a pause after reinforcement	fairly quick
fixed interval: reinforcement given after a fixed amount of time if response has occurred	being paid regularly for work	slow, speeds up when reinforcement is due	fairly quick
variable ratio: reinforcement given on average for a fixed number of responses	gambling	steady, high	very slow
variable interval: reinforcement given on average for a fixed amount of time; each trial is a different time, but overall average time may be set in advance	self-employed people receiving payment irregularly	steady, builds up with time after last reinforcement	very slow

such as moving the right hand towards the left in order to scratch. The right hand is then prevented from moving towards the left by engaging in another behaviour such as drumming on the table, for a count of about 30 seconds, which allows the scratching urge to lessen. The right hand is then taken to the left and engaged in non-scratching contact such as stroking, again for about 30 seconds. Repeated practice of this pattern is found significantly to reduce the urge to scratch and the scratching behaviour. This allows the skin to heal and become less inflamed and irritable, thus breaking the habit of scratching. Response prevention may also be taught to people with obsessional disorders in order to reduce the intrusion of unwanted thoughts, and with compulsive disorders to reduce ritualistic behaviours. See also aversion therapy.

Reward: something given as a consequence of behaviour that is perceived as intended to be pleasant and in recognition of a desired behaviour. A reward is not the same as reinforcement and may or may not result in the behaviour being repeated on another occasion. The term is essentially a cognitive one as it depends on beliefs and expectations and, as such, has no place in behaviourism. However, where something is given which meets a need of the recipient, it may both be perceived as a reward and serve as a reinforcer of the linked behaviour. Research with animals tended to be restricted to needs such as hunger, thirst and freedom from pain, whereas with people, any need, such as those given in *Maslow's* (1962) *hierarchy of needs*, may become involved.

Rewards can be related to intrinsic, that is inner, and extrinsic, that is outer, needs and interests. Intrinsic rewards for engaging in a task are those which stem from the task itself, that it is pleasurable in itself, either for the actual activity or for the satisfaction that completion brings. Extrinsic rewards are secondary to the task: engaging in the task will bring something else that is desired, such as praise, money or status.

In behaviour modification, the most effective reinforcers are those which are perceived as intrinsic rewards, in particular when successfully completing a step becomes a reward in itself. This will most readily occur where the patient wants to accomplish the activity for its own sake, is actively involved in choosing the intermediary steps and has already had a taste of success.

Extrinsic rewards, such as privileges, treats or token economies, are often employed in behaviour modification programmes, at least at first, but can lead to unpredictable or undesirable effects, especially if the patient does not readily comply or has difficulty managing the steps. The regular and predictable use of extrinsic rewards has been shown to lead to rapid extinction of the learned behaviour once the programme has ended.

Bruner points out that praising or otherwise rewarding good behaviour in children rarely results in exactly the same good behaviour being reinforced but in the children exploring new behaviours. As soon as cognitive processes are involved, basic behavioural principles no longer apply.

Sensitisation: the process by which emotions become associated with particular objects or events.

Social learning theory: an extension and development of behavioural principles that takes social interaction into consideration. Observational learning or modelling can lead to imitation or identification. Bandura (1965, 1977) drew attention to the difference between learning and behaviour. Not all learning results in observable actions. In pure behaviourism, it is believed that reinforcement works automatically with no element of free will; the human or animal is not required to assess or evaluate the effects of the behaviour. In contrast, Bandura believes that reinforcement serves as information and motivation. By 'informative', he means that the consequences of the behaviour tell the person in what circumstances it would seem wise to try a particular behaviour in the future; they improve

Reinforcement leads to new behaviour.

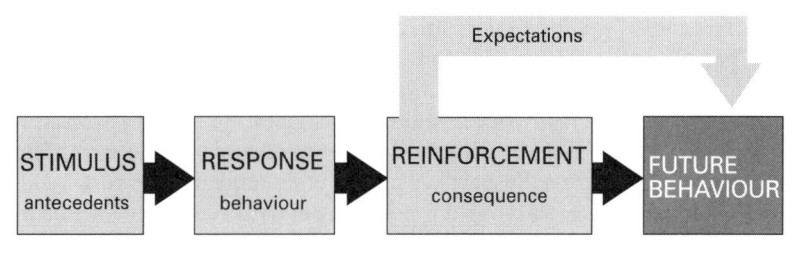

STIMULUS (antecedents) → RESPONSE (behaviour) → REINFORCEMENT (consequence) → FUTURE BEHAVIOUR

Expectations

Reinforcement serves as information and motivation, enabling free will and choice about future actions.

Figure 4.4 Social learning theory

the prediction of whether a given action will lead to pleasant or unpleasant outcomes in the future. People can learn from observing others (modelling and vicarious learning) since watching others can provide information on which kind of behaviour leads to which consequences. By 'motivational', Bandura means that more attempt will be made to learn the modelled behaviour if the consequences are valued. This approach implies that people can weigh up the disadvantages and advantages of behaviour and have a choice about what they actually do. See Figure 4.4, also Chapters 7 and 16.

Systematic desensitisation: see progressive desensitisation.

Time out: removing a person from a problem situation to prevent his or her behaviour being reinforced. For example, this can involve sending a child to another room, such as a bedroom, or using a 'naughty chair'. The child is held in the naughty chair, by force if necessary, until he or she promises to join in activities 'properly'. This procedure avoids the need for punishment and is recommended in some forms of behavioural programmes in family therapy where a child is persistently naughty.

Token economy: a method for strengthening or weakening existing behaviour, or for developing new behaviour, in which tokens are used as reinforcers. These tokens may then be exchanged for goods or privileges. As with behaviour modification schedules, the baseline is measured, the end goal is identified and intermediary steps are devised. Tokens are given as steps are achieved and behaviour is shaped until the end goal is reached. This kind of programme can be used with or without the full awareness and co-operation of the participant. Token economies are found to be useful in promoting the learning of new skills in people with learning difficulties and in rehabilitation programmes for people with enduring mental health problems.

Unconditioned response: a naturally occurring behaviour, such as a reflex or physiological process, that takes place automatically in the presence of a particular (unconditioned) stimulus and for which there is no apparent evidence of learning. Examples include the rooting and sucking reflexes of a newborn baby in response to stroking the cheek and putting an object in the baby's mouth, pulling one's hand away from a hot surface, salivation in response to having food in one's mouth and the startle response to sudden noises or gestures.

Unconditioned stimulus: the stimulus that evokes an automatic (unconditioned) response, apparently without any learning (or conditioning) having taken place.

Vicarious learning: a term used in social learning theory to refer to the ways in which people can learn by observing what happens to others. For example, a toddler may learn not to break plates by observing that a sibling is punished for doing so, or a young child learns to help in laying the table through noticing that a friend is praised for doing so. Vicarious learning differs from simple modelling in which any behaviour may be copied as it includes the assumption that the outcome of the behaviour (usually perceived as reward or punishment) has been observed. The terms 'modelling' and 'vicarious learning' may, however, be used interchangeably where outcomes are taken into account.

5 BIOPSYCHOLOGY AND PHYSICAL INTERVENTIONS

This is the perspective that helps us to understand behaviour and mental experience by examining what is happening physiologically in the body, particularly in the brain and nervous system. This approach has several different names, each of which links biology and psychology, such as biopsychology, psychobiology, neuropsychology, psychophysiology and 'the biological basis of behaviour'. This combination may be further linked with social psychology to give the biosocial and biopsychosocial approaches often referred to in health-care contexts.

This chapter gives some information on the brain and nervous system, the endocrine system and principles of genetics.

Definitions	
Glassman (1979)	The biological approach emphasizes the physical (or physiological) basis of behaviour, and the interactions between mind and body. The interactions work both ways: body can affect mind... and mind can affect body.
Green (1994)	Biopsychology studies... those changes in physiological systems that occur whenever behaviour changes. It has concentrated on individual psychological processes such as memory, attention, emotion, and motivation, and attempts to demonstrate how, for instance, learning a particular task is correlated with a particular change in activity in the brain.
Pinel (1997)	Biopsychology is the study of the biology of behaviour... [It] covers more than the neural mechanisms of behaviour; it also deals with the evolution, genetics and adaptiveness of behavioural processes.

> **Definitions (cont'd)**
>
> > ...[the term] denotes a biological approach to the study of psychology rather than a psychological approach to the study of biology.

Approaches, Arguments and Applications

Many mainstream psychologists today consider an understanding of biological processes fundamental to understanding psychological processes. The most comprehensive psychological theories, for example in learning, memory, emotion, sleep, pain and stress, are those which can be shown to relate psychological experience to known physiological mechanisms. This does not mean that biopsychology is necessarily 'reductionist' or is attempting to explain behaviour only in terms of the biology or reducing complex mental experience to a set of physical laws, but that for the psychological explanations to make proper sense, there should be a good match between what is observed psychologically and physiologically, with no significant contradictions. See also Chapter 12.

Key Terms and Concepts

Action potential: changes in the electrical composition of positive and negative ions on either side of the membrane of nerve fibres that generate impulses that carry signals from one part of the nervous system to another. See also nerve fibre and neurone.

Basal nuclei (previously known as basal ganglia): these consist of several clusters of cell bodies (nuclei) deep within the cerebral hemispheres. Names vary from text to text, but these nuclei are generally agreed to comprise the globus pallidus, lenticular nucleus and corpus striatum, which includes the caudate nucleus and putamen. The basal nuclei receive impulses from different parts of the cerebral cortex and are thus supplied with information relating to thoughts. The command signals sent out from the basal nuclei pass first to the thalamus and from there to many areas of the cerebral cortex, including the motor control area. They are important in co-ordination of movement and in related aspects of Parkinson's disease. The term 'nuclei' is now preferred for structures within the central nervous system, the term 'ganglia' for those in the peripheral nervous system.

Biofeedback: a set of techniques for helping people to gain some control over processes that are normally outside conscious awareness and control, such as muscle tension, heart rate, blood pressure and epileptic seizures (Phillips, 1991). The chosen process is monitored, usually by an electronic device, and connected to a computer or television screen that can give the person a visual or auditory signal of some kind. Through practice, a person learns to associate changes in the signal with something that he or she is doing and may eventually be able deliberately to create the desired changes.

In many cases, the person does not actually know exactly what causes the changes, only that feeling a certain way or willing the changes to happen will have the right effect. This is similar to how many activities such as walking, swimming or riding a bicycle, are learned through natural feedback from the surroundings. It was maybe not obvious how this was done, but it worked and improved with practice.

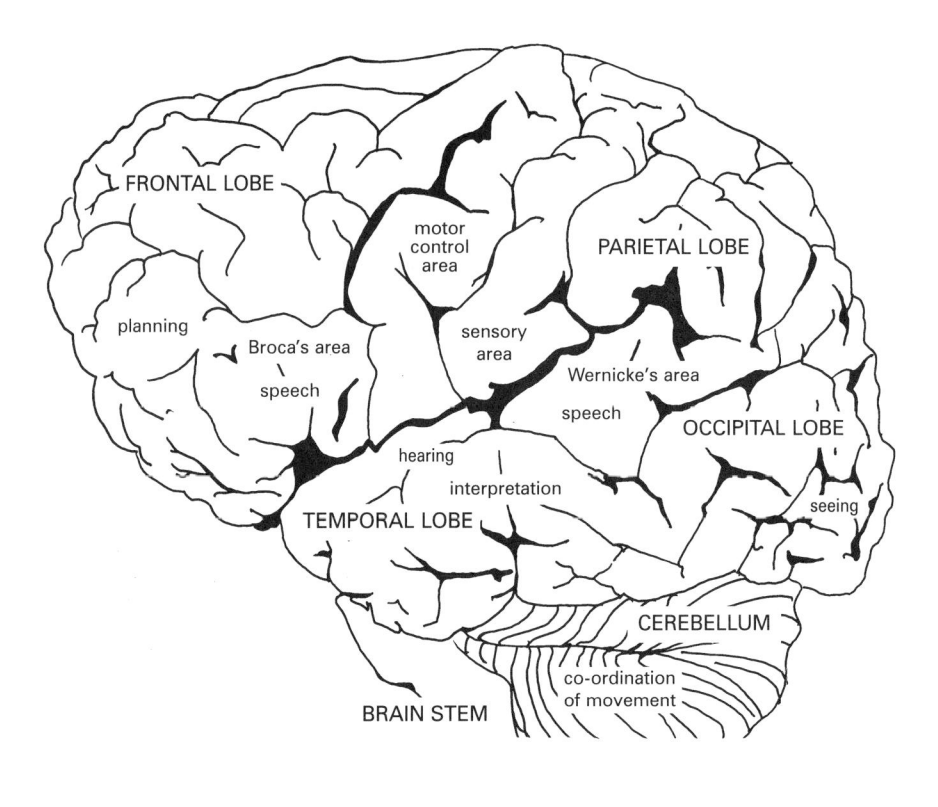

Figure 5.1 Left hemisphere of brain

Brain: the brain has the consistency of soft cheese and fits closely inside the top of the skull. It consists mainly of two types of cells: *neurones* and *glia*. Neurones are actively conducting cells. Glia cells are supportive and non-conducting.

The greyish outer layer of the brain is the cerebral cortex where most of the so-called 'higher' functions of the brain – thinking, perceiving, interpreting and so on – take place. This outer layer has many folds in it, rather like a sheet that has been crumpled up. It is estimated that if it were spread out, it would be like a sheet of foam rubber, 3–4 mm thick and about half a square metre in area. The nerve cells, or neurones, are arranged throughout this layer rather like the circuit boards in a computer. Estimates of the number of neurones range from a thousand million to about a million

million (10^{12}). It is as if the circuit board has been crumpled up into a ball, giving maximum area within minimum volume. The folds have been given individual names, and each area has traditionally been identified as being associated with a particular function (Figure 5.1).

The cortex consists of two cerebral (cortical) hemispheres ('half spheres') on the top, often referred to as the 'left brain' and 'right brain'. There is a fissure separating the hemispheres, running from front to back, but the two halves are connected by thick cables of fibres, in particular the corpus callosum, towards the centre of the brain.

The upper components of the brain grow outwards from a stem. The central part of the brain, whitish in colour and closest to the top of the brain stem, is the thalamus. This is the hub of communications for the whole brain, with a busy traffic of impulses flowing in all directions. The hypothalamus (below the thalamus) has a specialised role in the organisation of metabolism, the control of body temperature, the production and circulation of hormones and the mechanisms of being awake or asleep and of aggression. It is also active in sexual behaviour, and it controls the sympathetic and parasympathetic nervous systems in response to signals initiated by the cortex. The brain stem runs down to connect with the cables of the spinal cord. The cerebellum, or little brain, at the back, is concerned with learning and reconstructing skilled movements (Figure 5.2).

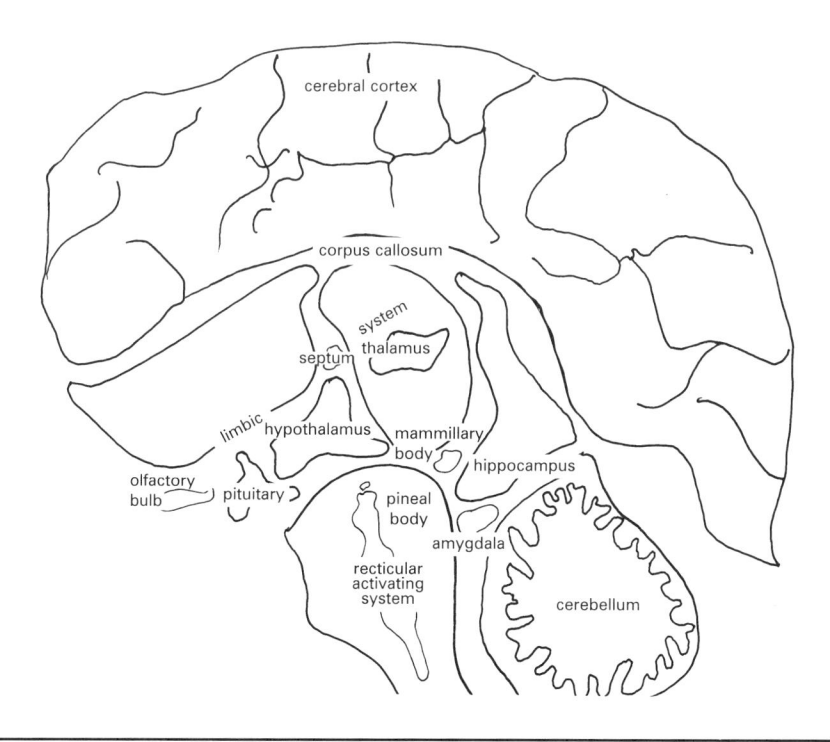

Figure 5.2 Inside the brain

A baby is born with all the neurones in place in the brain and central nervous system. Unlike other cells in the body, these do not divide and reproduce, and when lost through accident or disease, are not replaced. As the baby grows, the neurones enlarge and grow, the *dendrites* extend and spread further and the *axons* grow, and more connections are made between nerves. This kind of brain growth can continue throughout life and can be seen to correspond to the activities that a person undertakes. For example, there is some evidence that a person who regularly practises playing the violin will have a correspondingly greater number of nerve connections related to control of the muscles in the fingers. This correlates well with common knowledge and experimental evidence (Deliege and Sloboda, 1996) that regular practice, rather than merely theoretical knowledge and an understanding of music, is necessary for musicians. Learning a skill involves growing the necessary parts of the nerves, so it is not surprising that it is hard work and is unavoidable – there are no short cuts! There is also evidence that when one part of the brain is damaged, for example through a stroke, other parts of the brain can develop to take over the lost function if there is some kind of connection already available and sufficient practice is undertaken (see also brain damage).

The brain is active all the time, signals passing from place to place along well-established routes that have grown and developed according to the person's individual experience. Most of this activity takes place automatically without conscious awareness, as the brain monitors incoming information, matches it with previous patterns, assesses it for importance and activates relevant autonomic and motor systems or, occasionally, makes new connections between previously unconnected data. From time to time, snippets of data reach consciousness and we become aware that we are hungry or aching, or we have an idea. See also Chapters 12, 14, 16 and 17.

Brain damage: damage can be caused by direct injury or loss of blood supply in a stroke, or other means. Areas of damage can be identified with loss of particular functions. This does not necessarily imply that all the processing for a particular function takes place within that area, only that an essential piece is missing. This piece may simply be a significant part of the communication from one area to another. This can be compared with removing one component from a circuit board in a television, radio or computer. When the component is removed, the function of the set is altered, but it cannot be said that the lost function resided in that component, only that the component was necessary as part of the whole process. This comparison further enables us to regard the brain as a very special instrument. In most computers, a particular 'chip' will need to be replaced before function can be restored, whereas in the brain, other parts sometimes seem to be able to take over functions, so that if one part is damaged, skills can be relearned by using other parts.

The implications for caring for people following a stroke are that repeated practice of an activity may eventually result in some improvement, even if the brain is locally badly damaged. More research is needed to help to indicate when it is worthwhile persevering. An alternative approach is to look for a related function that will achieve a similar purpose. For example, a person who loses the ability to read because the part of the brain that processes visual recognition of letters and words is damaged, but who can still see, may learn to read in a new way. By tracing out the shape of letters with a finger, it is possible for 'muscle memory' in the fingers and hand to associate a pattern of movements with the name of each letter, using a previously unused and undamaged area of the brain. This method is slow and requires the same sort of continuous practice as playing a violin but might be considered worthwhile.

Brain scans: there are a number of techniques, such as computed tomography (CT), positron emission tomography (PET) and magnetic resonance imaging (MRI), for scanning the brain, each of which gives a different kind of information. When all this information is processed together by computer, all these images can be combined to give very detailed three-dimensional models of the brain or other organs of the body. Computer operators can rotate this three-dimensional image on the screen, explore different aspects of it, cut it open, look inside and roam through it. This has provided highly accurate data on the location of specific areas of injury affecting human function. Surgeons can simulate the effects of different approaches and, in effect, practise different cuts or techniques on a particular patient's organ, working out the best technique before the actual surgery. Computers are also available to many surgeons during surgery so that they can follow their actions on the screen. This enables surgeons to work deeply inside an organ without making a large incision.

CAT scan: see CT.

Chromosome: threadlike structures in the nucleus of each cell that transmit genetic information. There are 46 chromosomes in humans, which occur as 23 pairs, one chromosome in each pair being inherited from each parent. They are numbered 1 to 22 (autosomes), the last pair being the sex chromosomes XX or XY.

Each chromosome is a combination of protein and DNA (deoxyribonucleic acid). The DNA consists of two long strands that coil around each other forming a double helix. These strands can be thought of as the sides of a twisted ladder and are composed of sugar and phosphate. The strands are joined by bases which act like rungs of a ladder. There are four principal kinds of base: adenine, cytosine, thymine and guanine. Along the whole chromosome, individual sections of DNA can be identified, each of which is a discrete amino acid that can consist of up to 1000 pairs of bases. These individual sections are the genes. The order in which the bases are arranged in each gene is known as the genetic code and is important in heredity and in what is known as genetic engineering.

Chromosome mutations: in some cases of abnormalities, an alteration to the whole chromosome, or part of a chromosome, can be identified. Down's syndrome is associated with an extra chromosome 21, so that the person has three of these chromosomes instead of the usual pair. This occurs during cell division, an extra division taking place. Unlike inherited genetic codes, this abnormality can occur without either parent having any family history of Down's syndrome. In other instances, fragments of chromosomes can become lost, attached to the end of another chromosome, inverted or inserted into another chromosome. Mutations of the X and Y chromosomes give rise to unusual sexual characteristics (see sex).

CT or CAT images (X-ray computerised tomography or X-ray computerised axial tomography): these are computer-generated images of tissue density produced by measuring the absorption of X-rays in body tissue. The X-rays are passed through the tissue, for example the brain, as a fine beam sweeping through many different angles. This provides a succession of pictures or representations of slices of the tissue. The word tomography comes from the Greek word '*tomos*', meaning 'cut', as in appendec*tomy* and a*tom*. From these slices, a three-dimensional picture can then be generated on the computer monitor. The work on X-ray CT images in the early 1970s stimulated research into other kinds of imaging such as positron emission tomography (PET) and magnetic resonance imaging (MRI), which became available in the 1980s. See also brain scans.

Dopamine: this is one of the chief neurotransmitters that seems to be closely related to psychological experiences. Dopamine is produced at the synapses between particular kinds of neurones, known as the dopaminergic neurones, which occur only in the midbrain. One subgroup lies within the basal nuclei, which control co-ordination of movement. The other subgroup is in the limbic system, including the amygdala, which links with parts of the cortex dealing with the highest cortical functions, such as memory, intellect and personality. These dopaminergic neurones also receive impulses from regions of the brain involved in motivation, learning and rewarding mechanisms (see Figure 5.2).

In Parkinson's disease, there is a shortage of natural dopamine in the basal nuclei, which results in a lack of control over motor activities, tremor and rigidity. This can be treated with L-dopa, a synthetic form of dopamine. L-dopa has also been used (Sacks, 1991) in the treatment of patients with 'sleepy sickness', who appear to be in a sort of coma with very limited responsiveness to the outside world. It may also be used with other similar sorts of coma-like withdrawal.

There appear to be high levels of dopamine associated with the symptoms of schizophrenia and, in many instances, it seems that there is too much brain activity or that aspects of psychological functioning (as listed above) may be affected. It is known that disruption of the hippocampus can stimulate the overproduction of dopamine, and such disruption is implicated in some forms of schizophrenia (Srivastava, 1995). An alternative view is that the levels of dopamine may be within normal limits but cannot be tolerated. It is not clear whether the altered brain chemistry is a cause or effect of symptoms. *Antipsychotic* drugs act on those areas of the brain which are associated with dopaminergic neurones. Newer ones such as clozapine selectively block dopaminergic receptors. This leads to a reduction in psychotic symptoms and does not produce the Parkinsonian-type movement disorders associated with other medication. See also Chapter 12.

ECT (electroconvulsive therapy): also known as ECS (electroconvulsive shock), this is a technique for treating a variety of mental disorders, particularly depression. An electric shock is given to the brain by applying a voltage between two electrodes placed on the surface of the scalp. This is done under anaesthesia and with muscle relaxants to prevent the risk of fracture or injury during the generalised seizure produced. ECT has the effect of temporarily disrupting normal activity in the brain and can be quite effective in many cases in reducing depression. Gregory *et al.* (1985) compared real and simulated ECT (controls were given anaesthetic and muscle relaxant only) and found that unilateral and bilateral ECT were both effective. However, its use is controversial as there is no theoretical basis to justify it and it may produce permanent brain damage, particularly loss of memory and cognitive impairment, although there is little clear evidence of this (Gregory, 1987). In the 1970s there was a popular rumour that ECT was given as a punishment, without anaesthesia, to disruptive patients in long-stay institutions (for example, Kesey, 1976; Piercy, 1976). Breggin (1993) discusses the advantages and disadvantages of ECT compared with other interventions. When applied unilaterally with both electrodes applied to the non-dominant hemisphere, memory impairment is reduced. Modern methods (brief pulse, moderate or low dose) have less pronounced effects than early methods (sine wave or high dose) (Calev *et al.*, 1995).

EEG (electroencephalograph): the tracings of brain activity obtained by attaching electrodes to the scalp and measuring the variations in voltage produced by the brain. These voltages are tiny compared with familiar electricity obtained from batteries or the domestic mains: they are in the range of approximately 0.000 05 V (50 millionths of a volt or 50 μV).

Spots are selected beside the participant's eyes, on the temples and at the side and back of the head. The process is not painful, and the electrodes do not penetrate into the scalp (although in some special cases fine electrodes passing into the brain may be used). The colour-coded wires are drawn together at the top of the head like a multicoloured ponytail. The wires are linked to a recorder, together with readings for breathing, heart rate and pulse, blood pressure and body temperature. Up to about 16 channels may be used. The recorder has several pens that draw the traces.

Variations in the traces occur with the state of arousal of an individual and can be used to diagnose unusual or irregular brain activity such as seizure disorders and focal lesions. Their use is particularly noteworthy in sleep studies (see Chapter 12) and in measures of *evoked potentials*. Electroencephalography may be used with *biofeedback*, in investigating hypnosis, in attempting to find correlations with intelligence, in measuring the effects of tranquillisers and in investigating brain activity of all kinds. There has been some attempt to use these traces alongside *galvanic skin response* (GSR) in so-called lie detector tests on the assumption that telling lies increases arousal, but such use is unreliable.

Eugenics: 'the study of human genetics from the point of view (i) of encouraging breeding for good characteristics and (ii) of eliminating or reducing harmful characteristics' (Mackean, 1973: 99). There are no grounds for supposing that any planned programme of eugenics for a nation would have any noticeable effect. It can be tempting to think that preventing people with a harmful or undesirable characteristic from having children would eliminate these characteristics from the population. However, since most characteristics are caused by a combination of genes and many of these genes are 'recessive', which means that they can be carried unknowingly, even a complete ban on people with a known condition would have little effect on the population as a whole. Even wiping out a whole subdivision of the population, as Hitler had hoped to do by killing all members of various ethnic groups in Germany, would have only a short-term effect on the variation of genotypes.

According to Mackean (1973), several Scandinavian countries had introduced laws early in the 1970s that allowed for abortions to be induced for eugenic reasons. While now legal in the UK, there is considerable controversy over whether this is morally right or advisable. Some groups point out that it is more morally acceptable to allow all variations that have been conceived to survive and that we ought to be putting our collective resources into making sure we provide proper care and social support. Additionally, restricting the right to abortion focuses more attention on the prevention and treatment of conditions by other means, which may in the long term be more desirable for the future of society. Furthermore, if we allow any abortions, even if we draw the line initially at anything less than very harmful conditions, it might become too easy to slip into providing abortions for all undesirable characteristics. However, this view does not take into consideration whether there are sufficient resources for providing proper care for individuals with severely disabling conditions or the pain and discomfort experienced by some people who are born with crippling conditions.

Eugenics is not a simple issue of what is available technically but a social and psychological issue involving very complex moral and ethical considerations of what is right for each individual and what is right for society as a whole. See also genetic counselling.

Evoked potentials (EVs): small variations in voltages in the brain and nervous system produced by incoming stimuli such as flashes of light or touch. These can be difficult to detect as they are usually masked by the overall brain activity (for example, Springer and Deutsch, 1989) but can be isolated through computer averaging. Evoked potentials can be used to detect the specific areas in the brain that process incoming information and also measure the speed of transmission through the nervous system. This latter feature helps in the diagnosis and monitoring of conditions such as multiple sclerosis in which the loss of myelination slows down the transmission of action potentials along the nerves. Visual evoked potentials can also be used to assess visual function in apparently blind people (Towle et al., 1985).

Galvanic skin response (GSR): a measure of the electrical conductivity of the skin, usually the palm of the hand. Moisture in the skin can conduct electricity, and this alters with the saltiness or sweatiness of the skin. GSR has been widely used to study emotional reactions to stimuli, based on the assumption that a sudden emotional reaction will increase autonomic arousal and hence the sweat and salt content of skin on the palms of the hands.

Gamma rays: see X-rays.

Genes: sections of DNA, each of which is a discrete amino acid chain containing up to 1000 'bases' (adenine, cytosine, thymine and guanine) arranged in a specific order or code. Painstaking genetic labelling has resulted in many genes having been identified at known positions on the relevant pairs of chromosomes. Genes may be dominant or recessive, the recessive gene remaining 'silent' when paired with a corresponding dominant or active gene. Each gene that is passed on remains unchanged from generation to generation except where accidents or mistakes (mutations) happen during replication, repair or cell division, but the mix of genes that any individual receives is unique. Each gene contributes something towards one particular feature in the genotype or overall pattern of inherited characteristics.

In order to explain the principles of inheritance, it is sometimes helpful to talk as if each gene contributed one characteristic on a one-to-one basis, but most characteristics are influenced by a combination of genes. Examples of single-factor inheritance involving recessive genes include red hair and red–green variations in colour vision. Eye colour is determined to some extent by single genes, as illustrated in Figure 5.3. Conditions such as haemophilia can occur as a result of variations in any of the several genes responsible for blood coagulation.

If one parent is brown-eyed with two dominant genes (homozygous) and the other parent is brown-eyed with one dominant and one recessive gene (heterozygous) then all children will be brown-eyed with an even chance of being homozygous or heterozygous.

If both parents are brown-eyed with one dominant and one recessive gene (heterozygous), then a child may be brown-eyed with two dominant genes (homozygous), or brown-eyed with one of each type of gene (heterozygous) or blue-eyed. Blue eyes are always homozygous with two recessive genes.

If one parent is brown-eyed (heterozygous) and the other is blue-eyed, then there is an even chance that a child will be brown-eyed (heterozygous) or blue-eyed.

If one parent is brown-eyed (homozygous) and the other is blue-eyed, then all children will be brown-eyed (heterozygous).

KEY
● dominant gene ○ recessive gene
●● homozygous, dominant characteristic shows
●○ heterozygous, dominant characteristic shows
○○ homozygous, recessive characteristic shows

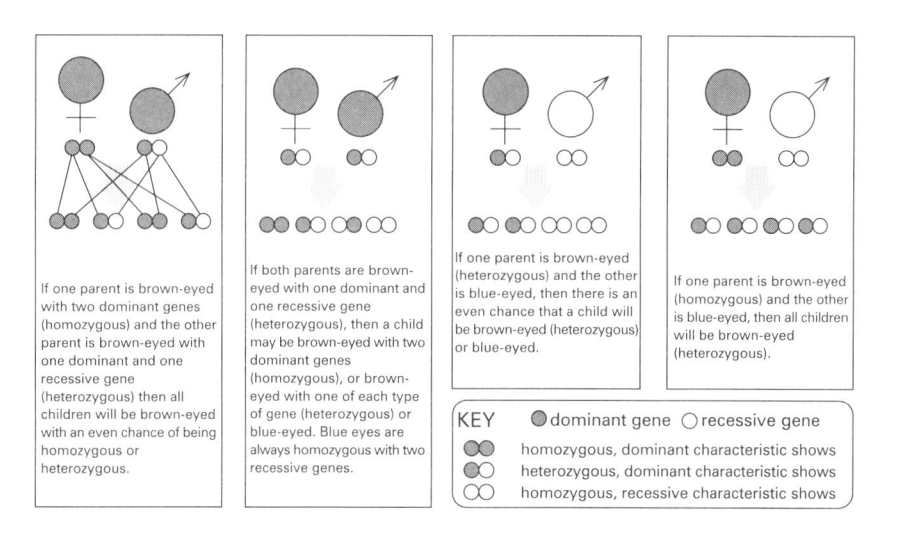

Figure 5.3 Inheritance of eye colour or other single-gene characteristic

Genetic counselling: in individual cases, genetic advice can help parents to make decisions about the way in which they plan their family. This may entail testing a person for known genetic variations that are likely to create problems for any offspring and providing supportive counselling. There are considerable ethical problems associated with genetic counselling, and parents, or prospective parents, face very difficult decisions related to whether to have children or to continue with a particular pregnancy. Counselling can be undertaken before marriage or before starting a family to point out any difficulties that might arise.

Most inherited conditions involve more than one gene but, for simplicity, the risk factors outlined below assume a one-to-one relationship similar to that for some aspects of eye colour inheritance, as described above. If a condition is caused by a dominant gene and if both parents have the condition, all the children will inherit it. If one parent has the condition, there is a one in two chance of the baby having the condition.

There is special risk where the potential parents have recessive genes in common that could give rise to undesirable characteristics in the baby, since the risk is not obvious without testing. If the condition is caused by a recessive gene, one parent having the condition and the other being a carrier, there is a one in two chance of the baby having it. If the other parent is not a carrier, the condition will not be passed on, although all the children will be carriers. If both parents are carriers, there is a one in four risk of the child having the condition and a two in four risk of being a carrier. After conception, the fetus can be tested for the presence of particular genes to see whether the recognised condition will develop. See also eugenics.

Genetic engineering: deliberate manipulation of genes in order to affect the next generation. This is common in the farming of animals and plants in order to produce new varieties that are resistant to disease, provide a greater yield or are interesting.

Genotype: the sum total of all the genes; the genetic constitution or inherited characteristics of an individual or group. These may or may not be outwardly apparent. For example, where genes are recessive or 'silent', the related characteristics will not be outwardly visible. Thus a person may have brown hair but carry the gene for red hair. It is possible for two people with brown hair to have a red-haired child if the child inherits the recessive gene from each parent. It can be quite startling and amusing if a naturally brown-haired woman who regularly dyes her hair red gives birth to a red-haired baby! See also phenotype.

Glia: also known as glial cells, neuroglia or satellite cells. These are non-conducting and serve as support cells to provide substance and packing between the neurones in the brain. This increases the insulation between neurones and contributes to the carrying of nutrients within the brain. There are several different types, including Schwann cells, oligodendrocytes and astrocytes (for example, Clegg, 1986: 204).

Hemispheric specialisation: the two hemispheres of the cerebral cortex are mirror images but not exactly symmetrical. The left hemisphere generally controls movements on the right side of the body and vice versa. Thus the right hand, arm, leg and foot are controlled by the left hemisphere and the left hand, arm, leg and foot by the right hemisphere (Figure 5.4). However, some movements, such as those of the trunk, shoulders and hips, can be controlled by either side. With vision, information from the left field of view crosses to the right hemisphere and information from the right field of view crosses to the left hemisphere (Figure 5.5). Auditory pathways are partially crossed (Figure 5.6).

In the majority of people, the left hemisphere is dominant, which results in the right hand being the preferred hand for many activities. The incidence of left-handedness is difficult to measure as it depends on how it is defined, seeming to vary from society to society. Figures vary from 4 per cent to 36 per cent (Gregory, 1987). Moreover, this dominance is not absolute, and many people have mixed hand preference and foot preference across a variety of actions such as picking up an object, catching, throwing, grip strength, lifting, kicking and jumping. Once a preference has been established, it is likely to be reinforced by habit.

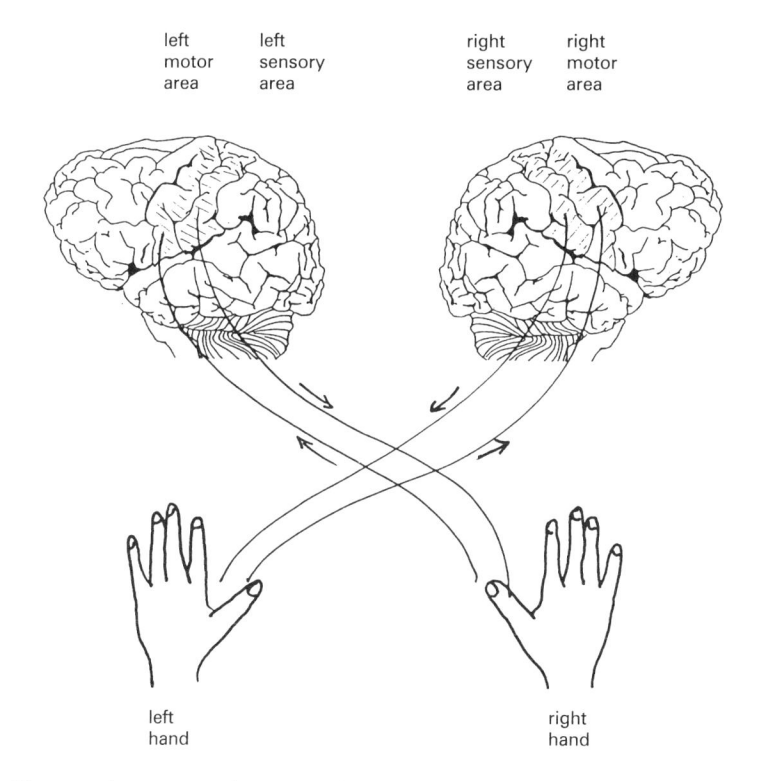

Motor and sensory pathways are almost completely crossed so that each hand is served primarily by the cerebral hemisphere on the opposite side

Figure 5.4 Motor and sensory pathways

Language is processed in the left hemisphere in the majority of left- and right-handed people. In a minority of left-handed people, whose brains are an exact mirror image of a typical right-handed person, the language centres are in the right hemisphere. According to Gilling and Brightwell (1982), 5 per cent of left-handers have language in the right hemisphere, but more recent experiments using the Wada test indicate that 15 per cent of left-handers have speech centres in the right brain and 15 per cent on both sides (Springer and Deutsch, 1989, 1993; McCarthy and Warrington, 1990). Also, 5 per cent of right-handers have speech centres on the right or on both sides of the brain.

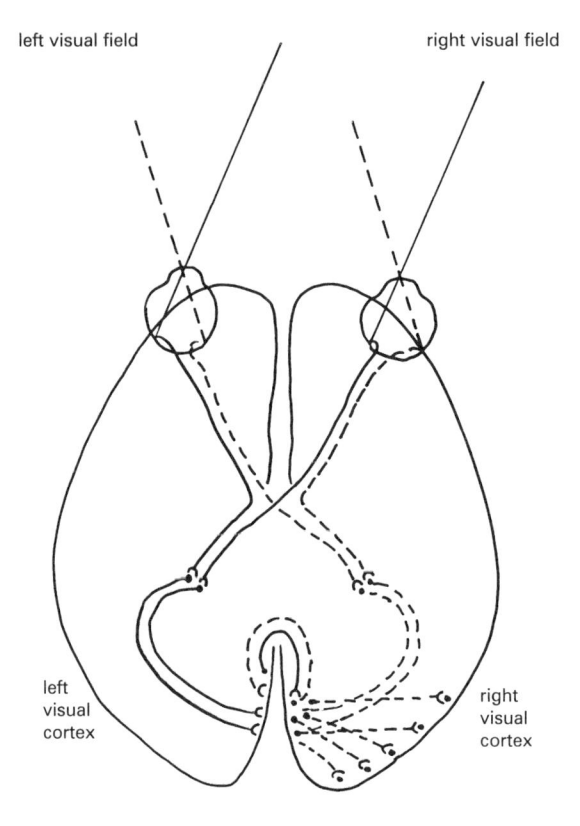

Brain from above

Information from the left field of view crosses to the right hemisphere and information from the right field of view crosses to the left hemisphere

Figure 5.5 Visual pathways

It is popularly reported that left-handers are more likely to have problems with reading and writing and show aspects of dyslexia. Furthermore, people who choose to specialise in mathematics and science may be thought to do so because of a dislike of, or difficulties with, language-based subjects and that this is related to hemisphere dominance and aspects of dyslexia. This speculation is fuelled by notions of conflict between right and left brain specialisation and dominance. However, there is as yet little evidence to substantiate this view. Dyslexia appears to be distributed throughout the population irrespective of intelligence, hand preference or subject preference.

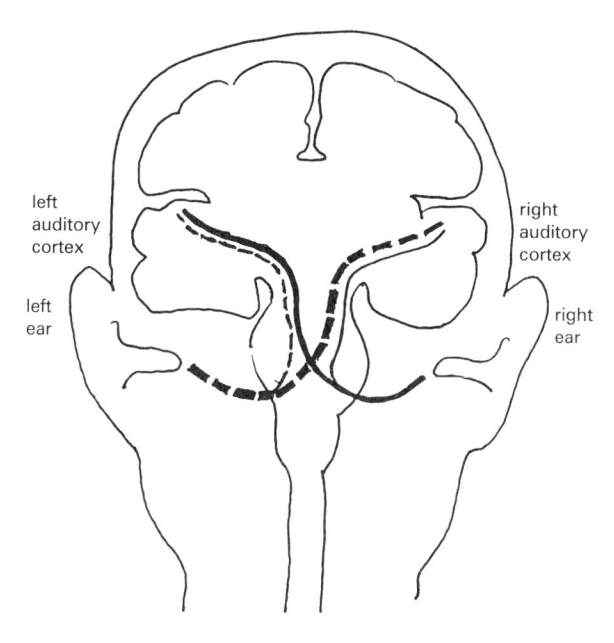

Brain from behind

Auditory pathways from the ears to the cerebral auditory areas are partially crossed. Although each hemisphere can receive input from both ears, the neural connections from one ear to the opposite hemisphere are stronger than the connections on the same side. When inputs compete, it is thought that the strong opposite side input inhibits the same side input.

Figure 5.6   Auditory pathways

The right hemisphere controls certain skills, for example spatial abilities such as drawing, map-reading and finding one's way around. The left hemisphere is popularly identified with the analytical scientist and the right hemisphere with the creative artist, but as Gilling and Brightwell (1982) point out, there is little scientific evidence for this. Even though the different regions are specialised, the hemispheres are normally in contact and there is no reason to suppose that it is hemisphere dominance as a whole that determines a particular person's mix of skills. It could be argued that a dominant left hemisphere may suppress an attempt by the right hemisphere to communicate in words (Gilling and Brightwell, 1982; Edwards, 1992). However, it is also likely that specialisation or discouragement early in life results in neglect of certain skills. With practice and perseverance, most adults can develop whatever skills they choose, from mathematics to drawing (Edwards, 1992).

On the other hand, there are differences between men and women that are documented and that can be related to hemisphere specialisation and the ways in which the hemispheres are connected. For example women are, on average, found to have a greater facility with verbal language (the spoken and written use of words), whereas men score more highly on tests of spatial ability. Women tend to have a thicker corpus callosum and hence more connection between left and right. There is some suggestion that a more complex corpus callosum is also found in some homosexual men. A detailed account of left and right brain specialisation is given in Springer and Deutsch (1993). See also topography.

Heterozygote fitness: a judgement about whether the corresponding genes in a zygote will produce desirable or undesirable characteristics.

Heterozygous: used in reference to a specific pair of genes on the corresponding pair of chromosomes. This occurs as a result of the fertilisation of an ovum with a sperm containing different genes relating to a particular characteristic. For example, a person can be called heterozygous for eye colour if the corresponding genes relate to a different colour of the eyes. As the gene for brown eyes is dominant, such a person will have brown eyes (see Figure 5.3 above). For other genes, the resulting characteristic will depend on which gene is dominant and whether several genes are involved in determining the characteristic.

Homozygous: as with heterozygous, this term is used in reference to a specific pair of genes on the corresponding pair of chromosomes. In this case, it occurs as a result of the fertilisation of an ovum with a sperm that contains matching genes for a particular characteristic. For example, a person can be called homozygous for eye colour if both corresponding genes relate to the same colour of the eyes (see Figure 5.3 above).

Language centres in the brain: two language centres have been identified in the brain: Broca's area and Wernicke's area. In most people, including the majority of those who are left handed, these language centres are situated in the left cortical hemisphere (see also hemispheric specialisation). Broca's area is towards the front of the brain, Wernicke's area further back (see Figure 5.1 above).

Damage to either of these areas causes aphasia or dysphasia, which means disruption of speech. This commonly follows a stroke affecting the left side of the brain, where the language centres are situated, and may be associated with right side paralysis of the body. There is no formal distinction between the terms 'aphasia' and 'dysphasia' and they are used interchangeably in the literature in relation to speech disorders. The prefix 'a' means 'without' or 'lacking'; 'dys' means that something is not functioning properly or that there is a problem. The particular type of speech disruption depends on whether Broca's area or Wernicke's area, or both, is affected and how deep into the brain the damage extends. Gilling and Brightwell (1982) give detailed accounts of patients with damage to these areas.

It appears from study of people with strokes in these areas that Broca's area processes use of grammar and the rules of language. This is usually noticeable as an 'expressive' disorder. Speech may be slow and require enormous effort and sounds are poorly produced. Patients leave out the little words such as 'if', 'but' and 'to', or lose endings such as plurals or verb tenses, so that sentences sound like a telegram. Writing may also be without grammatical rules. On the other hand, patients may be able to sing a melody well and may be able to sing words they cannot speak. There may be failure to understand complicated sentences, but in many patients understanding is not impaired. This adds support to the argument that potential for learning the rules of language is 'hard-wired' into the brain. That is, there seems to be a natural ability to learn language and follow rules in a way that is independent of intelligence or culture, even though the particular rules for different languages may bear little relation to each other. It is noticeable that this applies only to spoken language; learning the special rules for writing requires considerable motivation and effort.

In contrast, damage to Wernicke's area usually results in rather rapid speech with a normal flow and correct grammar but enormous difficulty in finding the right word, an experience commonly known as 'word-blindness' (receptive dysphasia). Wernicke's area appears to be responsible for holding the bulk of vocabulary, rather like a dictionary, so that the right word for an object or action can be found when wanted.

Children who sustain damage to the left hemisphere before the age of about 7 or 8 usually develop or recover language as the right hemisphere has the potential for language and appears to take over.

Limbic system: this consists of a number of structures around the central core of the brain, including the thalamus, hypothalamus, hippocampus and amygdala. It has a role in regulating emotional and sexual behaviour and often inhibits aggressive responses. Damage, surgery or cerebral atrophy may result in an increased incidence of aggressive behaviour.

Micrograph: a photograph obtained using a microscope, nowadays usually referring to the image obtained using a scanning electron microscope (SEM). This uses a beam of electrons rather than light, can magnify to a much greater extent than an optical microscope and can produce a three-dimensional image, but it cannot be used with living specimens.

MRI: magnetic resonance imaging, also known as nuclear magnetic resonance (NMR) or nuclear magnetic resonance imaging (NMRI). Like X-ray CT images, MRI images can be used to give anatomical data of the brain and contribute to a detailed three-dimensional computer model. Finer detail is possible than with X-rays, but different structures show up, so both techniques are needed for a full picture. The technique was first discovered in the 1940s (see Gregory, 1987) and came into widespread medical use in the 1980s. NMR is based on the observation that the nuclei of some atoms behave like miniature bar magnets when placed in a magnetic field. They can be lined up in a magnetic field and then manipulated by a controlled radio signal. As they recover from the radio disturbance, they emit radiofrequency signals that give information about the surrounding atoms. This provides a picture of how all the atoms in a particular region are arranged. In the brain tissue, the abundant hydrogen nuclei (which are simple protons) respond the most strongly to the magnetic and radio disturbance; for this reason, the technique may also be referred to as 'proton NMR'. See also brain scans.

Nerve fibre: the axon of the nerve with its surrounding membrane. Large fibres may extend more than a metre between the spinal cord and the extremities of the body. A nerve fibre conducts a group or volley of electrical impulses in one direction only by exchanging positive and negative ions across the membrane. At rest, there is a small resting potential across the membrane. The nerve impulse comprises a sudden, rapid, short-lived change in the membrane that allows ions to cross the membrane, creating an *action potential*. A change in the next part of the membrane occurs just ahead of an action potential and thus the impulse moves along the nerve fibre.

There are two main types of nerve fibre: myelinated and unmyelinated. Myelinated fibres have layers of myelin, a lipoprotein, folded around the axon. The myelin sheath is not continuous but has little gaps at intervals, called the nodes of Ranvier, where the interchange of ions can take place. One effect of the myelin sheathing is to increase the speed and efficiency with which action potentials can nerves. In multiple sclerosis, the travel along the nerve and prevent accidental connections with other myelin is progressively destroyed.

Nervous system: the nervous system consists of the brain and all the nerves that make up the communication system within the body. It is usual to call the brain and spinal cord the central nervous system (CNS), and everything else the peripheral nervous system (Figure 5.7).

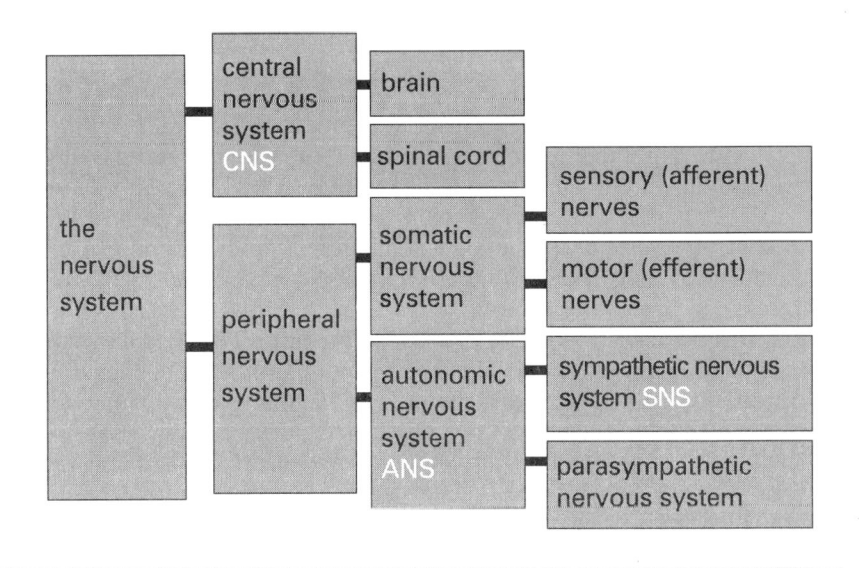

Figure 5.7 The nervous system

The peripheral nervous system, comprising 43 pairs of nerves, can be seen as consisting of the afferent or sensory nerves (carrying messages *to* the brain from the senses receptors) and the efferent or motor nerves (carrying messages *away from* the brain to the muscles, internal organs and glands). Most cell bodies lie within the brain or the spinal cord, only the extensions being spread out through the rest of the body. The nerve supplying an arm or leg muscle, for example, has its cell body and nucleus inside the spinal cord, with the axon extending down the limb. Within the spinal cord, the only way the peripheral nerves can connect with the central nerves is via chemical synapses: there is no physical connection. Nerves serving the muscles can be called somatic (*soma* = body) and are experienced as being under voluntary control. The nerves serving the internal organs and glands make up the autonomic nervous system (ANS), which is not usually felt as being able to be voluntarily controlled, except in special conditions such as through yoga, biofeedback and hypnosis. The autonomic nervous system is separated into the sympathetic and parasympathetic systems. The parasympathetic nervous system maintains or restores normal functioning such as heart rate, digestion, emptying of bladder and sexual activity, whereas the sympathetic nervous system (SNS) prepares the body for sudden action (fight or flight) at times of stress.

Neurone (or neuron): the nerve cell, which has a cell body with a nucleus and many extensions. The main extension is the axon; the others are dendrites. In motor (efferent) nerves, the axon is usually involved in carrying impulses away from the cell body, away from the CNS, towards the next neurone, while the dendrites pick up incoming signals from surrounding neurones. In sensory (afferent) nerves, the direction is in reverse, the axon normally carries impulses to the cell body, towards the CNS, and the dendrites pass on signals to the surrounding nerves. Individual brain cells fire electrical impulses, or action potentials, intermittently.

The action potentials are normally triggered by a change in the environment. An action potential in one nerve can either excite or inhibit the next nerve, depending on the nature of the *synapse* between them. Many factors have an influence on the firing of a neurone, including its threshold of excitability, the local chemical environment and the sum of excitatory and inhibitory impulses it receives at any time. There are various different kinds of neurone, and all possible directions of signal are possible – dendrite-to-axon is most common, but it is also possible to have axon-to-axon and dendrite-to-dendrite connections. Neurones do not undergo cell division or replicate themselves but they are continually manufacturing new protein that is continually lost or destroyed. According to some sources, nearly all the protein in the brain is renewed every 3 weeks.

Neurotransmitters: the chemicals that carry messages across the synapses between neurones. Different cells use different transmitters. These include noradrenaline, serotonin, dopamine, GABA (gamma-amino butyric acid) and acetylcholine. Alteration to neurotransmitter systems and their receptors are thought to account for some illnesses. See antidepressants, dopamine and serotonin.

NMR, NMRI: see MRI.

PET (positron emission tomography): like CT imaging and MRI (see above), PET images can be used to provide a picture of the brain. Unlike the other two techniques, however, PET scanning gives functional rather than anatomical information, that is, it shows what is actually happening chemically in the brain rather than just where things are. The technique involves giving a person a radioactive substance such as radioactive glucose and then detecting where that substance goes in the brain. Since brain activity depends on using glucose, regions that show up as having a high level of radioactivity can be assumed to be most active.

The radioactive atoms in the glucose have very short half-lives of a few minutes, and the radiation consists of positrons, which can be thought of as positive electrons or positive beta (β) rays. When an emitted positron interacts with an electron in the brain tissue, photons of gamma (γ) radiation are emitted, which can be picked up by the detectors that are usually arranged around the head in a circular fashion. PET images can be used to show areas of abnormal brain function and also to illustrate real-time brain activity during perception and problem-solving activities. PET images can be combined with X-ray CT images and MRI scans to give very detailed three-dimensional computer models of the brain and other organs. See also brain scans.

Phenotype: the sum total of all the observable characteristics of appearance and behaviour, whatever their origins, of an individual or group. At a basic level of inheritance of genes, there may be a genetic difference between people with identical outward characteristics. For example, two people with brown eyes may have different genes: one may have a *homozygous* arrangement with both genes contributing to brown eyes, the other may be *heterozygous* with the dominant gene for brown eyes on one chromosome in the pair but the recessive gene for blue eyes on the other. See also Figure 5.3 above.

Other characteristics may have been determined by the inherited genotype or affected by environmental factors or by a mixture or interaction of the two. A person with blonde hair may appear blonde partly because of the genes which determine fair hair and partly because of natural or artificial bleaching, or completely by artificial bleaching. With hair colour, it is relatively easy to determine what is inherited and what is added. However, with other characteristics such as personality, intelligence and mental health disorders, the distinction is not so clear. Such complex characteristics are most probably determined by the interaction of genetic inheritance with upbringing and experience. Where similarities are seen across families or cultural groups, speculation arises as to whether the observable phenotype is due more to shared inheritance or cultural patterns of behaviour. This kind of speculation has given rise to what is now referred to as the nature – nurture debate.

Resting potential: the electrical potential across the membrane of a nerve fibre while it is not firing.

Serotonin: also called 5HT or 5-hydroxytryptamine. This is a neurotransmitter thought to be implicated in depression. See Chapter 2.

Sex: strictly speaking, this refers to the biological designation of male or female. In most cases, it is decided on the basis of physical characteristics (morphology), usually depending on visible characteristics at birth.

The basic biological determinant of sex is the arrangement of chromosomes: generally, males have two different sex chromosomes, X and Y, the X inherited from the mother, the Y from the father, whereas females have two similar ones, X and X, one inherited from the father, one from the mother. All ova have only an X chromosome, while spermatozoa can be either X or Y. Thus it is the father who contributes the basic sex to the fertilised embryo. However, the development of the embryo is also influenced by the levels of hormones available. The presence of the Y chromosome may tip the balance in favour of maleness but the XY embryo will only develop male characteristics if there is sufficient androgen in the uterine environment, so a baby who is chromosomally male could develop (morphologically) as a female (for example, Ruse, 1990).

Genes for male and female characteristics may be scattered fairly evenly throughout all the chromosomes. Secondary sexual characteristics such as a bass voice, beard and muscular physique in males, breasts and a wide pelvis in females, are not the result of sex-linked genes but of the different expression of the same genes present in both sexes. Both sexes carry genes controlling the growth of hair, mammary glands and penis, but in the presence of male or female hormones, they have different effects. A person with fully developed male and female physical characteristics or functioning sex organs of both sexes is usually referred to as hermaphrodite, but the term 'bisexual' is sometimes used (see also Chapter 15).

There are also some rare chromosome variations that arise because the sex chromosomes fail to separate during meiosis (cell division) (Simpkins and Williams, 1987: 380). Some ova develop with an extra X chromosome or more, others with none, whereas some sperm develop with an extra X or Y chromosome. If the ovum has no X chromosome and is fertilised by an X sperm, the zygote will be XO and develops into a girl with Turner's syndrome. She will be infertile with no menstruation or breast development. If a normal X ovum is fertilised by a sperm containing two Y chromosomes, the zygote will be XYY. Some men with this arrangement have been found to be tall and aggressive, and, as featured in the movie *Aliens 3*, 'Double Ys' have been thought to be largely criminally insane. However, more recent studies have not upheld this belief. When an XX (or XXXX) ovum is fertilised by a Y sperm, the XXY (or XXXXY) zygote develops into a male with Klinefelter's syndrome. These men tend to grow taller than average, have incomplete infertile testes and may develop small breasts. Since sex is of such primary importance in society, special counselling would seem to be needed for people with unusual inheritance. Medical and biology books that describe these abnormalities rarely give any indication of what it feels like for these people. See also Chapter 15.

Split-brain: it is possible to separate the two hemispheres of the cerebral cortex by cutting the *corpus callosum*. This operation has been performed on a few patients since the 1940s in an attempt to reduce the effects of epileptic seizures. Some patients have gained a measure of relief without many obvious detrimental effects apart from a certain strangeness. From a psychological point of view, the few detectable changes are very interesting and contribute to the debate about where consciousness resides. One patient reported that when she intended to reach for an object with her right hand, her left hand might suddenly take control and grab something different even though she knew this was unsuitable (Gilling and Brightwell, 1982). Selective experiments with vision indicate that, in most cases, only an image available to the left brain can be named. Any other image is not apparently recognised, although it can sometimes be drawn by the left hand. It is only after making such a drawing and viewing it with both sides of the field of

Synapse: the microscopic area between neurones in which messages pass from one cell to another in the form of chemicals. According to Gilling and Brightwell (1982), the word 'synapse' is derived from the Greek word for handclasp, which evokes an interesting picture of a message being transmitted through the meeting of one set of extensions with another, although it must be remembered that, in synapses, the nerves do not physically touch. In more general terms, the original Greek simply means junction. When the action potential in one neurone reaches the synapse, the presynaptic cell endings manufacture and release a chemical substance that diffuses across the gap to the next (postsynaptic) cell, where it is taken up. Each nerve cell has thousands of synapses, and each synapse connects between many cells. According to Simpkins and Williams (1987), there are about $10^{2\,783\,000}$ synapses in an average brain. The synapses that converge on a cell all contribute to whether or not the cell will fire. Some are excitatory, which will cause the cell to fire, others inhibitory, which will prevent firing. If more excitatory synapses act, the cell will fire; if more inhibitory, it will not. There is no simple relationship between particular chemicals and excitation or inhibition: chemicals that excite some cells inhibit others. Any surplus chemical is reabsorbed by the presynaptic neurone (reuptake) or broken down by an enzyme, ready for synthesis again. Surplus chemicals would interfere with subsequent firing or inhibition. The rate of uptake by the postsynaptic cell and reuptake by the presynaptic cell determine the frequency with which a synapse can respond to incoming action potentials.

View that the patient can name the stimulus object. It appears that the image can be mentally processed and a drawing made without any conscious awareness. This may indicate that our experience of consciousness is closely connected with our capacity for language, but it is not possible to derive any general conclusions from a few isolated and unusual cases. See also Chapter 12.

Topography: the study of the areas of the brain. Some areas of the brain, for example the motor control area, or motor strip, are said to be arranged topographically such that particular functions can be related to specific areas in a clearly mapped out and unchanging way, (Blakemore, in Barlow *et al.*, 1990). The word comes from 'topology', a branch of mathematics concerned with the properties of figures, surfaces and spaces. Similarly, deeper inside the brain, it is possible to label distinct areas and give an indication of their main functions in relation to psychological experiences (see Figures 5.1 and 5.2 above). However, localisation does not exactly match the visible shapes, and there is increasing evidence that other areas can take over functions. Although such labelling is useful as an introduction to brain function, there is an increasing trend away from a topographical approach. See also hemispheric specialisation.

Twins: babies who develop together in the uterus. Twins can be either monozygotic (from one zygote or fertilised ovum that has divided into two within one amniotic membrane) or dizygotic (two separate zygotes in separate amniotic membranes). Monozygotic twins are identical and necessarily the same sex. Dizygotic twins are no more alike than any siblings and can be either the same or a different sex. Twin studies are useful in psychology as they help to distinguish between which characteristics are more likely to be due to genotype and which to upbringing and personal experience.

X-rays and gamma (γ) rays: these are short-wavelength, high-frequency, high-energy invisible rays belonging to the extreme end of the electromagnetic or light spectrum. They cover a range of frequencies known as 'soft' or 'hard'. They can penetrate solid matter, and the different frequencies may be used either for taking photographs of bones or other organs within the human body (soft X-rays) or for irradiating and destroying tumorous tissue (hard X- or gamma rays). They are identical except for the precise range of frequency. The distinction is made for historical reasons as they were identified separately and come from different parts of the atom. Gamma rays are produced naturally from the nuclei of atoms in radioactive materials such as cobalt-60. They are also produced by the collision of positrons and electrons. X-rays are generated by very high-voltage X-ray machines that stimulate the electron shells of atoms. X-rays are also naturally radiated from the sun but are absorbed by the atmosphere before reaching the earth.

Zygote: the initial stage in fertilisation when male and female gametes fuse, that is, when the sperm first joins with the ovum. After fertilisation, the zygote undergoes cell division and growth, and develops into an embryo and later a fetus. The term 'zygote' is also used at all stages of the lifespan in relation to specific characteristics that are determined by the initial fertilisation. Twins are described as monozygotic or dizygotic. All genetic characteristics can be identified as heterozygotic or homozygotic (see above).

6 COGNITIVE PSYCHOLOGY AND COGNITIVE THERAPIES

Cognitive psychology is chiefly concerned with experimental investigation of those mental processes to do with knowing and understanding that can either be brought readily into consciousness or revealed experimentally through the careful manipulation of variables.

Areas for enquiry include attention, perception, memory, thinking, problem-solving and language, which are discussed separately elsewhere. This chapter introduces some of the basic principles of cognitive psychology, explores ideas about the relationship between cognition and emotion and gives examples of how cognitive concepts have been developed within therapeutic techniques.

Definitions	
Drever (1964)	Cognition. A general term covering all the various modes of knowing – perceiving, remembering, imagining, conceiving, judging, reasoning. The cognitive function, as an ultimate mode or aspect of the conscious life, is contrasted with the affective and conative – feeling and willing... [Emotion is]... a complex state of the organism, involving bodily changes of a widespread character – in breathing, pulse, gland secretion, etc. – and, on the mental side, a state of excitement or perturbation, marked by strong feeling, and usually an impulse towards a definite form of behaviour.
Rubin and McNeil (1983)	Emotions set the tone of our experience and give life its vitality and, like motives, they are internal factors which can energize, direct and sustain behaviour. (Cited in Gross, 1996)
Stratton and Hayes (1993)	[Emotion is] the experience of subjective feelings which have positive or negative value for the individual... Most current theories

Definitions (cont'd)

	regard emotions as a *combination* of physiological response with a cognitive evaluation of the situation... Some definitions would reserve the term emotion for fairly intense and fairly brief experiences... [Affect is] a term used to mean emotion, but covering a very much wider band of feeling than the *normal* emotions. Affect includes pleasurable sensation, friendliness and warmth, pensiveness, and mild dislike etc., as well as the extreme emotions such as joy, exhilaration, fear and hatred. Broadly speaking, affect refers to any category of feeling, *as distinct from* cognition or behaviour [emphases added].
Williams *et al.* (1988)	Discussions of the relationship between cognition and emotion tend to focus either on the effects of emotion on cognitive processes or on the role of cognitive processes in the genesis of emotional states...
Robinson (1996)	Cognition and affect are not separate processes but all cognitions are emotionally coloured which gives a sense of urgency to the cognition.

Approaches, Arguments and Applications

Cognitive psychology, a part of cognitive science, represents one of the three most important mainstream perspectives in psychological enquiry, alongside biopsychology and social psychology. It has largely replaced behaviourism or behavioural science as the dominant approach in the UK.

Traditionally, theories of emotion and cognition see these as separate entities or domains but somehow influencing each other. The words 'emotion', 'affect' and 'mood' are often used interchangeably to refer to our feelings or passions, and it is difficult to be precise about their meanings. The word 'emotion' is derived from words meaning movement and suggests a stirring or agitation. 'Affect' comes from the same root as affection and was introduced in the nineteenth century, when Kant suggested that all psychological processes could be classified as *cognitive, conative* or *affective*, that is, thoughts, acts of will, volition or choice, and emotions. This has led to conceptions of thoughts and emotions as separate processes rather than as different aspects of the same process. Gross (1996: 119) illustrates this separation when he says, 'it is the richness of our emotions and our capacity to have feelings *as well as* to think and reason which makes us unique as a species' (emphasis added). Stratton and Hayes (1993), as can be seen from their definitions given above, demonstrate the difficulty in making this separation between behaviour, affect and cognition. They state, on the one hand that emotion is a combination of physiological response and cognitive evaluation, and on the other that affect is distinct from cognition and behaviour. They make a working distinction between emotion and affect suggesting that the term 'emotion' is most usefully applied to extreme basic or primary emotions, which they call *normal* emotions.

Fraser Watts (1992) argues that older theories of emotion have often seen emotion as dysfunctional and that many clinical approaches also make this assumption. This has led to current theories focusing on 'excess' emotion. Watts (1992) says that cases of poor or blunted emotion have scarcely been considered in cognitive psychology, although they are more adequately treated within psychodynamic or humanistic perspectives.

Early biopsychological studies of emotion, such as that by Cannon (1929), concentrated on extreme or high emotions, such as fear and anxiety, and emphasised peripheral physiological reactions, for example increased heart rate, sweating and goosepimples. Milder feelings, referred to as *moods*, were studied independently in psychodynamic approaches, with separate studies for short-term and long-term moods. Cognitive models of emotion centre on the question of whether, when faced with an emotionally arousing situation, the cognition or the emotion comes first. For example, does recognising something as dangerous make you afraid, or does being afraid make you realise something is dangerous?

The traditional split into domains of cognitive (knowing), affective (feeling), and conative (willing) is compelling, and until recently most psychological approaches have assumed that such separateness is fundamental to a study of human experience. However, recent trends in all fields towards eclecticism and integration are leading to changes even at this most basic level. The main debate is still the one outlined by Williams *et al.* (1988), as quoted above, concerning whether cognitions lead to emotions or vice versa, but some researchers, for example Robinson (1996), are questioning whether this split is meaningful and instead argue that cognition and emotion cannot be separated. Taking this view, emotion can be viewed as an abstract concept, an artefact of the development of language, rather than anything psychologically identifiable or measurable in its own right. That is to say, perhaps we do not have separate thoughts and emotions but emotionally coloured thoughts. It can be argued that, faced with a dangerous situation, our perceptions are fear-coloured, which gives an urgency to our decision about what to do next.

Cognitive therapy is based on the earlier assumption that emotion and cognition are separate, that *cognitive appraisal* comes before emotion, rather than the other way around, and that *cognitive restructuring* will alter the emotional experience. That is, if you believe that a situation is harmful, you will feel anxious, but if you gain new information so that you can judge that the situation is not harmful, your anxiety will fade.

Key Terms and Concepts

Affect: a general term that can be used either to refer to all levels of emotion from mild to strong or to only the milder end of the spectrum. Affect can be a more useful word than emotion when referring to inner feelings where there are no facial or other non-verbal clues to indicate the feelings or where there is a discrepancy between what is felt and what is displayed.

In some cultures, the social consensus is that overt emotional display, such as of jealousy, anger, sorrow or jollity, is not helpful to normal social functioning. In common experience, it may be noticed that people who believe that such emotional display is wrong also tend to believe that emotions interfere with rational decision-making. At least some of the dispute about the acceptance of emotions may be a result of the tendency to define emotion only in terms of excess, high or strong feelings. In contrast, the word 'affect' can be used to include milder forms, such as warm feelings, mild regret or amusement. Mood has traditionally been regarded as quite separate from emotion, but both could come under the general heading of affect. Evidence suggests that some affect, far from preventing rational thought, is actually essential to decision-making in certain situations. Rational thought permits a person to set out all the possible alternatives and work out what the outcomes will be, but deciding which outcome is the *better* one often requires feelings that give a sense of *value* to the different outcomes.

Affective: anything relating to affect, mood or emotion.

Affective disorders: disorders of mood and inner feelings. This medical diagnosis usually refers to depression or 'negative' affect but can also be used for mania, bipolar mood disorder, seasonal affective disorder (SAD) and other affective or emotional states. See also Chapter 2.

Arbitrary inference: a type of cognitive distortion in which a conclusion is drawn from irrelevant or insufficient evidence, for example 'Everyone is avoiding me because I have a pimple on my face.'

Artificial intelligence: the use of 'thinking machines' and computer modelling to simulate human behaviour in an attempt to increase understanding. Early thinking machines (see Turing, 1936, cited in Gross, 1996) were used in carefully controlled situations in which the typed responses of the machine were compared with those of a human given the same question. It was argued that, if an observer could not tell whether the response came from the machine or the person, the machine could be said to be thinking. Whether or not that conclusion is valid, the early work has given rise to some interesting speculations.

Through the analysis of the questions and answers that are typical of a diagnostic interview, various computer programs have been devised that simulate a clinician's responses and assist in diagnosing a client's main areas of concern. Naturally enough, the use of this is increasing as it saves money. Happily, clients report some satisfaction with the arrangement and sometimes feel more at ease typing in responses at a keyboard than talking to a therapist.

Other lines of investigation simulate problem-solving behaviour and seek a greater understanding of neural processes.

Basic emotions: several authors have classified emotions, based on various types of evidence, such as photographs of facial expressions or actors' demonstrations. For example, Gross (1996) cites Ekman and Friesen (1975), who list six primary emotions, and Izard (1977), Oatley (1989) and Plutchik (1980), who name eight. Five are common to all the lists:

- pleasure
- anger
- fear (or anxiety)
- distress (or sadness)
- disgust.

These five, in particular, seem to be basic emotions that are universally recognisable from facial expressions and postures. During evolutionary processes in which an organism was becoming capable of dealing with environmental emergencies, these would have formed a useful set of response patterns, directing an animal towards or away from situations with varying degrees of urgency. Moreover, it is possible to identify a corresponding underlying physiological system for each of the five. Each is linked to an area of the *limbic* system, which has many connections upwards into the *cortex*, where cognitive processing takes place, and downward into the *peripheral nervous system* and the effectors of bodily adjustment. The feeling or emotion of pleasure can be viewed as linked to the 'pleasure centres' of the brain (Olds and Milner, 1954). Fear is linked with anxiety, and stress with the production of adrenaline, anger with aggression and the hypothalamus and amygdala, disgust with the centre that precipitates vomiting, and sadness with the system that precipitates tears. Furthermore, it has been claimed by Ekman and Oster (1979) that these are innate systems.

It seems reasonable to suppose that these five basic emotions need not, and usually do not, act alone. Everyday experience is usually a mixture of these, which are closely combined with cognitions.

Belief: Morgan and King (1971) define a belief as 'the acceptance of some proposition'. It can be argued that most knowledge consists of beliefs rather than facts, in that many so-called facts are simply widely held beliefs for which there is consistent empirical evidence. Plato distinguishes between three types of knowledge or belief: (1) things for which there is little or no empirical evidence or rational argument and which require faith, such as confidence in the efficiency of free market economics or the existence of fairies or Father Christmas; (2) things that are true according to widely held belief, perhaps because they always happen that way or they can be shown to happen through scientific investigation, such as that the sun will rise tomorrow or that touch is an important aspect of communication; and (3) things whose truth is a matter of irrefutable knowledge, for example 'by definition', such as that a triangle has three sides. It is argued that some scientific findings can be considered irrefutable, provided that the conditions under which things always occur can be precisely defined. Later philosophers make this kind of distinction by talking of 'grammar' (Wittgenstein) or 'sense' and 'reference' (Frege). That is, the choice of words used to refer to things and the 'rules' for the use of particular words determines how the truth about those things is communicated. Putting free market economics next to fairies in a sentence, as above, possibly suggests something about the writer's beliefs.

A distinction needs to be made between 'believe about' and 'believe in'. A young theologian faced repeatedly with the question 'Do you believe in sex before marriage?' (which is the sort of question people ask young theologians) might be tempted to reply, 'Well, it is more likely than Father Christmas.'

Bottom-up processing: a term that has a variety of meanings, depending on the context. In general, it means working upwards from basic information or raw data towards a higher mental process. This can be compared with notions of induction in thinking and problem-solving. In perception, this refers to awareness of the world that is determined solely by the incoming sensory information. This is also known as data-driven processing and involves initial recognition of all the basic elements in order to match the incoming stimuli with previous experience. These elements can then be synthesised into a complete whole.

Catastrophising: a type of cognitive distortion that involves thinking the very worst of a situation; for example 'I've failed my first assignment – I'm obviously hopeless at study' or 'I've eaten a chocolate and ruined my diet.'

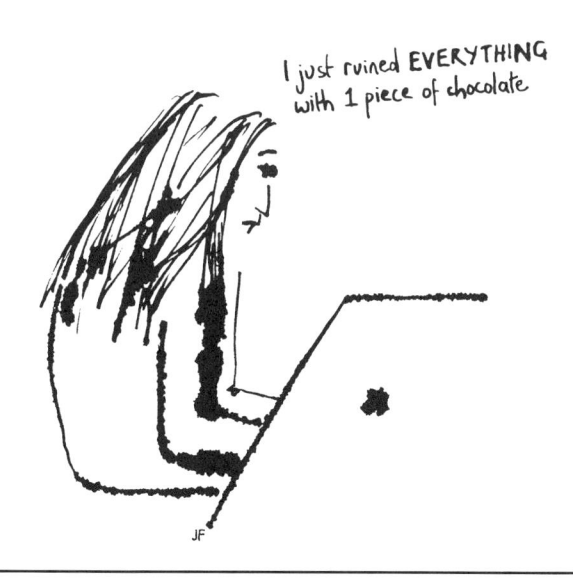

Figure 6.1   Catastrophising *(Jacky Fleming, 1991)*

Chaos theory (also known as catastrophe theory): a new approach to solving complex scientific problems that began in the mid-1970s with the work of Feigenbaum (cited by Gleick, 1988). Classical physics had provided useful solutions for ordered processes, but these could never quite be applied to situations that appeared to be disordered, such as when smooth water flow suddenly becomes turbulent when its speed increases. Feigenbaum and others began to see similarities in the ways in which different complex systems developed into disorder and found a way of expressing the disorder, or chaos, in mathematical terms. The most familiar items from this approach are the 'butterfly effect', 'fractal curves' and 'strange attractors'. It is suggested that chaos effects can be compared with a butterfly flapping its wings in one part of the world and setting in train a sequence of events that can create a storm somewhere else. Fractal curves produce beautiful and intriguing pictures. Strange attractors, through minute influences, affect how the next tiny change will take place.

Chaos theory has been applied to various biological processes and to certain aspects of conditions such as schizophrenia. Gleick (1988) describes how Huberman (c. 1986) examined the eye movements of schizophrenic patients. It has been known since 1908 that some people diagnosed as having schizophrenia, and their relatives, have difficulty tracking the movements of a pendulum. Their eyes jump about disruptively in small jerky movements, overshooting or undershooting the moving target. Huberman made accurate measurements of the movement of the pendulum and the eye movements, and ran them for hours on a computer, changing the parameters and making graphs of the resulting behaviours. He found a mixture of order and chaos. Some of the disorder was exactly the same as that obtained from other areas of exploration into chaos in physics. Huberman suggested that the erratic behaviour had nothing to do with the outside signal but was instead related to too much 'non-linearity' in the system. This pointed to a genetic explanation for schizophrenia and can be linked to further discoveries of the unusual processing of dopamines now associated with schizophrenia. The ways in which nerves and blood vessels branch into successively smaller and smaller channels, each branch seemingly random but the overall effect following a recognisable pattern, can be analysed using 'chaos' mathematics.

Cognitive appraisal: a mental summing up of a situation that takes into account all knowledge, beliefs, memories and perceptions. This process can be a mixture of conscious and unconscious mental activity.

Cognitive appraisal theory: a model from Lazarus (1982) for the relationship between cognition and emotion, which suggests that the ability to put a name to an emotion and talk about it, and hence the emotion itself, follows cognitive appraisal. This appraisal includes both the situation and an awareness of the state of physiological arousal (Figure 6.2).

This assumption, that emotion depends on cognitive appraisal, forms the basis of much cognitive therapy since it can be argued that if the cognitive appraisal alters, the emotion will also alter. That is, if a person can be persuaded to view the situation in a different light, a change in emotional state will automatically come about. The level of arousal may stay the same, but interpretation of the situation will affect whether the arousal is judged as a positive or a negative emotion.

```
STIMULUS  →  COGNITIVE APPRAISAL  →  EMOTIONAL EXPERIENCE
              ↑              ↑
         Unconscious and conscious processes
```

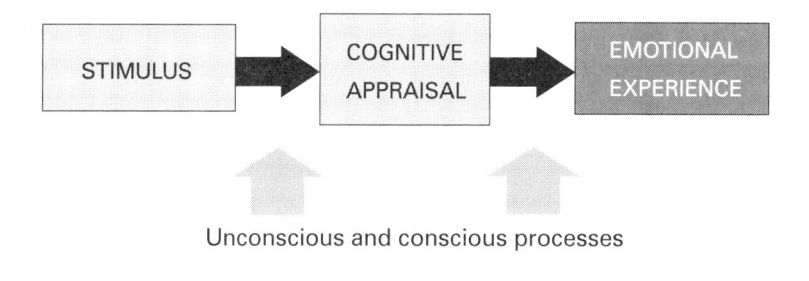

Figure 6.2 Cognitive appraisal model *(derived from Lazarus, 1982)*

If someone is approached from behind and kissed, without being able to see who is there, he or she might experience a sudden rush of adrenaline but will not know whether to be pleased, disgusted or angry until the perpetrator is known. Initial pleasure might soon turn to dismay on fuller cognitive appraisal. When clients with bipolar disorder experience a sense of arousal, they tend to interpret the arousal according to environmental cues. Cognitive therapy seeks to help people alter their perception of themselves and of events so that emotional arousal is reinterpreted in positive terms.

Cognitive behaviour therapy: a combination of cognitive therapy and behavioural techniques.

Cognitive approaches are often combined with a behavioural programme that includes set tasks for the client to complete at home. This is a *didactic* approach in which the emphasis is on education, feedback and support.

There are four basic assumptions in this approach (Dryden and Rentoul, 1991):

- All behaviours can be viewed along a continuum from little or none to excessive
- Individuals can move along this continuum
- Learned behaviour can be analysed and modified
- There are good reasons for continued unwanted behaviour even if the individual is not aware of what these are.

The cognitive-behavioural view is based on the expectations a person has about the outcomes of his or her behaviour, the value the person places on those outcomes and the nature of the situation in which the person is behaving. Assessment techniques include standardised questionnaires, monitoring of behaviour, interviews, physiological measures and the analysis of all of these. Interventions include addressing clients' expectations, dealing with ambivalence, giving information, focusing on clients' goals, helping clients to restructure cognitions, teaching clients new skills, providing a range of strategies, thinking ahead and anticipating problems and their solutions.

Therapy involves performance, practice or rehearsal and 'homework'. The client is given tasks to carry out that are designed to lead progressively to a reduction in the unwanted behaviour. At first, these steps are carried out under supervision, but then the client practises them at home and reports back to the therapist at the next visit how successful they have been.

Cognitive-behavioural therapy is thought to be effective with behaviour such as smoking, alcohol or drug dependence and eating disorders. The chief limitation with most cognitive-behavioural programmes is that, although 'homework' is given, the therapist does not follow or accompany the client into the client's customary environment. Since the environment is recognised as one of the chief factors in precipitating or maintaining behaviour, the effect of therapy can be lost soon after the completion of a programme. In some drug rehabilitation programmes, this difficulty is recognised, and the therapist continues to work with clients in situations that are seen to put the clients at risk of resuming unwanted habits. This has limited application owing to resource implications.

Cognitive distortion: negative or distorted thoughts and beliefs, often associated with problem behaviour or feelings of low self-worth. These may include:

- dichotomous reasoning
- selective abstraction
- arbitrary inference
- overgeneralisation
- catastrophising
- *excessive reliance on the words 'should' and 'must'.*

Cognitive restructuring: analysis of cognitive distortions and replacement with positive beliefs and thoughts more appropriate to the reality of the situation.

Cognitive science: a global term for an approach to understanding cognitive processes that includes cognitive psychology, neurological approaches, philosophy, linguistics, artificial intelligence (AI) and other aspects of cybernetics and computer modelling. Leiber (1991) argues that cognitive science approaches questions about thought and thinking, about consciousness and computation, according to the assumption that whatever the human brain does can be done by other materials.

Cognitive therapy: one of the main 'talking' therapies, cognitive therapy is concerned with analysing clients' beliefs and understanding of themselves and their situation. It is based on the assumption that problems are often caused or exacerbated by limited or inaccurate knowledge and distorted perceptions and beliefs. It is a *didactic* or teaching approach aimed at improving knowledge and restructuring beliefs. Cognitive therapy has always been concerned with confronting reality rather than simply substituting positive thinking for negative or distorted thinking. When reality is itself bad (as with a serious illness), therapy becomes concerned with making the negative thoughts explicit so that they can become accepted rather than hidden or associated with shamefulness or contributing to feelings of low self-worth. Cognitive therapy tends to be best known as an effective method for treating depression but is also used with people who are anxious, distressed by physical ill-health, suicidal, obsessional or hypochondriacal, or as an alternative to cognitive-behavioural programmes for clients with smoking, eating, drug or alcohol problems (Scott *et al.*, 1991). Derivatives of cognitive therapy include rational-emotive therapy, solution-focused therapy and neurolinguistic programming.

Cybernetics: the science of systems of control and communication. The applications within cognitive science involve modelling of cognitive processes using special purpose models that can be analogue, mathematical, statistical or of other kinds, which can be carried out by computer programs. Automata or robots may also be used. One of the most useful approaches in relation to health issues has been in the use of neural nets, which parallel the interactions between neurones. This can assist in exploring the possible effects of having different numbers and types of synapse. Each system to be studied is said to be 'complex, dynamic, capable of "learning" and has feedback, feedforward or both' (Paritsis and Stewart, 1983: xi).

Dichotomous reasoning: dichotomous means cut in two. Dichotomous reasoning means seeing things in terms of two extremes or thinking in extreme and absolutist terms, for example 'I need to hide my anger completely, because once I start getting angry, I'll totally lose control.'

Dysfunctional cognition (cognitive impairment): as a student translated, this means an 'inability to think straight'. The prefix 'dys' is used to mean not functioning properly or presenting a problem. Dysfunctional cognition is a term associated with brain damage following an accident or stroke or with a patient's inability to take in new information because of anxiety, depression, lowered self-esteem or information overload.

Emotion: as mentioned in the introduction, the word 'emotion' is derived from words meaning movement and suggests a stirring or agitation. Emotions can be seen as passions or disturbances, and most words for emotions convey a sense of strong feeling. A person described as 'emotional' is someone who displays strong emotion. Early studies of emotion, such as that by Cannon (1929), concentrated on extreme or high emotions and emphasised peripheral physiological reactions, such as increased heart rate, sweating and goosepimples.

Some studies of emotion (see basic emotions above) are based on what is visible to others and derive systems for describing basic emotions from the interpretations of photographs of facial expressions or from actors' portrayals. Again, these tend to refer only to strong feelings.

Emotions can be faked or play-acted by adopting suitable facial expressions and other body language or verbal expression in order to hide one's true inner feelings. This makes explicit the realisation that the outward expression may not be the same as the inner feeling. In addition to deliberate acting, we also find that there can be a considerable difference between what we feel inside and what we show to others, either because we have not developed sufficient social skills in recognising and displaying our emotions, or because these emotions are repressed. See also affect and expression of emotion.

Emotional colour: an idea explored by Robinson (1996) that cognition and affect are not separate processes but that all cognitions are emotionally coloured: emotion and cognition are inextricably bound together, rather than one occurring before the other. In our everyday experience, there is no separate thing called remembering that can be distinguished from the sadness or the gladness. One does not remember first and then add the emotion afterwards. The cognition of remembering is built in a particular emotional colour, which imparts a level of urgency to thoughts and perceptions that influences decisions about what actions to take.

This fits well with the physiological viewpoint, since it can be argued that the *limbic system* in the brain, which is active in emotional arousal, interconnects with the *cortex* via the *thalamus* and suffuses the whole brain and nervous system with emotion-related hormones. This influences the whole of cognitive processing, what is involved both with the individual's present concerns and with recording in memory of its past concerns. This imparts a bias of cognition, that is, a sort of colouring.

Robinson argues that the idea of 'colouring' is more helpful than, for example, flavouring, since it leads to an analogy with colour perception that may be found useful. One way of sorting colours is to think in terms of three dimensions: hue, saturation and brightness. Hue relates to frequency or wavelength, the basic hues being the colours that can be readily distinguished in a spectrum (see Chapter 14). This might correspond to the five (or more) basic emotions such as pleasure, anger, fear, sadness and disgust. A fully saturated hue is a 'primary' colour that looks as if it is pure and unmixed, and saturation can be defined as the mix of hues or the tendency towards a neutral grey. This would be the equivalent of the mixture of emotions. Brightness is the perceived intensity of light, which can be seen as an analogy for the intensity of emotion. Using this analogy, thinking jealously about a rival for a loved one might be analysed as involving a mixture of angry, fearful and sad memories, perceptions and expectations, in varying degrees.

This approach allows a more complex analysis of cognitive restructuring than the *cognitive appraisal model* suggests. Cognitive therapy may give rise to the introduction of new cognitions with a different emotional colouring. These do not automatically replace previous cognitions but need to be taken into the individual's scheme of looking at things. In Piagetian terms, the newly coloured cognitions can be assimilated alongside, or accommodated with, existing schemas. Otherwise, they may be rejected and soon forgotten. See also Chapter 16.

Excessive reliance on the words 'should' and 'must': a type of cognitive distortion in which the client can be observed to speak primarily in terms of what she or he should or must do, such as 'I must exercise for at least an hour each morning', 'I should take the children to the park every day', 'I must not eat chocolate.' Pressures may be generated by the failure to achieve such self-imposed targets. Cognitive therapy aims to restructure beliefs so that the client is directed towards an increased range of choices, expressed in terms of what the client would like to and can already do.

Expression of emotions: the outward display or representation of feelings in verbal (word) or non-verbal (non-word) forms. There is an ongoing debate about whether the expression of emotion helps to dissipate the distress or whether it fuels and encourages more negative affect. There is evidence that the control or suppression of emotion, particularly of anger, can contribute to illness (see Chapter 7). Health interventions, both mainstream and complementary, are now likely to encourage 'getting in touch with one's feelings' and are aimed at helping people to express them. Cognitive and psychodynamic therapies work on the assumption that awareness of affect will lead to a reduction in problems. Forms of expression may include vocalisations, such as crying and laughing, together with facial expressions, postures and gestures, or may be through the spoken or written word in conversation, poetry, story-telling and so on. William Blake illustrates attitudes to expressing anger in his poem 'A Poison Tree', which starts:

> I was angry with my friend;
> I told my wrath, my wrath did end.
> I was angry with my foe;
> I told it not, my wrath did grow.

However, there is a difference between awareness and actual expression. If expressing emotion involves shouting and tears, having rows and *being* angry, rather than just stating that you are angry, the outcome is less predictable. The psychodynamic approach usually leads to the conclusion that an outburst leads to *catharsis* and that this can be cleansing and healing. In contrast, the behaviourist approach leads to the conclusion that any pleasure felt in giving vent to feelings will reinforce that behaviour, so that it becomes a habit, making outbursts more frequent, and will therefore worsen the anger rather than alleviate it. Cognitive therapeutic approaches generally favour the unemotional, rational discussion of emotion in preference to its actual display, but some cognitive-behavioural styles (for example, Crowe and Ridley, 1990) may include *paradoxical* interventions such as deliberately initiating rows at set times of the day. Creative arts make it possible for the expression of strong emotions using non-verbal means, such as painting, music, mime and dancing. Drama combines verbal and non-verbal forms of expression. The effects of these art forms can often be more immediate than talking, and it is possible to allow for extreme emotional expression to take place in a safe contained environment (see Chapter 17). See also Chapter 1.

Gestalt school of psychology: a German approach within cognitive psychology that sees the whole as greater than the sum of the parts. See also Chapter 14.

Gestalt therapy: a style of therapy that was developed by Frederick Perls in the 1950s. Perls (1969) was influenced by orthodox Freudian psychoanalysis, existentialism, ideas of *self-actualisation* and the theatre, as well as by the Gestalt school of thought. He strove to achieve an holistic approach that integrated the body, cognitions and communication patterns. Partlett and Page (1990) describe the Gestalt approach to balance and imbalance in the individual as a cycle of awareness, suggesting that whenever an imbalance occurs, the cycle can be interrupted and self-regulation re-established. Therapy may involve theatrical techniques for re-enacting a situation, for example the 'empty chair' experiment in which a client speaks to 'someone' in the empty chair and then moves to the chair and replies. Alternatively, the therapist may be 'used' as the other person, with whom the client can carry out a desired conversation. Artwork, fantasies (guided or unguided) and dreams may also be used. A key assumption is that a person has developed self-defeating behaviours that prevent goals being reached. In all cases, the emphasis is on being in the imagined situation right now and enacting it in order to gain insight, self-awareness and acceptance, and try out new patterns of interaction.

Information processing: an approach within cognitive science that developed through comparing the human mind with the way in which computers operate. Many psychologists see this as the 'dominant *paradigm* within cognitive psychology as a whole' (Gross, 1996: 262). Many explanations of attention and memory rely on the information processing approach and describe the carrying out of mental operations as serial or parallel processing, or as bottom-up or top-down processing.

Mood: in the 1950s and 60s, when the word 'emotion' applied only to extreme states, mood was regarded as something less than emotion. For example, Drever (1964) defined mood as 'An affective condition or attitude, enduring for some time, characterised by particular emotions in a condition of subexcitability, so as to be readily evoked, for example, an irritable mood, or a cheerful mood.' However, few modern textbooks list mood in the index or discuss mood separately from emotion. It is probably most useful simply to define mood as the prevailing emotional state at any given time. Evidence suggests that mood influences perception and the memory of events. Williams (1984), cited by Williams *et al.* (1988), describes a patient whose experience of swimming was interpreted differently depending on her mood. When she was in a good mood, she recalled the swimming as a pleasurable experience. Later, when rather depressed, she described particular parts of the swimming event that she had not liked, mostly those affecting her self-esteem.

Negative affect: unpleasant or distressing feelings, expressed through characteristic facial expressions, postures or actions.

Neurolinguistic programming (NLP): a therapy developed by Bandler and Grinder (1975, 1976) from their analysis of what makes other therapies work: the 'structure of magic'. NLP takes what it sees as the effective elements that therapies have in common and refines and redefines these. NLP is based on a number of principles that include distinguishing between *primary representation* of the world, which is our immediate perceptual experience, and *secondary representation*, which is how we talk about that experience in words.

According to Robbie (1988), the client is viewed not as damaged or broken but as working perfectly although succeeding at the 'wrong' things, things that the client does not want. Therapy is seen as enabling the client to bring to consciousness and articulate what he or she wants in the way of change. The therapist is trained to become sensitive to subtle responses in the client's use of words to describe feelings and understanding, and to respond to minute aspects of body language such as eye movements or an alteration in the thickness of the lips. This leads to developing a flexible way of asking questions that enables the client to become aware of what he or she wants, how both client and therapist will recognise when this has been achieved, the context in which the change is desirable and what else is likely to change. As with many psychotherapies, NLP has evolved a register or jargon of its own that tends to lend it an air of mystique, but the terms are intended to provide clarity and precision for what are otherwise seen to be vague or intuitive behaviours. This enables techniques to be learned systematically during training rather than arising chiefly from the charismatic personality of the therapist. A novel that describes non-verbal signs in the same kind of minute detail is *Oscar and Lucinda* by Peter Carey (1988).

> Her face changed subtly. You could not say what had happened – a diminution of the lower lip, a flattening of the cheek, a narrowing of the eye [perhaps]. But there was no ambiguity in her intention. She had withdrawn her trust from him abruptly. (p. 374)

Overgeneralisation: a cognitive distortion in which it is concluded from one negative event that another negative event is likely to follow, such as 'I was late for my appointment last week, so something is bound to go wrong next time.'

Parallel processing: a way of carrying out a complicated process in which several operations are carried out at the same time.

Positive affect: feelings of pleasantness or well-being, expressed through characteristic facial expression, postures or actions.

Primary representation: a term used in neurolinguistic programming (NLP) to refer to our 'raw' experience of the world derived from our senses. NLP identifies five representation systems, based on the senses, labelling these visual (V), auditory (A), kinesthetic (K), gustatory (G) and olfactory (O). The kinesthetic system includes the sensation of touch and feeling (which is linked directly to emotion) and does not distinguish between the experience of touch arising from receptors on the surface of the body (which respond to external stimuli) and from muscle receptors (which provide data about the body's position and movement). These do not correspond exactly to biological classifications (see Chapter 14), and NLP does not include any specific mention of the vestibular sense (sense of balance). Other usage suggests that this would be included in the kinesthetic representation system as part of how one 'feels'. Bandler and Grinder (1975, 1976) argue that people are born with equal sensitivity in each of the primary representation systems but by the age of 5 or 6 years old show a preference for describing the world in terms of one system. How these descriptions are formed in words is called secondary representation. See also Chapter 14.

Problem-lumping: Thelan *et al.* (1994) describe how critically ill people have a tendency to lump all their problems together. They may worry equally about the mortgage and not being able to cut the grass. Care can help to sort out priorities and identify friends and family who can help.

Rational-emotive therapy: an approach developed by Ellis (1973) and Ellis and Grieger (1977) that is based on an individual's failure to assume personal 'responsibility' for feelings and actions. A central concept is that people have the potential to be highly rational. Problems are thought to emerge when people engage in thinking that is irrational, 'magic-orientated', superstitious or impossible to validate empirically. Ellis suggests there are 10 common and basic irrational ideas that create unpleasant emotions. These can be compared with the *cognitive distortions* recognised by most cognitive therapists:

- It is an absolute necessity for an adult to have love and approval from peers, family and friends
- You must be unfailingly competent and almost perfect in all you undertake
- Certain people are evil, wicked and villainous, and should be punished
- It is horrible when people and things are not the way you would like them to be
- External events cause most human misery; people simply react as events trigger their emotions
- You should feel fear or anxiety about anything that is unknown, uncertain or potentially dangerous
- It is easier to avoid than to face life difficulties and responsibilities.

Techniques of confrontation and action orientation are used to encourage risk-taking and the trying out of new behaviours, with the aim of facilitating self-acceptance and behaviour change. Ellis's approach is aggressive and attacking and may be considered to violate humanistic principles.

Rationalisation: giving a rational explanation for something that is not really explainable; 'inventing' a plausible explanation for irrational behaviour or when the reasons are not known. This can be seen most clearly with post-hypnotic suggestion. Participants who carry out 'daft' activities tend to offer sensible-sounding explanations, seen as a face-saving activity or avoidance. Rationalisations are often used to cover embarrassment or situations in which it is difficult to recognise and express the underlying emotions.

Repertory grid: a way of collecting data from individuals that preserves their individual *personal constructs* or beliefs of how they see their world, without imposing any theoretical concepts or constructs. It combines cognitive and phenomenological principles. It is formally structured, following a set pattern of collecting responses to questions, but content free. The repertory grid was invented by George Kelly (1955) as a therapeutic technique and further developed by Bannister (for example, 1971) as part of personal construct theory. It is particularly known for the way in which it can be used to reveal individuals' implicit notions about personality. It has many uses in therapy, education and research for exploring peoples' ideas and helping them to manage their lifestyles effectively. See also Chapters 8 and 15.

Secondary representation system: the way in which words are used to describe the world as it has been perceived. This term has been refined by the founders of neurolinguistic processing (Bandler and Grinder, 1975, 1976) in their attempt to describe accurately the difference between what we perceive and how we communicate these perceptions to each other. In NLP, this difference is called 'slippage'. Much of this therapy is concerned with assisting the client to develop appropriate language for articulating experience.

    At all times, we are constrained by the language we have, and by the language which has developed historically for our society or others we know of. Further constraint is applied in each individual's choice of language on a day-to-day basis. It can be seen that there is a further 'slippage' between those words which are known and those which are regularly used. Therapy can assist either in recognising the language used by the client and linking this to cognitions and emotions that have been so far unexplored, or in increasing the range of language available and introducing new concepts.

Selective abstraction: selecting some parts of a situation and ignoring others, such as thinking, 'If only I had thinner thighs, I would be more attractive.'

Serial processing: a step-by-step sequence in any cognitive process, for example perception, memory or problem-solving, in which the steps of the process are carried out separately, one after the other.

Signal detection theory (signal detectability theory): a theory, fashionable in the 1960s and 70s, which is useful in the study of sensation, perception and memory. It is based on the measurable responses to varying levels of stimulation and in particular shows how weak signals can be detected even when there are distracting stimuli. According to Robinson (1996), its main achievement was to separate a participant's sensitivity to a stimulus from the mental 'preparedness' to acknowledge it. Participants were more likely to detect a signal when they were expecting it or when they attached some value to detecting it.

Solution-focused therapy: a form of brief therapy, developed by de Shazer (1985, 1986), in which the focus of a session is not on a fixed problem but on changes that the client will be able to make. Conversation is directed towards 'non-problem talk', 'complaint talk', exceptions, goals and tasks. The client and therapist talk about general problems in the client's life, not through asking what each problem actually is, but by attempting to gauge the severity, frequency, number of people affected and so on in measurable terms. Clients are then encouraged to give examples of exceptions, that is, less severe occasions, and look for the differences. This then leads to an identification of goals by asking such questions as 'When you have this problem sorted out, how will things be different?' A specific technique used by de Shazer (1985) is asking the 'miracle' question: 'When you wake in the morning, the difficulty you came here with no longer exists. What will be the first thing you notice, and what next? What else would you notice? What would other people see that's different?' In this way, the clients are guided towards recognising what they want. When goals are more clearly identified, these are then expressed in measurable terms and tasks are set that help to focus on areas of strength and exceptions and lead to changes that can be identified and measured.

Top-down processing: a concept linked with bottom-up processing that refers to starting with a higher mental process, hypothesis or schema and working downwards towards recognising the basic elements or examples. In thinking and problem-solving, this can be compared with deductive processes. In perception, it refers to identifying an object by reference to a previously formed synthesis or concept of a class of objects or expectations. It is also known as concept-driven (or conceptually driven) processing.

Value: the judgement that a person places on the desirability, worth or utility of obtaining some outcome. This is an important concept, of significance particularly in relation to mild emotions or the lower end of the spectrum of affect, but it does not fit well with other aspects of cognitive function. Much work in cognitive psychology and philosophy has been concerned with the rational aspects of decision-making, and humans have been found to be, in formal terms, only partly rational decision-makers. Historical beliefs about rational thought and emotions are not easy to reconcile. However, in the light of the *emotional colouring* approach, this is of no surprise as all cognitions can be seen as emotionally coloured or biased. When trying to discover exactly how or why a human decision-maker strays from rationality, it is necessary 'at least to try to set the affective scene in which the decision is being made' (Robinson, 1996). A person wishing to travel may work out all the options and calculate which method of travel is quicker and which is cheaper. The rational choice would appear to depend on whether the person places a higher value on time or cost. However, the final decision may be to take the route that is most pleasant. This may not be based on rational or conscious processes but on merely that it feels right and can be seen to be related to aesthetic or comfort values.

The findings of Damasio (1994) support the notion that affect should be included in the concept of value. He describes at length the plight of a patient with frontal lobe damage. This man's disability was confined to a very narrow section of total psychological function but one that proved to be of crucial importance. His management of most aspects of his life was normal, but when given a complex decision-making task in which he had to weigh up a number of factors bearing on the decision, he entirely failed. It was not that he came to the wrong decision: he was not capable of coming to any decision at all. Damasio attributes this to a failure of the patient's cognitive processes to engage affect and thereby to evaluate the urgency of the factors in the decision.

Damasio goes on to make the case that affect is an indispensable component of rational thought. His view is compatible with the notion of cognition as a continuing process of changing of purpose. 'Such a process will usually reshape moment by moment with the advent of new major and minor purposes and it is inconceivable that an organism could select a productive route through the possibilities without the guidance of affect' (Robinson, 1996).

7 HEALTH BELIEFS, LIFESTYLE AND HEALTH PROMOTION

The origins of many health problems are found in the lifestyle of the sufferer, linked to the person's beliefs about herself or himself.

In promoting healthy behaviour, health education and illness prevention strategies can be utilised. These may range in scope and potential influence from personal teaching to the use of legislation.

Definitions

Kasl and Cobb (1966)	Health behaviour is… an activity undertaken by a person believing him/herself to be healthy for the purpose of preventing disease or detecting it in an asymptomatic stage.
	Illness behaviour is… any activity undertaken by a person who feels ill, to define the state of health and to discover a suitable remedy.
	Sick-role behaviour is… activity undertaken for the purpose of getting well, by those who consider themselves ill. It includes receiving treatment from appropriate therapists, generally involves a whole range of dependent behaviours and leads to some degree of neglect of one's usual duties.
Kiger (1995)	Health represents a condition of mastery in which the extent of growth and the direction of potential lie with the individual.

Approaches, Arguments and Applications

It is easy to assume that if the lifestyle risk factors associated with health problems can be identified, those at risk will be motivated to change their behaviour in order to prevent the occurrence or deterioration of the health problem.

However, simply encouraging those at risk to change their behaviour may be ineffective as the links between a person's health beliefs and health behaviour is a complex one. Although health beliefs can be influential in determining health behaviour, a number of factors beyond the control of individuals can hinder them in taking responsibility for their own health.

Such factors include the social, cultural, environmental and economic framework around which the lifestyle of an individual is based. The individual may be powerless to influence these factors, but such factors can exert a profound influence over the choices available to people and may be regarded by them as having priority over the attainment and maintenance of health.

Additionally, and perhaps more importantly, it has recently been realised that many decisions relating to health and lifestyle are not based on rational choices but are linked to an individual's *self-concept*. New approaches now include a consideration of *self-efficacy*.

The concept of health is a complex one. A person's health is commonly understood to have a number of dimensions, such as physical, psychological, social and spiritual. Some of these are interdependent. Table 7.1 illustrates some of the dimensions involved in a young person's decisions about whether to engage in sexual behaviour and whether to use a condom. The analysis helps in identifying some of the elements involved in making a decision, but it can quickly be seen that the elements cannot be regarded separately.

Approaches to health tend to reflect different assumptions:

- A person's health may be placed somewhere on a continuum from wellness to illness
- Health has a number of different dimensions and means more than the absence of disease or infirmity
- Health is dynamic
- If adults are to take responsibility, when appropriate, for their own health, they must be made aware of the possible effects of their lifestyle choices
- Not all behaviours are founded on conscious decisions; they may be habits
- Health-care professionals must accept some responsibility for promoting health-related issues
- Attempts at health promotion must take into consideration the beliefs, values and attitudes of the people being targeted
- Health promotion is aimed at improving the quality of life of the whole population.

Phillips (1990) notes that it is important for health-care providers and consumers to share similar views about health, otherwise conflicting goals may result in poor adherence to care plans. In relation to health promotion, a number of different strategies can be identified. These tend to fall in the following categories:

- preventive: behaviour responsible for ill-health is targeted
- educational: information is provided to enable a person to make an informed choice about behaviour
- empowerment: confidence and self-esteem are raised to enable a person to exercise control over his or her health

Table 7.1 Dimensions of health: some examples of issues involved in a young person's decisions about sexual behaviour, for discussion

Social	Affective	Cognitive	Spiritual	Behavioural	Biological outcome
peer pressure to engage in sex	pleasure, excitement, arousal, love and affection	values with regards to dependence and independence	wanting to do what's right	having (or not) intercourse	pregnancy or disease (or not)
parental pressure not to engage in sex	fear of pregnancy, disease and punishment	perceptions of parents' attitudes	wanting to fulfil parents' hopes	using (or not) condoms	
partner's pressure not to use condoms, for example selfishness, power, entrapment	fear of losing partner if not complying with his/her wishes	perceptions of partner's attitude	feeling a sense of duty towards partner	using (or not) other contraception	
	embarrassment about visiting GP for contraception	knowledge and beliefs about menstrual cycle, conception, contraception and risks of disease	having a sense of wholeness and personal fulfilment		
	embarrassment about buying condoms	belief that condoms interfere with spontaneity	trusting in fate		

- radical/social change: health issues are influenced at social, political or economic levels.

Different teaching and learning styles can also be identified and the following contrasts made:

- behavioural versus cognitive
- gradual development versus insight
- concrete versus formal/abstract
- product versus process
- discovery versus guided
- field dependent learner versus field independent learner
- surface versus strategic versus deep learning.

For all types of learning to be effective, teaching has to consider each learner's individual needs and abilities (see also Chapter 16).

Cognitive approaches: these emphasise the role of the learner's own thinking processes in the beliefs formed about health and the lifestyle decisions that have been made. A person's understanding of health issues depends on the ability to see how the various components of the knowledge to be learned are related to each other. This is influenced by the learner's perception, memory, imagination, judgement, reasoning and problem-solving skills. See also Chapters 11 and 16. The role of the health-care professional involves presenting information in such a way that the learner is able to make informed choices about lifestyle.

Behavioural approaches: these are concerned with the health behaviours of people and the way in which they learn these behaviours by making new associations between events occurring in their environment. The process of association is known as *conditioning* and involves the identification of an event's components as *stimulus* or *response* (see Chapter 4). This approach assumes that if an unhealthy lifestyle has been learned, it can be unlearned, and a person can be helped to develop new behaviours that are beneficial to health or at least not harmful. A healthy lifestyle is seen as desirable, and the role of the health-care professional involves encouraging and reinforcing healthy behaviours.

Humanistic approaches: these help people to make choices that reflect their own interests and values about health. The role of the health-care professional involves giving people information and enhancing their skills so that they are empowered to take control of their lifestyle. The lifestyle choices made by a person must be respected even if they are unhealthy ones.

Social learning theory approaches: these, based on behavioural concepts, consider that much of a person's lifestyle is learned through observing the behaviour of others and noting whether they are rewarded or punished for their health actions. A person is more likely to engage in healthy behaviour if he or she expects to be reinforced for the behaviour and values the reinforcement (Rotter, 1975). The media provides a forum for direct role-modelling, and health promotion campaigns tend to use attractive role-models who have desirable lifestyles. The message being conveyed is 'engage in this behaviour and you too will look good, feel great and have an exciting lifestyle' (see Chapter 4). Health-care professionals can also be effective role-models of undesirable as well as desirable behaviour.

Biopsychosocial, social context or social cognition models: these explore the interrelationships between health-damaging and health-enhancing behaviours. A variety of models have been devised to explain the adoption of health-related behaviours. They try to explain the health behaviours of people by exploring beliefs about the behaviour and its consequences, the seriousness of the health risk and the perceived threat to the individual. The following figures, given in chronological order, demonstrate a significant change from the late 1980s onwards as the concept of self-efficacy is introduced and the gap between intention to act and actually acting is emphasised. In these figures, each model has been adapted to illustrate an example of health-related behaviour.

These can be directly compared with the precaution adoption model of Weinstein (1988) (see changing risk behaviour) and with the social learning theory model of Bandura (1977) (see Chapter 4). Comparisons and criticisms of models are given in Schwarzer (1992), Messer and Meldrum (1995) and Stroebe and Stroebe (1995).

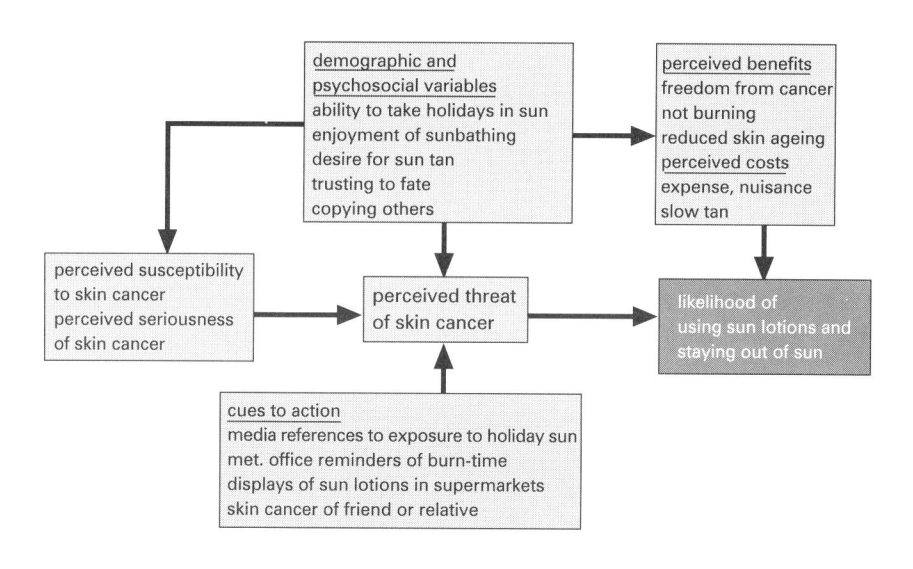

Figure 7.1   Health belief model (*adapted from Becker and Maiman, 1975*)

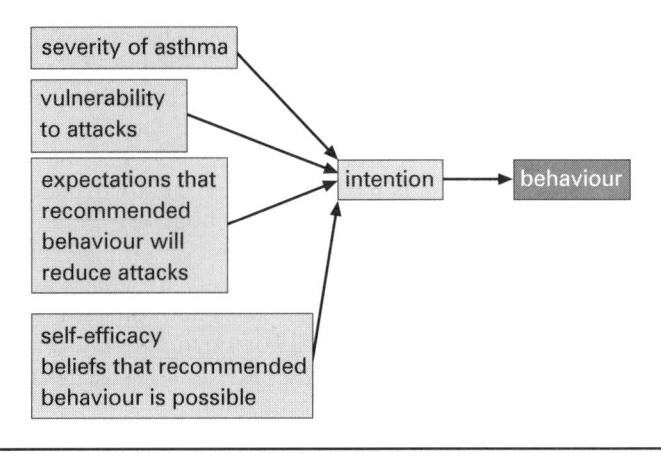

Figure 7.2 Protection motivation theory (*adapted from Rogers, 1975*)

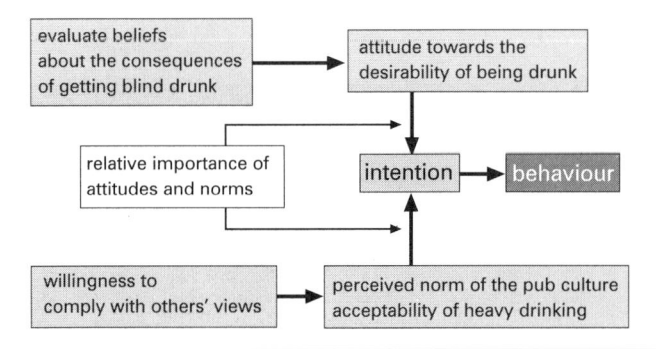

Figure 7.3 Theory of reasoned action (*adapted from Ajzen and Fishbein, 1980*)

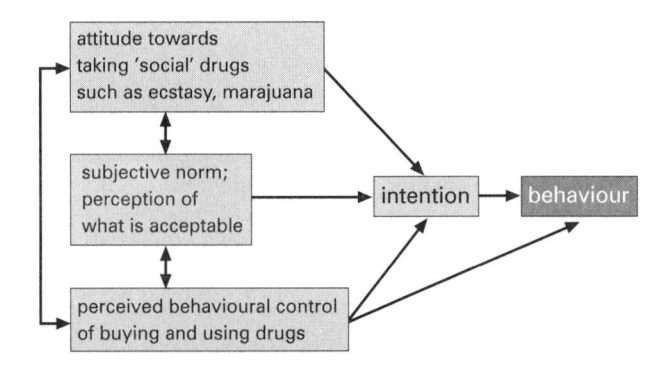

Figure 7.4 Theory of planned behaviour (*adapted from Ajzen, 1991*)

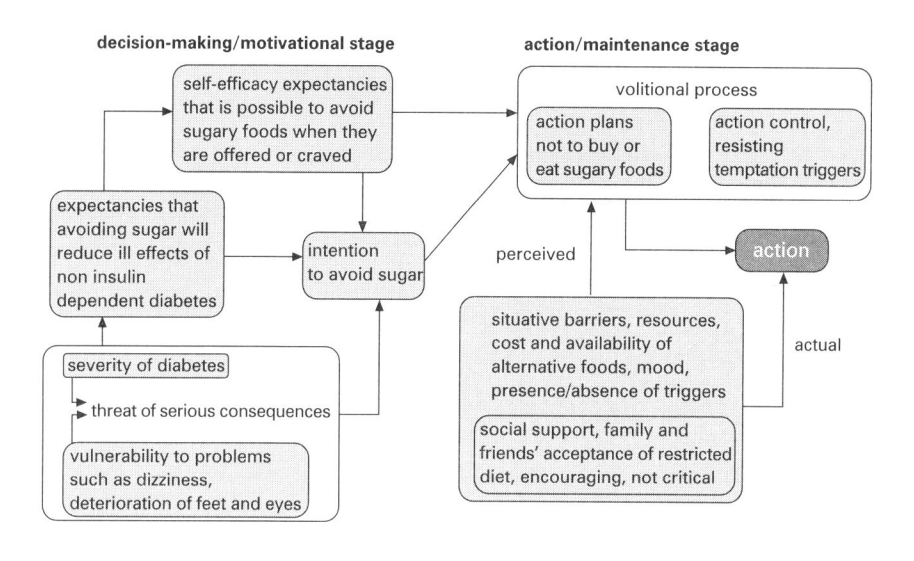

Figure 7.5 Health action process approach (*adapted from Schwarzer, 1992*)

Key Terms and Concepts

Advance organisers: these may be used to provide a link between old and new material when teaching and are recommended by Ausubel (1968), who favours a sequential approach. Ideas that are similar to the material to be learned but are more generalised are introduced in advance of the new material in order to provide an anchor for it. Thus the learner can be helped to discriminate between old and new ideas and prepare for learning. For example, in applying Ausubel's method, the health promoter might explain the principles of a healthy diet before initiating discussions about cholesterol and heart disease. Thus a *deductive* approach to learning is adopted. Sometimes an advance organiser deliberately presents a problem, such as a case example, for which the learners cannot provide adequate solutions. This alerts them to the need for learning.

Attributions: how people explain events such as why they become ill: what they attribute their illness to. See Chapter 15.

Barriers to behaviour change: Rosenstock (1974) defines barriers as physical, psychological or financial distress associated with any form of action. Physical barriers or costs include the complexity, duration and side-effects of the treatment regime. See health belief model.

Benefits of behaviour change: Rosenstock (1974) defines benefits as the potential to be gained from a particular course of action to reduce a health threat. See health belief model.

Changing risk behaviour: a person's motivation to change any behaviour that is associated with a risk to health has been considered in the context of a number of stages by several writers. Weinstein (1988) proposes a precaution adoption model for examining the adoption of precautionary health behaviours. This suggests that the patient:

- has heard of the hazard
- believes that others are susceptible to the hazard
- acknowledges personal susceptibility
- decides to take action
- takes precautions.

Weinstein argues that particular factors will be influential in helping a person to progress through each stage. For example, in the early stages, information about the nature of the health risks is useful. Information about personal risk is pertinent during the middle stages, while during the later stages, information about how behaviour may be changed is relevant.

Prochaska *et al.* (1992) acknowledge that the process of behaviour change may not be a smooth one as a person may 'relapse' or revert back to their original behaviour before finally adopting the new one. They propose a number of stages, which are not necessarily encountered in a linear sequence:

- precontemplation
- contemplation
- preparation
- action
- maintenance.

During the precontemplation stage, change is not being considered. This may be due to apathy, denial or lack of awareness that the behaviour has the potential to cause health problems. Health promotion strategies at this stage will aim to help the person acknowledge the links between health behaviour and outcomes, be these real or potential. Analysis of the costs and benefits of maintaining or altering the behaviour takes place during the contemplation stages, so it may be appropriate to teach the person how to use problem-solving techniques at this stage. During the preparation stage, the benefits of changing behaviour are perceived as outweighing the costs, and change is seen as worthwhile and possible. Helping the person to prepare for change might involve teaching them new coping skills. Help with goal-setting, the provision of support and the use of reinforcement will be appropriate during the final stages, when behaviour change takes place and relapse prevention is considered.

The model proposed by Weinstein and Sandman (1992) is particularly relevant to modern approaches:

- unaware of issue
- unengaged by issue
- deciding about action
- deciding to act
- acting
- maintenance of action.

The problem facing psychologists is to find explanations for how people move from 'deciding about action' to 'deciding to act'. Models that include the concept of self-efficacy, as in the theory of planned behaviour (Ajzen, 1991) and the health action process approach (Schwarzer, 1992), go some way towards providing an explanation.

Chronic conditions: these include the outcomes of inherited conditions, injuries, diseases, pain and stress. Research questions in relation to chronic conditions include:

- What are different people's expectations about recovery, rehabilitation and quality of life?
- Are there stages or phases of recovery?
- Are personality profiles or mood changes associated with particular chronic conditions?
- How can interventions assist?

Helping people with long-term conditions can be improved through knowledge and understanding of:

- models of reactions to diagnosis and prognosis (see Chapter 10)
- wider issues, including who, besides the patient, may be involved, for example the family and care team
- models of intervention and coping.

Coping and intervention models: there are a large number of different models that have been designed to illustrate the components of coping processes. These include Lazarus and Folkman (1984), Moos (1986) and Danish and D'Augelli (1982). A discussion is given in Niven (1994). Other models that are designed to deal specifically with loss and grief are described in Chapter 10.

Lazarus and Folkman (1984) define two categories of coping:

Problem-focused	**Emotion-focused**
advice	denial, avoidance
information	relaxation therapy
feedback on progress	turning to others for support
	opportunity for expression
	humour

Moos (1986) adds *appraisal*-focused coping, which suggests an additional set of strategies to assess the situation in total. This gives three categories:

- **appraisal-focused**: developing skills to modify and comprehend the threat of a situation
- **problem-focused**: actively confronting *problems* and dealing with the consequences
- **emotion-focused**: developing *skills* for the management of feelings.

In order to address these issues, Moos suggests that people need to carry out a number of *tasks* and that this can be done through coping responses. The role of the carer is to assist in carrying them out effectively.

Moos' five sets of adaptive tasks
- Establish the meaning and significance of the situation
- Confront reality (*confrontation*)
- Sustain relationships with friends
- Maintain a reasonable emotional balance
- Preserve a satisfactory self-image.

Moos' nine coping responses
- logical analysis and mental preparation
- cognitive redefinition (restructuring)
- cognitive avoidance and denial
- seeking information and support
- taking problem-solving action
- pursuing alternative rewards
- affective (mood) regulation
- emotional discharge (expression, catharsis)
- resigned acceptance.

Danish and D'Augelli (1982) propose a personal competency model of lifespan development that can be applied to any life event or change or adopted as a continuous process of adjustment throughout life:

1 goal assessment
  1.1 identification
  1.2 importance
  1.3 attainment
2 knowledge acquisition
3 decision-making
4 risk assessment
5 creation of social support
6 planning of skill development
  6.1 definition
  6.2 rationale
  6.3 criterion
  6.4 model
  6.5 supervised practice
  6.6 continued practice
  6.7 evaluation

Costs: see barriers.
Critical illness: Thelan *et al.* (1994) list signs that can indicate when a person who is or has been critically ill is not coping:

- negative verbalisation
- problem-lumping
- projection
- displacement
- denial
- non-compliance

- suicidal thoughts
- self-directed aggression
- failure to progress from dependence to independence.

Cues to action: Rosenstock (1974) defines cues to action as stimuli that trigger appropriate health behaviour. They can be either internal (perception of bodily states) or external (advice or reminders from others or the mass media). Cues to action may include the individual's level of motivation, the influence of significant others, sources of information, for example media campaigns, magazine articles or health promotion leaflets that enhance the person's knowledge of health issues, or a change in circumstances. See health belief model.

Didactic: pertaining to instruction or teaching. Within health promotion, this is usually regarded in the light of giving information in a structured way, both instructor and instructed taking an active role in a partnership (see teaching and Chapter 9). It need not imply an authoritarian or overbearing attitude on the part of the instructor, although some dictionary definitions indicate that this is the normal usage of the term.

Factitious illnesses: a term for all illnesses in which there is thought to an element of 'make-believe' on the part of the patient. This can be subdivided into 'dissimulation' (in which the illness is false) and 'somatising' (which involves a belief that one is ill). 'Malingering' is a form of dissimulation in which symptoms or illness are exaggerated or faked in order to gain material benefits. Examples include prisoners who fake illness in order to go into hospital, where conditions are better, drug addicts who feign pain to obtain narcotics and those who fake illness to obtain social security benefits. There have been recent reports in the press of people faking conditions such as arthritis in order to obtain medication for their pets without having to pay the high veterinary fees. Munchausen's syndrome and Munchausen's by proxy are serious dissimulation conditions in which a person fakes illness in himself or others so that this becomes the focus of life. These are thought to be related to deep-seated emotional disturbance. Somatising includes *health anxiety, hypochondria* and some aspects of *psychogenic* illness (see Chapter 20). A suspicion that a person is faking can create impatience and frustration on the part of carers, which may lead to a reduced quality of care. Understanding the underlying factors may lead to increased *empathy* and more choice of care options.

Fear: images that arouse fear are sometimes used in health campaigns to promote a change in attitudes towards health. They are intended to frighten people into changing their behaviour. However, too much fear can be counterproductive and result in people rationalising their risky behaviour by ignoring, denying or minimising the health threat. Fear-inducing messages often lack two factors that Sarafino (1990) claims are necessary if attitude change is to result in changed behaviour. These are specific instructions or practical advice for performing the preventive action, and strategies to support confidence. See also persuasion in Chapter 3.

Health action process approach: a model devised by Schwarzer (1992) that builds on earlier health belief models and incorporates important new elements (see also Messer and Meldrum, 1995). Schwarzer believes that there are two distinct stages in moving towards carrying out health-related behaviour, these representing a vital shift from 'deciding about action' to 'deciding to act' (see also precaution adoption model). Deciding about action involves the decision-making/motivational stage, shown on the left-hand side of Figure 7.5 above. Deciding to act is the action/maintenance stage, shown on the right-hand side. Schwarzer argues that there are three key elements in the adoption and maintenance of health behaviour:

- self-efficacy
- outcome expectancy
- risk perception

and that, of these, self-efficacy expectations are the most important ingredient in making the shift from planning to action. See Figure 7.5 above.

Health anxiety: this refers to concern about health in the absence of pathology, or excessive concern where there is some degree of pathology (Lucock and Morley, 1996). In extreme cases, the diagnosis of hypochondria may be made. Dysfunctional beliefs about illness, arising from past experiences, may lead to the misinterpretation of symptoms, and beliefs may persist despite medical reassurance. Lucock and Morley (1996) have devised the Health Anxiety Questionnaire, based on a cognitive-behavioural model of health anxiety, which can be used to predict response to reassurance following medical examination.

Health belief model: there are various different models concerned with health beliefs but the one usually referred to as 'the health belief model' is that by Becker (1974), developed by Becker and Maiman (1975) and shown in Figure 7.1 above.

This early model is based upon the assumption that people *value* health and will want to engage in health-related behaviour. It makes the assumption that behaviour is goal directed and influenced by perceptions of the value of the goal and estimation of the degree of success. In the context of health-related behaviour, the goal is usually regarded as being the attainment of health or the avoidance of ill-health. The model was originally devised in order to try to explain why people fail to take advantage of preventive health services such as screenings and inoculation (Becker, 1974; Rosenstock, 1974). Becker (1974) argues that the perceived costs and benefits of a health-related behaviour will influence people. Factors that influence the likelihood of taking preventive action include:

- the person's perceived susceptibility or vulnerability to a disease or injury
- the person's perception of the seriousness or severity of that disease
- the perceived association between behaviour and disease
- the benefits of engaging in preventive behaviour
- the barriers or costs of engaging in preventive behaviour
- demographic and sociopsychological (*psychosocial*) influences
- cues to action that act as reminders to engage in particular health behaviour.

The model suggests that people are more likely to adopt health-related behaviours, such as complying with medical advice or taking preventive action, if they feel susceptible to disease, believe that the consequences of the disease will be serious if not treated, and believe that the costs (drawbacks) of the preventive action are outweighed by the benefits.

A health promotion programme based upon this model would need to identify a link between the target behaviour and disease, emphasise the severity of the disease and suggest alternative non-risky ways of behaving that are relatively inexpensive and easy to follow.

The model fails explicitly to acknowledge that apparently health-related behaviours may be influenced by factors other than a desire to achieve the health-related goal, although these can be included in the perceived benefits. For example, a person may join a gym to meet new people, diet to gain social approval or use suntan lotion to avoid premature ageing of the skin rather than skin cancer. The boxes and arrows in Figure 7.1 above do not appear to be positioned in the best way. For example, 'cues to action' might be better towards the right, feeding directly into 'likelihood of taking action'. Furthermore, the model does not acknowledge that an individual's lifestyle is not always the outcome of rational decisions but may be influenced by *unconscious* processes related to *self-concept* and *self-efficacy*.

Although this model remains a useful foundation for understanding health-related behaviour, it has been superseded by later models. Self-efficacy represents a new area for research and is likely to give rise to a continued increase in understanding.

Health education: the use of health education strategies is founded upon the belief that it is possible to influence the health of people by either persuading them or assisting them to change their behaviour. The aims of health education are to:

- ensure that individuals are able to exercise informed choice when selecting the lifestyle that they adopt (Department of Health, 1992)
- reduce or limit the drain on the public purse created by ill-health that could be prevented by changes in the behaviour of individuals (Kiger, 1995: 23).

Health education programme: seeks to change personal habits and behaviour and thus prevent disease by providing information and education (Naidoo and Wills, 1994). The following provide a useful format for a programme:

- Explore clients' health beliefs
- Reinforce positive attitudes to health
- Challenge health myths and negative attitudes
- Explore the costs and benefits of both behaviour change and non-change
- Devise a plan of action with the client to suit his or her needs and lifestyle.

Many mass media health education campaigns seek to provide information aiming to persuade people to change their attitudes. These campaigns often work on the notion that behavioural change will follow attitudinal change. This premise has been challenged by empirical research showing that appropriate attributions do not cause a consistent behaviour change (see Chapter 3).

Health of the Nation: this White Paper (Department of Health, 1992) set targets in five key areas of health associated with behavioural and social risk factors: coronary heart disease and stroke, cancers, mental illness, HIV/AIDS and sexual health, and accidents. In setting the targets, the government appears to assume that rational thought governs health behaviour and, in doing so, ignores the emotional, social and economic forces that influence choice.

Hypochondria: usually defined as an excessive and unnecessary worry about health and a continuing belief that one is ill when medical opinion does not confirm this. This is currently referred to as 'paradise syndrome' when exhibited by people such as film stars who are constantly under scrutiny by the mass media. People accused of hypochondria who have become depressed because of distressing symptoms can be extremely relieved when finally diagnosed as having a condition such as multiple sclerosis. For some people, knowledge that they were not imagining symptoms can help to offset some of the difficulties involved in adjusting to living with a deteriorating condition.

Intention: what a person intends to do. Conner *et al.* (1996: 316) summarise intention as including three sets of factors:

- attitude towards the behaviour: a function of a person's beliefs about the likelihood and evaluation of wanted outcomes of the behaviour
- the subjective *norm* or perceived social pressure: motivation to comply
- perceived behavioural control: beliefs about the frequency of occurrence of the factors likely to facilitate or inhibit the performance of the behaviour.

Learned helplessness: Seligman (1975) demonstrated that animals that were subjected to unpleasant experiences over which they had no control tended not to take action in other situations in which the outcome was in fact under their influence. He initially used these findings to explain the passivity of people who were depressed and did little to try to help themselves. His ideas have been subsequently revised to include a cognitive element and developed into *attribution theory*.

Learning: 'learning occurs whenever one adopts new, or modifies existing, behaviour patterns in a way which has some influence on future performance or attitudes... This reasonably permanent change in behaviour must grow out of past experience and is distinguished from behaviour which results from maturation or physical deformity' (Child, 1986: 81).

An individual's ability to learn is affected by many different factors. Bruner (1971) identifies three variables that he feels must be examined by any individual who is engaged in teaching – the nature of:

- the learner
- the knowledge
- the learning process.

Each contains a number of factors that may affect an individual's ability to learn. Within the learner, factors include intelligence, memory and beliefs, as well as the learner's previous experiences, motivation and personality. The nature of the knowledge to be gained can influence whether the learner will be receptive to being taught. This highlights the need for the teacher to make the information interesting to the learner and of personal importance. The nature of the knowledge will also determine whether the learning objectives can be identified in observable terms, as advocated by Bruner (1971).

Where the objectives have a behavioural focus, for example developing practical skills, these can be clearly defined in observable terms so that achievements may be easily assessed. However, this principle is more difficult to apply to objectives with a cognitive or affective focus, as for example when developing interpersonal qualities. In such circumstances, the teacher may need to rely on the learner's self-assessment of achievements. The teacher is part of the learning process. The attitude, personality, motivation and communication skills of the teacher are likely to impinge on his or her ability to teach and affect the student's ability to learn. By establishing a rapport with a learner and by creating a supportive, *learner-centred* atmosphere, the teacher can foster an effective learning environment.

Locus of control: Rotter (1954, 1966, 1975) developed the construct of locus of control to explain differences in behaviour. This has now been adopted by many psychologists as representing a personality characteristic whereby those who expect that their behaviour will influence outcomes are defined as having a belief in 'internal control', while those who expect outside forces such as chance or powerful others to have greater influence have a belief in 'external control'. Studies suggest that, when confronted by health problems, those who have an internal locus of control engage in more adaptive responses than do those with an external locus of control (Kerr, 1986).

People with health problems may see themselves as being dependent upon the expertise of health-care professionals and may fail to see that they themselves have a part to play in achieving healthy outcomes. Studies have reported beneficial effects when clients have been encouraged and enabled to take control of their own care, for example controlling their own anaesthetic administration (Atwell *et al.* 1984, cited in Pitts and Phillips, 1991: 71). On the other hand, there may be an added problem for people with a strong internal sense of control. Some may feel that they are totally responsible for any illness or symptoms they experience. They may then feel frustration, guilt and shame when all their endeavours are unsuccessful in making them well, which could lead to depression. Those with a strong sense of control are also less likely to comply unquestioningly with medical advice.

This model is controversial, partly because the questionnaires designed to measure the locus of control are not considered to have either *face validity* in relation to health issues or consistent *construct validity*.

Motivation: it is generally accepted among psychologists that all behaviour is meaningful and purposeful, however unusual, incomprehensible or bizarre it may appear. Given this assumption, it should always be possible to find what motivated the behaviour and give a meaningful explanation for it.

Most people look for a rational explanation first, and it is nearly always possible to find some sort of plausible reason for ordinary behaviour. People know why they did something and can say so. It is, however, important to distinguish between admitted reasons and possibly different real reasons. People may lie or cover up their real reasons and give a reason which they think is more socially acceptable.

When the reasons are not known, or seem inadequate or inappropriate, particularly where the person is distressed abut his or her behaviour, it may be necessary to look for hidden causes, such as biological malfunction, early childhood experiences, stress, low self-esteem and so on.

Some psychologists regard all behaviour as striving towards the satisfaction of drives or needs to achieve a goal or comfortable end state. These needs may be purely biological in origin, such as needing food and water, or can be individual or social, such as needing approval, comfort or affection. Maslow (1962) devised a much-cited hierarchy of needs to illustrate that everything people do can be described as fulfilling a need of some kind:

- self-actualisation, reaching one's full potential
- aesthetic appreciation, of balance, order, form and beauty
- cognitive stimulation, through curiosity, exploration and learning
- esteem and regard, for oneself and others, a sense of competence
- love and belongingness, trust and acceptance in a group
- safety, freedom from physical and psychological harm
- physiological functioning related to the fundamental characteristics of living organisms – respiration, digestion, elimination, movement, irritability (sensitivity to surroundings) and reproduction – together with rest and sleep.

A useful distinction when talking about motivation is between *intrinsic* and *extrinsic* motivation. Intrinsic motivation includes all reasons, causes or needs that stem from *within* the person, such as eating healthily and exercising because it feels good. Extrinsic motivation includes all things that govern behaviour from *outside* the person, such as smoking to gain peer approval. These are things done in order to gain something else or to avoid unpleasant consequences.

Persistence of risky behaviour: the health risks associated with certain behaviours are well known, but people continue to engage in them. Bunton and Macdonald (1992) offer some explanations for this:

- Short-term gratification may have a greater influence on behaviour than the prospect of long-term harm
- Reinforcement of the behaviour may be intermittent, so the behaviour is resistant to extinction
- Unconscious mental processes such as denial may be operating to protect against any anxiety that stems from the knowledge that the behaviour is potentially harmful
- The consequences of not engaging in the behaviour are worse than those of engaging in it.

Personality patterns in health: applications of theories within health psychology tend to focus on specific aspects of lifestyle, learned behavioural characteristics and social skills rather than the uncertain concept of personality. It is assumed that there is a purpose to all behaviour, but much may be beyond conscious awareness, and that it can help to become aware of the development of behaviour patterns. Concern lies with the identification of specific maladaptive behaviours that are amenable to change rather than with attempting to provide a comprehensive all-embracing picture of personality. Peck and Whitlow (1975) distinguish between 'comprehensive' theories, which attempt to give a complete picture, and *narrow-band* theories, which are concerned with a more specific and restricted content area. Some of the most well-known theories used in health psychology, for example type A behaviour pattern, learned helplessness and locus of control, are narrow band.

Eysenck (1985) postulated a cancer-prone personality and argued that cancer is caused by a complex interplay of genetic, personality, lifestyle and stress factors. He coined the term type C personality (which he saw as being more or less the opposite of type A) to describe a combination of traits such as being co-operative, appeasing, non-assertive, compliant with external authorities, nice, sociable and conventional, tending to give way rather than fight, and non-expressive of emotions such as anger and hostility. This work sparked off some media interest in the 1980s and cancer patients were often portrayed as typical 'nice' people, inclined to be 'doormats' who 'allowed their cancer to take over'. It was suggested that cancer could be avoided, or even cured, by individuals becoming more *assertive*. Most research does not support this view, despite the intuitive belief that there is some truth in it, which dates back to ancient times. In 1994 Eysenck repeated his assertions, identifying four main personality types. Type 1 he called the cancer prone, the overly patient person, suppressing emotions and failing to cope with stress. Type 2 is the heart disease-prone type, angry and hostile, with a tendency to regard 'an emotionally highly important object as a cause of their unhappiness'. The other two were a mixed type with psychopathic tendencies and a healthy autonomous personality. His findings were greeted with scorn and astonishment by many academics but have awakened renewed interest in this approach. There may be some support for the suppression of anger and hostility as a factor in illness, and this is now seen as the most important single factor in type A vulnerability to coronary heart disease. It may well be found that the similarities, in relation to poor expression of anger, between type A behaviour pattern and Eysenck's type C (or type 1) are more significant than the differences. See also Chapter 15.

Placebo effect: a placebo is a harmless, inactive preparation in the same form as a drug under test. The word 'placebo' comes from the Latin for 'I shall be acceptable.' It is frequently found that people given placebos obtain relief similar to that given by active drugs. This indicates that beliefs and expectations about outcomes can bring about change. See also Chapter 13.

Precaution adoption model: see *changing risk behaviour.*

Prevention of disease: interventions intended to prevent ill-health may be categorised according to their focus (Naidoo and Wills, 1994):

Primary prevention: interventions may be applied to a generally healthy population or may target high-risk groups in an attempt to avoid the onset of ill-health. Examples are immunisation programmes and the fluoridation of water supplies.

Secondary prevention: interventions aim to eradicate or control existing health problems by focusing on the early detection, diagnosis and treatment of those problems, for example by setting up screening programmes.

Tertiary prevention: interventions aim to prevent the recurrence of cured disease or to minimise the effects of existing health problems by avoiding the needless progression of disease. They can prevent complications, for example by educating clients who have enduring mental health problems about the effects of their medication and by monitoring their compliance with treatment.

Protection motivation theory (PMT): a model of health behaviour from R.W. Rogers (1975) that can be directly compared with Becker's health belief model. See also Rogers (1983, 1985), cited in Schwarzer (1992) and Messer and Meldrum (1995). The theory is based on ideas of expectancy and value, and includes a person's perceptions of severity and vulnerability. To these are added expectations about the effectiveness of actions and self-efficacy. A key emphasis in on fear as a motivating factor, related to negative associations with illness, rather than positive association with feeling healthy. See Figure 7.2 above.

Rehabilitation: a period of adjustment or the creation of a new lifestyle following an enforced major change due to injury or disease. In common usage, the word 'rehabilitation' is often associated with restoring a person to a previous level of functioning through training, and as this is not always possible, it is important to explore the expectations of the patient, relatives and carers. Issues for consideration include patients' attitudes to themselves and their new and future state of health: changes in body image, self-concept and self-esteem; the expression of sexuality; and personality and mood (including anxiety, depression, locus of control and learned helplessness). Models of the stages or tasks of personal development following a major life change, with the support systems and styles of counselling considered beneficial for different needs, should be considered.

Self-efficacy: the belief in one's ability to achieved desired *goals*. This can be expressed as 'I personally have the capability to do something' (Schwarzer, 1992). For example, 'I am confident that I can perform a planned exercise even if I am tired, friends are visiting, the weather is bad and so on.' Schwarzer identifies three components – self-efficacy, outcome expectancy and risk perception – as contributing to the adoption and maintenance of health behaviours. He presents various arguments to try to determine the relationship between these components and health behaviour, citing several alternative models, which involve the following contrasting assumptions:

- All three components are of equal importance in determining intentions and subsequent behaviour
- Prior behaviour, or habit, is a better predictor of subsequent behaviour than are any of the three components
- Self-efficacy is the most important component and is outside voluntary control
- All possible paths contribute to behaviour, so deliberate planning can be seen to be important
- Intentions determine behaviour
- There is a jump to be made between *deciding about* action that could be taken and *deciding to act*.

Schwarzer suggests that all these components represent not independent variables but aspects of a process of achieving action. We imagine outcomes, and what we imagine depends on what we think we can do. He represents the key elements of moving towards health behaviour in his health action process model (Schwarzer, 1992). See Figure 7.5 above.

Severity: Rosenstock (1974) defines severity as the degree to which an individual *perceives* the *consequences* of having an illness to be severe.

Susceptibility: Rosenstock (1974) defines susceptibility as individuals' beliefs about whether they likely to contract an illness. See health belief model.

Teaching: 'a system of activities intended to induce learning, comprising the deliberate and systematic creation and control of those conditions in which learning does occur' (Curzon, 1985: 14).

Teleology: the doctrine or study of ends or causes, especially in relation to the belief that everything in nature has been designed according to some purpose. In the context of health beliefs and lifestyle, a teleological approach is based on the concept that a person's current behaviour is driven or motivated by goals. Adler took a teleological approach to personality and believed that an understanding of personality was only possible if an individual's goals were known. He believed that people strive towards fulfilment of their own personal potential; this can be compared with Maslow's (1962) notion of self-actualisation and his hierarchical model of needs (see motivation).

Theory of planned behaviour: this model from Ajzen (1988, 1991) adds perceived behavioural control (self-efficacy) as a predictor of behaviour to the theory of reasoned action. See also Schwarzer (1992), Messer and Meldrum (1995) and Stroebe and Stroebe (1995). Perceived behavioural control refers to the extent to which a person believes that it is easy or difficult to perform a specific behaviour. The theory of planned behaviour 'postulates that the most immediate determinant of a person's behaviour is behavioural intentions – what the person intends to do' (Conner *et al.*, 1996: 316). See Figure 7.4 above.

Theory of reasoned action: an earlier model than the theory of planned behaviour (Ajzen, 1991), which now replaces it. Ajzen and Fishbein (1980) suggested that the best predictor of a person's behaviour is the intention to engage in that behaviour. This intention is influenced by the person's attitudes about that behaviour and their perceptions about the attitudes of others (subjective norm). Attitudes about the behaviour will be determined by the expectations the person has about the consequences of the behaviour and the evaluation of these. A person's perceptions about the attitudes of others will encompass beliefs about how others expect them to behave and their motivation to comply with these expectations. The influence of others may be a significant factor in determining behaviour, and this highlights the potential value of role-modelling in health promotion. The underlying assumption upon which this model is based can be criticised as a person may not translate intentions into action (see self-efficacy). See Figure 7.3 above.

8 HUMANISTIC PSYCHOLOGY AND COUNSELLING

Humanistic approaches are also known as phenomenological, person-centred, client-centred, non-directive and facilitative. Phenomenological therapy focuses on the wholeness of experience and emphasises the searching for personal meanings and essences of experience. Behaviour and events are explored only from the point of view of the client. Therapy is not concerned with theory-driven interpretations of hidden or unconscious emotional dynamics or with quantitative measurements of behaviour.

Humanistic or person-centred approaches, based on the phenomenological paradigm, involve the application of psychological knowledge, awareness, intuition and counselling experience in working with clients in such a way that the relationship between therapist and client is one of an equal partnership.

This chapter focuses on counselling styles that are based on the humanistic approach or which integrate these principles with other strategies. Other counselling and psychotherapy approaches are described in Chapters 4, 6 and 17.

Definitions	
Rogers (1961)	It is the client who knows what hurts, what directions to go, what problems are crucial, what experiences have been deeply buried. It began to occur to me that unless I had a need to demonstrate my own cleverness and learning, I would do better to rely upon the client for the direction of movement in the process.
Burnard and Morrison (1991)	In client-centred counselling, the counsellor is not an expert in other people's problems but someone who enables or facilitates the problem-solving capacity of the other person.

Definitions (cont'd)	
McLeod (1993)	Humanistic psychology has always consisted of a broad set of theories and models connected by shared values and philosophical assumptions, rather than constituting a single, coherent, theoretical formulation... The common ingredient... is an emphasis on experiential processes... the here-and-now...
Silverstone (1993)	The theory is concise. The theory is so easy to understand intellectually, so difficult to incorporate into one's way of being. Very few of us have experienced a model in our upbringing in which the person knows best. So, it is like learning a new language.
British Association of Counselling (1990)	The overall aim of counselling is to provide an opportunity for the client to work towards living in a more satisfying and resourceful way. The term 'counselling' includes work with individuals, pairs or groups of people, often, but not always, referred to as 'clients'. The objectives of particular counselling relationships will vary according to the client's needs. Counselling may be concerned with developmental issues, addressing and resolving specific problems, making decisions, coping with crises, developing personal insight and knowledge, working through feelings of inner conflict or improving relationships with others. The counsellor's role is to facilitate the client's work in ways which respect the client's values, personal resources and capacity for self-determination.

Approaches, Arguments and Applications

It can be argued that although there are more than 400 distinct models of counselling and psychotherapy, there are three 'core' approaches – humanistic, cognitive-behavioural and psychodynamic – representing fundamentally different ways of viewing people and their emotional and behavioural difficulties (McLeod, 1993). These three approaches can be contrasted, as shown in Figure 8.1.

```
                    HUMANISTIC
                   client-centred
                    skills based


   PSYCHODYNAMIC              COGNITIVE-
                              BEHAVIOURAL
   therapist-centred             didactic
      theory based
                            theory and skill mix
```

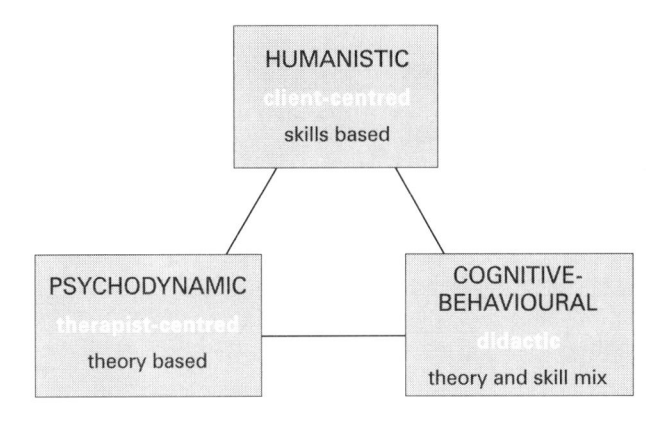

Figure 8.1   Styles of therapy

This diagram exaggerates the extremes. In practice, many counsellors or therapists integrate styles, and some cannot always say precisely what approach they are using at any one moment. However, the contrast enables different elements to be identified.

Humanistic psychology is primarily an applied field concerned with counselling and psychotherapy, developed in the first half of the twentieth century in response to dissatisfaction with the extremes of the psychodynamic and behaviourist approaches. Although there is a wealth of clinical experience, the absence of systematic, quantitative data based on hypotheticodeductive methods means that the approach remains outside mainstream psychology.

The principles of humanistic psychology underlie much of nursing theory and lead to the development of person-centred listening skills within nursing, which can be used instead of, or alongside, more directive advice and information-giving as appropriate.

Prominent figures in humanistic psychology have been Carl Rogers, Charlotte Buhler, Abraham Maslow and Sydney Jourard. These practitioners share a vision of therapy that will facilitate the human capacity for growth, creativity and choice. The image of the individual in humanistic psychology is of someone striving to find meaning and fulfilment in the world.

In the client–carer relationship, the client is encouraged to take control and the therapist encourages and assists the client in finding a sense of direction and moving towards whatever the client perceives as desirable.

Rogers (1961, 1980) argues that there are three basic principles of the client-centred or person-centred approach:

- genuineness (congruence)
- unconditional positive regard (unconditional regard, warmth, caring, acceptance, respect or prizing)
- empathy.

Rogers believes that the actual method or style used in counselling or psychotherapy may be a matter of preference for therapist and client but that no method can be successful unless it is based on the three basic principles. Moreover, in practice, only these three are needed; that is, they are the 'necessary and sufficient' conditions for effective therapy. Murgatroyd (1995) says that other researchers agree that they are necessary but argue they are not sufficient, and he mentions Robert Carkhuff, who identified three more basic conditions of helping:

- concreteness
- immediacy
- confrontation.

Murgatroyd (1995: 21) summarises all these essential features in the following way:

- A person in need has come to you for help
- In order to be helped they need to know that you have understood how they think and feel
- They also need to know that, whatever your own feelings about who or what they are, or about what they have done or not done, you accept them as they are – you accept their right to decide their own lives for themselves
- In the light of this knowledge about your acceptance and understanding of them, they will begin to open themselves to the possibility of change and development
- But if they feel that their association with you is conditional upon them changing, they may then feel pressurised and reject your help.

This identification of essential elements can be usefully compared with *neurolinguistic programming*, which also purports to have found what makes therapy work – what is called the 'magic' of therapy.

The chief drawback with a person-centred technique is that a counsellor who never asks questions or gives suggestions may be perceived by the client as unengaged or uninterested in the client. Such difficulties are most likely to result from a lack of understanding of the technique: a poorly trained counsellor is not using the techniques well, the method has not been explained to the client, insufficient time has been given for the client to move towards a position of control, or the technique is not suited to the client or the problem. Person-centred approaches tend to be most successful with educated, highly motivated people who have a natural tendency towards self-examination.

Key Terms and Concepts

Active listening: listening attentively to a client and providing *non-verbal* and *verbal* cues to the client that attention is being paid and an effort being made to understand what the client is saying.

Active listening is not an absence of speech on the part of the counsellor but a positive approach undertaken with a view to gaining a fuller understanding and allowing the client an opportunity to explore thoughts and feelings without direction from the counsellor. There are a number of useful techniques for achieving this. These include assuming an attentive listening posture, *mirroring* the client's words, and matching non-verbal aspects such as posture, head and hand movements, speed and tone of speech, facial expressions, laughter, sighs and so on. Robbie (1988) also gives a description of these techniques in his account of neurolinguistic programming and points out that the matching must be subtle and discrete, not obvious copying or 'parroting' which can be seen as sarcastic parodying.

Mirroring or reflecting words may take the form of a repetition of the client's own words or a rephrasing. Simple repetitions can be startlingly effective as the client hears the words and seemingly notices them in a new way. The client may not even realise that the words are a repetition but may imagine that the counsellor has found new words to express clearly what the client had thought was a jumbled muddle of thoughts. Where words are rephrased, care must be taken to check with the client that these do adequately express what the client was saying, for example 'What I think you're saying is..., is that right?' Neutral *empathy-building statements* such as 'I notice...' and 'I imagine...' can also be used to indicate attention and attempts to understand. Matching of non-verbal components of communication makes deliberate use of a natural tendency for this in ordinary conversation (see Chapter 9). Active listening may also involve the positive use of silence to allow the client time to collect his thoughts without feeling a need to speak.

Bridges and links: a technique developed in some uses of *person-centred art therapy* to help a client to see connections between the drawn image and everyday life situations (Silverstone, 1993). For example, if a client says that the picture represents an occasion on which the client was faced with carrying out a disliked activity, the counsellor might encourage the client to explore what that might mean now and make a link between the previous experience and the present situation.

Client–carer relationships: There is an infinite variety of ways in which a client and carer might interact, the styles varying from occasion to occasion or even moment to moment. This can apply to professional carers, *parenting styles* or family and friends. It can be helpful to identify the following hierarchy of styles:

- coercive: making others do as they are told by threats or other emotional pressure
- authoritarian: telling others what to do in a bossy or overbearing manner
- authoritative: telling others what to do in a friendly but firm manner
- persuasive: applying some emotional pressure to direct others towards action
- directive advice-giving: offering alternatives, indicating which is the 'better' choice
- didactic: teaching what to do and how to do it

- non-directive advice or information-giving: offering alternatives as equal choices
- facilitative: helping others to work towards what they want for themselves
- befriending: spending time together in a friendly supportive way
- *laissez-faire*: giving room to work things out, without interference
- neglecting: leaving others alone in an uncaring and unsupportive manner.

One method may be more appropriate on a particular occasion than another. For example, an authoritative approach may be necessary in an emergency or life-threatening situation. A mixture of information and teaching may be needed alongside a facilitative approach so that the client can make informed choices. A *laissez-faire* approach may be appropriate in some community nursing situations, in which families will function most effectively if left to work things out for themselves. However, they may be reassured to know that the carer is available when needed.

Concreteness: providing definite examples and helping the client to be accurate.

Confrontation: in the context of counselling, the term confrontation does not mean disagreement or using aggressive tactics, but helping the client to face up to discrepancies between what the client says and does, or between how the client views things and how the helper views them. Murgatroyd (1995) gives examples of the kinds of discrepancy that can arise when clients have an unrealistic view of their abilities and persist, for example, in applying for jobs that are either above or below their capacity. The task of the counsellor is to help the client towards a more realistic view. It can be argued that this is a judgemental approach as it is centred on what the helper sees as realistic. Confrontation can be compared with techniques in cognitive therapy that address what the therapist sees as the client's distorted cognitions.

Congruence: see genuineness.

Counselling skills: the British Association of Counselling (BAC) distinguishes between counselling and counselling skills, and provides a separate code of ethics for practitioners who are not trained counsellors but who wish to use counselling skills in their workplace. The *BAC Code of Ethics and Practice for Counselling Skills* (1989) states that:

> The term 'counselling skills' does not have a single definition which is universally accepted. For the purpose of this code, 'counselling skills' are distinguished from 'listening skills' and from 'counselling'. Although the distinction is not always a clear one, because the term 'counselling skills' contains elements of these other two activities, it has its own place in the continuum between them. What distinguishes the use of counselling skills from these other two activities are the intentions of the user, which is to enhance the performance of their functional role, as line manager, nurse, tutor, social worker, personnel officer, voluntary worker, etc., the recipient will, in turn, perceive them in that role.

McLeod (1993: 3) warns that although it would not be helpful to bar all these other professionals from counselling, it can be confusing or even damaging to a client when someone who is trying to help him becomes entangled in *role conflict*. This might happen, for example, through trying to be both counsellor and manager. It can also be worrying if a helper becomes involved in a situation which is beyond his or her training and competence. Part of the development of using counselling skills is learning when to refer to a relevant specialist and how to avoid inadvertently doing more harm than good.

Emotional Maturity Scale: a scale developed by Willoughby (cited by Rogers, 1961) to measure the quality of everyday behaviour. Items are concerned with whether a client characteristically appeals for help with problems, becomes angry with those who impede his or her progress (particularly car drivers), balances the recognition of demonstrated inferiority in some respect with the consideration of activities that show superiority, organises efforts and welcomes appropriate opportunities for sexual expression without being ashamed, fearful or preoccupied with this. An investigative study showed that clients who were judged to have made significant movement in therapy were judged by themselves, the therapist and friends to have increased in maturity. Interestingly, those judged by the therapist to have made least movement in therapy, and rated by observers as having deteriorated in maturity, showed a noticeable increase in their self-assessed score after therapy and at follow-up. Rogers suggests this seems to be clear evidence of a defensive self-rating when therapy has not gone well.

Empathic listening: the demonstration of empathy through active listening and reflecting skills.

Empathy: the word empathy came into English use in 1912 and is derived from the Greek *en* for in and *pathos* meaning feeling. As a concept, empathy appears to have originated from the German word 'Einfühlung' meaning 'feeling within' and refers to the projection of one's personality into understanding a situation. It is now used in counselling to refer to an understanding of what a situation or condition feels like for another person, or a demonstration of that understanding. This is also referred to as 'empathic understanding' and is particularly associated with the work of Carl Rogers. According to Rogers (1975), the use of empathy involves entering another person's perceptual world in an attempt to see and understand that world as if it were one's own.

Rogers (1980) describes an empathic way of being with another person as having several facets:

> Empathic understanding means that the therapist senses accurately the feelings and personal meanings that the client is experiencing and communicates this understanding to the client. When functioning best, the therapist is so much inside the private world of the other that he or she can clarify not only the meanings of which the client is aware but even those just below the level of awareness. This kind of sensitive, active listening is exceedingly rare in our lives. We think we listen, but very rarely do we listen with real understanding, true empathy. Yet listening, of this very special kind, is one of the most potent forces of change that I know (p. 116).

It means entering the private perceptual world of the other and becoming thoroughly at home in it. It involves being sensitive, moment by moment, to the changing felt meanings which flow in this other person, to the fear or rage or tenderness or confusion or whatever he or she is experiencing. It means temporarily living in the other's life, moving about in it delicately without making judgements; it means sensing meanings of which he or she is scarcely aware, but not trying to uncover totally unconscious feelings, since this would be too threatening. It includes communicating your sensings of the person's world as you look with fresh and unfrightened eyes at elements of which he or she is fearful. It means frequently checking with the person as to the accuracy of your sensings, and being guided by the responses you receive. You are a companion to the person in his or her inner world. By pointing to the possible meanings in the flow of another person's experiencing, you help the other to focus on this useful type of referent, to experience the meanings more fully, and to move forward in the experiencing (p. 142).

Rogers (1980: 146–50) cites research to support the following general statements:

- The ideal therapist is, first of all, empathic
- Empathy is correlated with self-exploration and process movement
- Empathy early in the relationship predicts later success
- In successful cases, the client comes to perceive more empathy
- Empathic understanding is provided freely by the therapist, rather than drawn from him or her
- The more experienced the therapist is, the more likely he or she is to be empathic
- Empathy is a special quality in a relationship, and therapists definitely offer more of it than even helpful friends
- Experienced therapists often fall short of being empathic
- Clients are better judges of the degree of empathy than are therapists
- Brilliance and diagnostic perceptiveness are unrelated to empathy
- An empathic way of being can be learned from empathic persons.

The development of an empathic approach towards clients can be viewed as involving two distinct phases of projection of oneself into the other person's position. One phase is the ability to imagine what that situation would feel like, putting oneself in the other's shoes. A more complex phase is being able to work out what it actually feels like for the other person, whose previous experience, needs, fears and worries might be very different.

Empathy-building statements: Philip Burnard (1994: 131, 132) outlines a number of statements that can be made by a counsellor to show empathic understanding. Burnard points out that many such statements involve 'reading between the lines' of what the client is saying and intuitively guessing what he or she means. Such conjectures, assumptions or interpretations can be either close or far from what the client is trying to say, and it is important for the counsellor to watch for verbal and non-verbal clues that indicate the client's response and then choose whether to continue such statements or return to non-directive listening and mirroring.

Liesl Silverstone (1993) encourages the use of relatively neutral statements such as 'I notice...' and 'I imagine...'. These statements demonstrate that the counsellor is making an attempt to understand but acknowledges the limitations of the counsellor's ability to guess what the client really feels like. Instead of saying, 'You sound angry with them' (Burnard, 1994: 132), Silverstone (1993) would recommend saying something like 'I notice you are saying people at work don't have a lot of time for you. I imagine you feel angry about that.' Silverstone argues that this approach gives the client more opportunity to disagree with the counsellor and find a way of expressing feelings. Moreover, phrasing the anger in connection with the people's behaviour (using the words 'angry about that') rather than the people themselves ('angry with them') also helps to promote regard for people, at the same time as being honest about disliking what they do.

Empowerment: giving the client control over a situation and the interventions that are available. Sully (1996) discusses how health-care professionals who try to empower patients may find themselves in conflict with other professionals or with patients and their families who expect a more directive approach.

Genuineness (congruence): Rogers (1980: 115) defines genuineness or congruence as:

> the therapist openly being the feelings and attitudes that are flowing within at the moment... The therapist makes himself or herself transparent to the client, the client can see right through what the therapist is in the relationship, and experiences no holding back on the part of the therapist. As for the therapist, what he or she is experiencing is available to awareness, can be lived in the relationship and can be communicated if appropriate. Thus there is a close matching, or congruence, between what is being experienced at the gut level, what is present in the awareness, and what is expressed to the client.

A counsellor or therapist who is perceived as honest and genuine may help clients to feel more trusting of their own feelings and may encourage their honesty and genuineness in relation to others.

One of the aims of the person-centred approach is to provide training that enables the counsellor to explore personal feelings and develop awareness. The more the counsellor can accept him or herself, the more likely he or she will be able to respond in a personal, honest way to the client.

Guided fantasy and guided imagery: the use of stories or descriptions to help someone imagine a scene or event. This may also include producing the image in art form, as in *person-centred art therapy*. See also imaging in Chapter 13, fantasy play in Chapter 16 and iconic imagery in Chapter 14.

Immediacy: keeping the focus of a counselling session on the client's immediate needs, dwelling neither on the past nor the future.

Integrative therapy: there are several distinct ways in which different psychological and therapeutic perspectives or schools of thought can be brought together to produce an integrated therapeutic programme. One approach is *eclectic blending*, which combines selected elements from a number of different approaches. This can be a blend of structure, *media, modes* of interaction and *theory* (Calisch, 1989). It can be done in a general way for all clients or be a special blend planned for a particular client. Difficulties lie in the choice and proportions of the different elements and in matching the blend to the attributes and interests of both client and carer. Sometimes the identity of the contributing elements may be lost. The therapist may not always know which approaches are being used, which may lead to confusion, contradictions or inefficiency.

An alternative method of integrating therapies is to design a *multimodal* programme. In this case, a number of clearly identified separate styles of therapy can be provided. During the programme, the client 'visits' each of these in turn. The hope is that, although all methods do not suit all persons, something may work well and the combination may prove fruitful. A typical programme might include cognitive-behavioural therapy, group therapy, occupational therapy, relaxation and exercise. Multimodal programmes are often used in *pain* and *stress management*. Windy Dryden (1992) provides accounts of integrative and eclectic therapies.

Metaphor: in the context of therapy, metaphor refers to any use of art, music, dance, mime, story-telling or other creative art with *symbols* and stories to represent issues from real life. Mayo (1996: 209), using group art therapy in palliative care, tells how they 'try together through art, music and story telling, to release the creative life within us which we may have been repressing'.

Personal construct therapy: an approach for investigating individual ways of seeing the self and others, based on a *phenomenological paradigm* and using repertory grids (Fransella, 1990). See Chapters 6 and 15.

Personal growth: humanistic theory adopts an optimistic view of human potential and theorists such as Maslow (1962) and Rogers (1965) believe that each person has an innate capacity for personal growth. Maslow (1962) uses the term 'self actualisation' for the process of realising one's full potential and argues that this can only be attained if basic physical and psychological needs have been satisfied (see motivation).

Relationship inventory: Barrett-Lennard (cited by Rogers, 1961) devised a relationship inventory designed to study five facets of the relationship:

- the extent to which the client felt him or herself to be empathically understood
- the level of the regard
- the unconditionality of the regard
- the congruence or genuineness
- the counsellor's willingness to be 'known'.

Different forms were used for the client and the therapist. Rogers reports that experienced therapists were perceived as having more of the first four qualities than those who were less experienced but less of the last quality. That is, inexperienced therapists seemed more willing to reveal their own thoughts and feelings but were perceived as less effective in the other ways.

Responsibility for self: humanistic or person-centred approaches encourage each individual to take responsibility for him or herself, working with the counsellor, carer or other partner only as needed in order to do this. This can be difficult at first for a person who is more used to being told what to do or to conforming to another's expectations or group norms. Much of a carer's task lies in helping a client to gain confidence and a belief in the ability to take responsibility and achieve personal goals (self-efficacy), that is, to move from being dependent to independent. Clients with a strongly developed so-called authoritarian personality who are accustomed to following or giving instructions in a rigidly controlled, hierarchical family or organisation may be at a particular disadvantage when a carer is adopting a person-centred approach.

Supervision: this is often understood to mean the process in which an experienced counsellor or therapist collaborates with a less experienced practitioner and assists that person in refining his or her practice, understand some of the personal and idiosyncratic components of his or her clinical work and work towards achieving the greatest possible personal and clinical understanding (for example, Calisch, 1989). However, many experienced practitioners continue to seek mutual supervision with colleagues in order to continue this process throughout a lifetime of clinical practice. The British Association of Counselling (BAC) and Person-centred Art Therapy Association (PCATA) codes of ethics make it clear that this is a requirement rather than an option. The BAC Code of Ethics (1990: B.3.1) stipulates that:

> It is a breach of the ethical requirement for counsellors to practise without regular counselling supervision/consultative support.

Therapeutic use of art: in addition to psychodynamic *art therapy or psychotherapy*, based on a clinical model, art can be used in many ways, with therapeutic benefits. Informal uses of art include giving access to a range of media (such as paints, crayons, clay or papier mâché) that can be used in a non-interpretative way. Carers may set a theme or project or leave clients to work independently. This can be beneficial with patients who cannot, or do not want to, talk but who value being able to express and communicate emotional experiences in a non-verbal way. Art may also be used simply as a distraction or a way of occupying time. This use is not trivial, and what may begin as idle playing can sometimes give rise to great satisfaction and benefit.

Art can also be used alongside person-centred counselling. This is gradually becoming more established as 'person-centred art therapy' but is still rather frowned on by some psychodynamically orientated institutes of art therapy, who view it as not academically rigorous enough. Person-centred training does not usually require a background in art, art history or psychodynamic theories but focuses on the experiential learning of counselling techniques (Silverstone, 1993). Artwork is used as a vehicle for expression that helps the client in finding his or her own meanings. The counsellor is trained to become aware of any tendency to interpret the client's pictures or ask direct or leading questions and must practise, under supervision, ways in which to avoid doing this.

The technique combines the person-centred counselling approach with the use of images in art form. Using readily available materials, the client is encouraged to produce a visible image of whatever mental images come to mind in response to a given situation, word or *guided fantasy*. The image may be drawn, painted or made out of clay, torn paper, 'found' objects or miscellaneous bits and pieces.

The counsellor uses techniques of *active listening, bridges and links* and other strategies to help the client towards a personal interpretation of the image and feelings or thoughts associated with it.

During training, the counsellor engages in regular role-play situations as counsellor, client or observer, in order to practise techniques and create a portfolio of personal images and reflections. Emphasis is placed on the counsellor's awareness of a personal style of communication and on learning to match this to the pace and form of each different client. Personal fears, worries, expectations, biases and assumptions that can interfere with listening are uncovered. Silverstone (1993) argues that the necessary learning for the counsellor does not occur through reading, writing or talking about how to counsel but through much personal work, which can be slow and painful.

Many uses of art therapy incorporate elements of humanistic and psychodynamic approaches (for example, Wadeson, 1980). Calisch (1989) describes eclectic blending in supervision.

Ziesler (1993: 107) describes how 'through art therapy, cancer patients may have an outlet for inner emotional pressure; an increased insight into their own situation; and a better mental balance that may lead to an improved quality of life'. Ziesler's approach is essentially humanistic but also acknowledges the importance of symbolism which may be interpreted by the carer.

There is a risk with the blending of approaches if practitioners lose sight of boundaries between different theoretical and personal constructs. When bringing interpretations to images, there may be confusion between personal meanings and those indicated by a particular theory. This may distract a client from searching for his or her own meanings.

Transactional analysis (TA): a multifaceted system of psychotherapy developed by Eric Berne (1910–1970) that stems from psychodynamic theories but 'values the importance of the person's subjective experience above any interpretation, prejudgement or preconceived theories or ideas' (Clarkson and Gilbert, 1990: 199).

Like others, Berne (1964) believes that life is basically hard and that everyone feels anxious. He suggests that various unconscious conversational devices or 'games' may be used to maintain control of a situation. These include adopting the *positions* of 'parent', 'adult' and 'child', which have developed out of childhood experiences. In particular, each of us may respond to a distressing situation by adopting a childlike or helpless position, or by attempting to be parentlike and controlling. By understanding our responses, we can learn to be more balanced and adultlike.

A parallel is sometimes drawn between Berne's use of 'child', 'adult' and 'parent' and Freud's 'id', 'ego' and 'superego'. However, Berne uses the concepts in a different way and has more in common with Melanie Klein's descriptions of positions than Freud's theory of instincts. Secondary sources are inclined to refer to transactional analysis as if it offers a means of interpreting other people's behaviour and hence move away from the person-centred perspective. The greatest danger lies in imposing one's own idea of what the terms 'parent' and 'child' stand for instead of appreciating that these are different for every individual.

Transference: Carl Rogers believes that the phenomena of transference and countertransference, so vital to psychodynamic therapies, have no place or relevance in client-centred therapy. Rogers (1965: 197) categorically states that 'Transference, as a problem, doesn't arise.' If the client and counsellor are in equal partnership, he feels that client and counsellor need not view each other in terms of previously encountered *authoritarian* or *role-related* relationships. He accepts that such attitudes occur in some degree in the majority of cases but argues that strong attitudes of transference rarely occur. See also Chapter 17.

Unconditional positive regard (unconditional regard): Rogers (1980) wrote that 'the therapeutic phenomenon seems most likely to occur when the therapist feels, very genuinely and deeply, an attitude of acceptance of and respect for the client as he is, with the potentialities inherent in his present state'. Words such as warmth, caring, acceptance, respect or 'prizing' may also be used to convey regard but the essential feature is that these are 'unconditional'. It is considered important that the client must not be made to feel that the carer's warmth or caring is conditional or dependent on some change taking place as a result of the relationship or therapy (Murgatroyd, 1985). Nor should any views about whether the client is a 'nice' or 'good' person be allowed to interfere with therapy. During training, a therapist is encouraged to explore personal feelings of insecurity or need associated with wanting to believe that he or she is being a 'good' counsellor and is causing the client to change. Real help will only occur when the therapist is not trying to make the client change.

9 Language and Therapeutic Communication

There are probably almost as many definitions of communication as there are writers on the subject, but accounts agree that communication is a basic non-stop human activity for getting and giving out information. This information is conveyed through organised systems or codes. These codes may consist of a relatively unstructured collection of signs or form a more elaborate language.

A distinction can be made between primary representation *of the world, which is our immediate perceptual experience, and* secondary representation, *which is how we communicate about that experience. Bandler and Grinder (1975) demonstrate that there is always a 'slippage' between the two.*

Within therapy, much of the therapeutic process is concerned with developing a shared means of communication between therapist and client and finding ways for communicating thoughts and feelings that have hitherto been inaccessible to the client's conscious awareness or are difficult for the client to express or articulate.

Definitions

Dance and Larson (1976) give 126 definitions of communication. The following are from their list (see Dance and Larson, 1976, for references):

Anderson (1959) — the process by which we understand others and in turn endeavour to be understood by them. It is dynamic, constantly changing and shifting in response to the total situation.

Barnlund (1968) — an 'effort after meaning', a creative act initiated by man in which he seeks to discriminate and organise cues so as to orient himself in his environment and satisfy his changing needs.

Definitions (cont'd)	
Berelson and Steiner (1964)	the transmission of information, ideas, emotions skills, etc., by the use of symbols – words, pictures, figures, graphs, etc. It is the act or process of transmission that is usually called communication.
Cherry (1966)	broadly: the establishment of a social unit from individuals by the use of language or signs. The sharing of common sets of rules, for various goal-seeking activities.
Corts and Richards (1970)	One mind so acts upon its environment that another mind is influenced, and in that other mind an experience occurs which is like the experience in the first mind, and is caused in part by that experience.
Mead (1963)	It is sometimes believed that conflict is a result of poor communication; that conflict arises because people do not understand each other. If communication means the ability to see another's point of view then some conflicts rooted in false perceptions may be eased by increasing communication.
Rodnick and Wood (1973)	Communication competence can be defined, then, as mastery of an underlying set of rules, determined by the culture and the situation, affecting language choices in interpersonal communication events.
Wilden (1972)	All behaviour is communication.
Schramm (1982)	the tool that makes societies possible.

Approaches, Arguments and Applications

Historically, communication has been studied either as a *process* by which signs are encoded, produced, transmitted and decoded with some effect, or as a social activity during which people create and exchange *meanings*. These two approaches, known respectively as process approaches and semiotic approaches, traditionally give very different interpretations of communication.

Process approaches tend to look at acts of communication with mathematical or telecommunications models. Semiotic theories focus on the products or texts, based on literature, art, music, dance and so on. It can be difficult fully to integrate the two approaches but between them, the various theories of communication help us to look at different ways of communicating, the purposes and effects of communication, the nature of the communicators, the context in which the communication is taking place, language and meanings that can be read into texts.

A text does not have to be written: in this context, the term can refer to any form or product of communication such as a conversation, including body language, a painting, photograph, film, piece of music or dance sequence. The meanings will depend on the social reality in which both texts and people exist, that is, the culture and individual knowledge, interests and needs.

Most communication is considered as happening between people (interpersonal), but much activity occurs within ourselves (intrapersonal), purely for our own benefit without involving anyone else. Even in sleep, the mind rearranges thoughts and memories that sometimes come to awareness in the form of dreams. Processes and meanings may be engaged consciously or unconsciously. Whatever the intentions, it is probably true to say that 'one cannot not communicate'.

Robbie (1988: 256) describes how, in neurolinguistic programming (NLP), it is believed not only that one cannot not communicate, but also that one cannot not respond to others and that the therapist has a responsibility for the responses given by the client:

> it's a principle of NLP that a person can't not respond... NLP believes not only that you can make people feel, but also that you will always elicit some response – and that elicitation is something you are responsible for.

Robbie (1988: 263) goes on to say that whether a therapist notices a response from a client depends on how sensitive the therapist is to subtle and minute changes in choice of words and non-verbal expressions, and that effective therapy depends on the therapist being as flexible and sensitive as possible.

One of the most important shifts in process models is towards the realisation that the 'receiver' or 'consumer' plays an active part in all communication and is not merely passively receptive.

Study of communication in health care is important in helping to design effective communication and in understanding and recognising when things go wrong. It is relevant to establishing therapeutic relationships, describing procedures, advising, counselling, health promotion and education and all other health-care contexts.

Key Terms and Concepts

Barriers to communication: anything that interferes with or prevents a message being received and understood in the way it was intended. Four types of barrier can be described:

- mechanical
- semantic
- psychological
- organisational.

Where some meaning gets through and is perceived with difficulty, the terms 'interference' or 'noise' may be used. 'Noise' and 'interference' are readily described for mechanical barriers, where a clear distinction is defined, but are also used in a general way for semantic, psychological and organisational barriers.

Mechanical barriers include faults in the communication channel and can be subdivided, using technical terms from communications industries, into noise, interference and breakthrough. In this sense, noise refers to relatively low-level undifferentiated background sounds such as the constant humming of machinery, traffic sounds or the buzz of conversation, which can all contribute to making communication seem like hard work and even reduce the willingness to help others (Mathews and Canon, 1975). 'White noise' is heard as a distinctive hiss and is sometimes used to block out unwanted sounds. It may also be used to simulate conditions of hearing loss, such as the background noise sometimes associated with hearing aids or conditions such as tinnitus in order to give carers an indication of what a sufferer hears. The term 'noise' may also be extended to refer to visual impairment and, in the widest sense, to other sensory impairments such as skin conditions that would make touch difficult or unpleasant.

Interference refers to higher-level intermittent sounds. In a hospital context, this may include distant alarms or low flying aircraft, which temporarily prevent speech being heard clearly but do not themselves require attention.

The term 'breakthrough' is used to refer to sudden meaningful sounds that totally replace the current communication. Technically, this could include, for example, police messages coming through on the radio and crossed telephone lines. In conversation, it includes being distracted by a different conversation, nearby event or alarm that demands attention. Interference and breakthrough can also be extended to refer to all sensory channels.

Semantic barriers involve problems of encoding and decoding meanings. If, for whatever reason, two people who are engaged in a conversation do not attach the same meanings to the signs being used, they will not understand each other. This may be a simple case of not sharing the same language but would also refer to the use of regional dialects, subcultural slang and specialist *registers*. A doctor or nurse who uses medical terms unfamiliar to a patient will put up semantic barriers. It is sometimes difficult to remember that professional vocabulary that has become second nature is still new to a patient (or trainee nurse). A senior nurse once confessed (personal communication) that when she started training, she thought that the room labelled 'MI Recovery' was intended for victims of road accidents on the nearby M1 motorway.

Psychological barriers include emotional ones such as anxiety, depression or loss of self-esteem, which alter perceptions, concentration, comprehension and memory. Many factors, for example expectations, previous experience, attitudes, stereotypes, prejudices, beliefs and values, can be barriers that affect perceptions, attention and judgements and alter the way in which messages are communicated.

The fourth barrier to communication has to do with the structure of organisations themselves. One mark of a good organisation is that it has clearly defined and smoothly operating channels of communication between its different members and various departments.

Body language: the aspects of non-verbal communication that directly involve the body. See non-verbal communication.

Categories of communication: this term is often used for classifying communication according to how many communicators, and of what nature, are involved. The main categories are intrapersonal, interpersonal, medio, group, mass media and extrapersonal. See individual entries.

Channel: the physical means of transmitting communication. At a human level, this refers to the sensory channels: hearing, vision, smell, taste, touch and *proprioception* (see Chapter 14). More fundamentally, it refers to physical sound waves, light waves and chemicals, and to neurological pathways. In communication study, it is sometimes also useful further to distinguish between channel and carriers so that, for example, sound waves are carried by air, water or solid materials such as wood. Sound travels very well through solids, which is why it is possible, with practice, to hear far-off traffic by putting an ear to the ground, or to make a 'telephone' out of two tin cans and a piece of string. This explains why deaf people can still feel the vibrations of sounds in their bodies. Beyond the human senses, use can be made of channels such as radio and microwaves, ultrasound and X-rays, which enable signals to be carried over long distances or through materials.

It is important to know and understand what channels are available and how to make the best use of them. People with sensory loss may have to learn new methods of communicating to compensate. For example, in the rare condition of loss of proprioception, individuals no longer have the intrapersonal awareness of where the parts of their body are. They may need to use mirrors to watch themselves all the time in order to be able to move (Sacks, 1985). Technological developments in alternative channels have led to, among other things, echo-sounding sticks for blind people, touch-telephones for deaf people and the interesting scientific exploration of converting touch to vision in people with an intact optical cortex but impaired eyes. For people with impaired voice production, devices can be used which pick up vibrations in the throat and reproduce these as speech. Where a person is unable to speak at all, such as is the case with a sufferer from motor neurone disease, computer simulation can be used to convert small movements, via a keyboard, into recognisable speech.

Code: The term 'code' is used in a number of different ways. Most commonly it refers to systems like Morse code and semaphore, which provide a way of encoding words into a form that can be transmitted over long distances through either sounds or flag signals. Secret codes can be used to translate words into signs, the meaning of which is known only to the sender and to a receiver who has the cipher. These codes are all based on words and are therefore restricted to a particular language.

In communication theory, the word 'code' can be used to refer to any collection of signs or symbols (word or non-word) that can be used to convey meaning. A code may consist of a relatively unstructured collection of signs, such as roadsigns, that are linked according to a few basic rules or constitute a more elaborate *language* with a recognisable grammar.

Communication skills: a communication skill is an ability to *encode* or *decode* information effectively. With encoding, this needs a suitable medium, knowledge the rules of the language relevant to that medium, awareness of the possibility of inadvertent or hidden meanings, knowing the other person and his or her needs and making good use of *feedback*. When speaking, it is important to choose words and a sentence structure familiar to the listener, to know when to pause and take turns and how to use eye contact and other non-verbal communication to advantage, to avoid sending mixed signals and so on. Decoding relates to making sense of what someone else is trying to communicate. The most important decoding skills are probably listening, the interpretation of body language and reading. The term 'skill' is used because it has been realised that these abilities are learned through experience and can be deliberately improved with training, perhaps through the use of video recordings.

Communication with children: effective communication with children follows similar rules to that with adults: it requires listening for the patterns that the child uses and reflecting these. Various theories of child development make different recommendations about the kinds of explanation that are appropriate at different ages or stages (see Chapter 16), but a summary of all the findings suggests that careful listening to a child's preconceptions and then building a simple account in the child's own language that addresses these preconceptions is what is required.

Decoding: 'reading a *text*' or making sense of a set of signs and signals that appear to carry meaning according to some system or language.

Encoding: turning thoughts and mental images into a recognisable form or text.

Extrapersonal communication: communication with anything that is not a person, for example animals, plants and computers, including the Internet and the Web, where there is no direct communication with another person. It could also include occult communication, such as telepathy and spiritualism, or attempts to send signals to extraterrestrial beings. It might also include religious communication such as prayer, although it could be argued that prayer can also be seen as either interpersonal or intrapersonal according to individual beliefs. Most formal study has been with communication with computers, looking at the 'languages' available and at ways to make the programs more user-friendly.

Eye contact and gaze: Argyle (1983) describes how when two people engage in conversation, each looks at the other from time to time, particularly in the region of the eyes; he refers to this as 'gaze'. Looking at each other's eyes simultaneously is eye contact or mutual gaze. It is found that each culture has patterns of acceptable types and durations of gaze, mutual gaze and turn-taking. According to Morris (1978) and Argyle (1983), in typical English exchange, each person looks at the other 25–75 per cent of the time and the length of glances varies from 3 to 7 seconds, or longer where the individuals know and like each other. On the whole, a person will tend to look nearly twice as long while listening as while speaking: glances are longer and away-glances briefer. This enables the listener to make use of the visual signals that are part of the speaker's body language and to indicate that attention is being paid.

Facial expressions: the way in which the face is able to express emotions or the emotional 'colouring' of thoughts. The work of Thayer and Schiff (1969), illustrated in Gill and Adams (1992), with cartoon faces suggests that it is mainly the positioning of eyebrows and mouth that gives rise to different expressions. Most research supports the view that facial expressions relating to extreme forms of the basic emotions (see Chapter 6) are universally recognisable, which would indicate that such expressions are innate rather than learned.

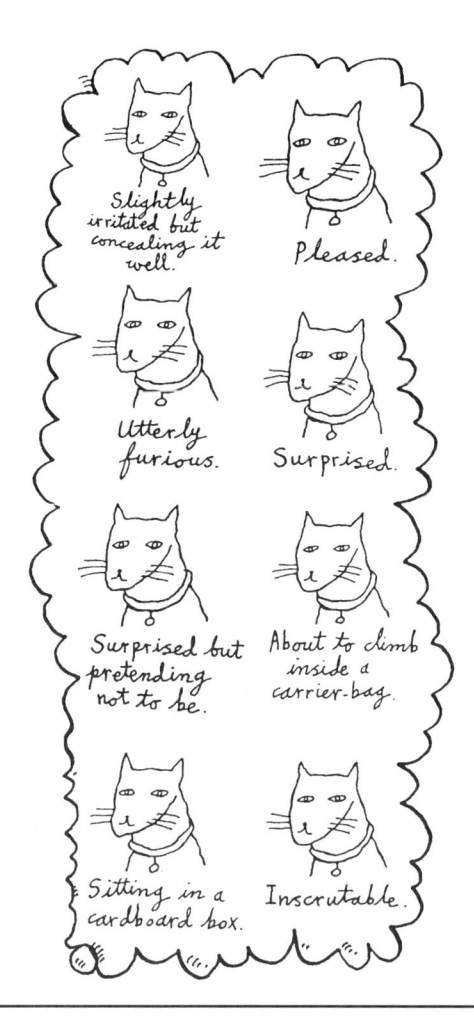

Figure 9.1 Facial expressions *(reproduced from Appleby, 1996)*

However, this argument tends to be rather circular, since the identification of some of the basic emotions is based on responses to facial expressions. Complex mixtures of emotions, such as jealousy, fiendishness and sheepishness, or subtle or milder forms of emotion, are probably subject to cultural or individual variations, which may lead to misinterpretations. For example, there is a type of smile that can be recognised as indicating smouldering anger, and another smile that suggests fear or appeasement. Recognition may depend on whether the smiling person is deliberately making the expression and can therefore exaggerate the distinctive feature and whether this is known and understood by the observer. Otherwise, an inadvertent smile may be taken at 'face value' as indicating pleasantness or friendliness, and the hidden emotional message may be missed.

Feedback: in the communication process, feedback refers to a particular kind of response of one person to another, which gives some idea of how the message is being received and thus whether some modification would be beneficial. Feedback can be positive or negative. In the technical sense, positive feedback increases or reinforces the existing conditions, whereas negative feedback modifies or reduces them. For example, if a teacher finds that students are attentive and ask relevant questions, this can serve as positive feedback that an appropriate style of teaching is being used. If, on the other hand, the students look bored and interrupt with irrelevant questions, this is negative feedback, indicating that a change is needed. Positive feedback is not necessarily a good thing. At a party, people can incite each other to more and more noisy and wild activities, which can soon get out of hand. Negative feedback is not necessarily bad: a patient who has had sufficient painkillers can tell that a reduction in dosage is required.

Form: the form of the communication refers in a non-technical way to the type of text or product, such as speaking or gesturing, a leaflet or book, sculpture, dance, music, painting or photograph. When choosing the form that a particular communication should take, it is necessary to look at what channels, media and codes are available or appropriate. A leaflet is probably the most common form of communication for reminding a mother-to-be what to bring into hospital. This is appropriate if the medium (system for designing and printing) is available, the woman can use the channel (can see) and this code (read the language chosen for the leaflet). Alternative forms might include leaflets in various languages, typed and in Braille, leaflets with pictorial (iconic) illustrations, an audiotape or videotape, or having a sample set of the required items that can be shown to the mother. This last, concrete, form (combined with conversation) may be best for facilitating questions, assisting understanding of unfamiliar items and aiding memory – but the mother cannot take it away with her. A mixture of forms is often the best solution.

Group communication: in addition to interpersonal skills used in a group situation, the special features of communication within groups can be identified. There are differences between small and large groups and between the kinds of network available for communication (see Chapter 19). In small groups, there is a greater possibility for open communication and flexibility in changing from one network to another. In large groups that rarely meet as a whole at any one time, it may be necessary to settle on one pattern of communication and keep to it until certain tasks are accomplished. This avoids the confusion that can arise if changes do not reach all members of the group at the same time. See also Chapter 19.

Iconic imagery: Barlow (in Barlow *et al.*, 1990) makes a clear distinction between those images in the outside world (before the eye) and those which are in the mind (behind the eye). Images in the outside world include paintings, drawings, photographs, television and video pictures, films, shadows and reflections. It is often difficult to communicate mental images and reproduce them in an outside world form.

The artist M.C. Escher (1967: 7) describes how he learned to communicate through visual images:

> Ideas came into my mind... which so fascinated me that I longed to communicate them to other people. This could not be achieved through words, for these thoughts were not literary ones, but mental images of a kind that can only be made comprehensible to others by presenting them as visual images... Yet a mental image is something completely different from a visual image, and however much one exerts oneself, one can never manage to capture the fullness of that perfection which hovers in the mind and which one thinks of, quite falsely, as something that is 'seen'. After a long series of attempts, at last – when I am just about at the end of my resources – I manage to cast my lovely dream in the defective visual mould of a detailed conceptual sketch. After this, to my great relief, there dawns the second phase, that is the making of the graphic print; for now the spirit can take its rest while the work is taken over by the hands.

Much of cognitive, humanistic and psychodynamic therapy is concerned with helping people to develop the forms needed to articulate images and feelings. Music can have tremendous effect without the need for words; most other therapeutic techniques involve a combination of words and non-word forms.

Interpersonal communication: communication between people. This term is typically used for face-to-face interaction in any context where two or more people have the opportunity to communicate directly with each other. The communication that takes place will depend on the communication skills and background of the individuals, the channels available, the situation or context and the code or codes used. Berlo (1960) provides a useful model of the ingredients of interpersonal communication and gives a list of principles, based on behavioural theory, of effective communication that will reduce the effort required by the 'receiver' in responding to the message. These include the amount of reward that was perceived as a consequence of the response, the time lag between making the response and receiving the reward, and the amount of effort that the receiver found to be necessary in making the response. These early ideas of reward in communication have been developed in many modern approaches to counselling (for example, Dickson, 1993).

Intrapersonal communication: a term used to categorise communication that is 'within' the individual, that is, purely for the individual's own purposes and not intended to be shared with others. This includes unobservable behaviour such as thinking and dreaming and also any observable means, such as writing notes, shopping lists, singing to oneself or laughing out loud while reading, which may be picked up additionally by other people and serve as interpersonal communication. For example, singing in the bath, which is primarily intended as intrapersonal communication, may convey to another person that there is someone in the bathroom and may also give some idea of the mood that person is in.

Jargon: see register.

Language: According to the *Concise Oxford Dictionary* (1982), language is 'the whole body of words and the methods of combining them used by a nation, people or race, a 'tongue''. In the social sciences and *ethology*, the term 'language' may be used instead of 'code' to refer to any collection of signs (iconic or symbolic) that can be seen to have a structure or system of rules for combining them. Language in this sense can include sign language, body language and the languages of art, dance, bees and computers.

Leakage: a term used for the situation in which body language gives away clues to inner feelings where a person is trying to convey a different emotion or lack of emotion.

Means: see channel, code, form and medium.

Medio: a specialist term for interpersonal communication that makes use of large-scale communication networks such as postal and carrier services, telephone, fax, the Internet and e-mail. This differs from the mass media in that it refers to situations in which the messages are sent by individuals without editing by the networking system.

Medium (plural media): a term that is used in various different ways depending on the context but which usually refers to the means or materials used for communication. In art, this refers to the type of paint and other materials used to create a picture; in physics, it is related to the physical material (also known as the carrier) through which communication signals are transmitted. In communication studies, it is usually used to refer in more general terms to the system for communication, such as speech, dance or photography.

The term 'medium' is closely related to 'channel' but is used in subtly different ways, so that 'channel' refers to the basic physical characteristics, and 'medium' to the system. For example, it would be appropriate to say that where the medium is speech, the channel is sound. We can distinguish between the channel of radio and the medium of radio, the channel consisting of the radio waves travelling through air or space, which can be compared with other channels such as optical fibres, the medium being the broadcasting system, which can be compared with other media such as newspapers. However, some authors often use 'channel' and 'medium' interchangeably or variably according to context.

In a health-care context, it may be important to know what media are available for communication or whether these differ from normal and need special attention. People with learning difficulties or mental health problems that result in restricted speech may function well in a medium such as dance, mime, music or painting.

Medium (plural mediums): the name given to people who believe they can communicate with people in the afterlife or in other worlds.

Metacommunication: awareness of one's own communication skills and styles.

Non-verbal communication: in common usage, this refers to the combination of body language, *paralanguage* and silence that complements spoken words. In this sense, the abbreviation NVC is often used. These non-verbal signs can carry information about emotion. For example, fidgety hand movements, together with silence, rapid speech or a loud voice, may indicate anxiety. Where this is unintentional, it may be referred to as leakage. NVC has been identified by Argyle (1983) and others as:

- eye contact and gaze
- facial expression
- posture
- gesture
- orientation
- touch and bodily contact
- proximity
- territoriality and personal space
- clothes and appearance
- paralanguage
- silence.

Since many people find it difficult to express emotions in words, either because the feeling is new and they simply do not know how to find the words, or because they believe they should not complain, non-verbal signs can be important clues to how a person is feeling. Books on non-verbal communication, such as that by Weitz (1979), indicate how non-verbal signs can be identified and what sort of interpretations are most likely.

Weitz comments wryly on the way in which non-verbal signs came to be viewed in the 1970s as more reliable than words for conveying true attitudes, with the conclusion that verbal communication could not be trusted. She quotes from Fast (1970, 1977), who talks of:

the rather disturbing vision of a world populated by detectives each busily reading the body signs of the other, while disregarding the intentional words spoken, and all the while trying to disguise their own verbal and non-verbal displays so that equally skilled readers cannot discover each other's true ploys.

Such a view has been fuelled by popular books such as *The Naked Ape* and *Manwatching* by Desmond Morris (1978), which are based on the ethological belief that non-verbal signs are genetically based and that meanings are universal. This may be true of some basic facial expressions, such as opening the eyes wide in surprise or baring the teeth in anger in order to bite (Argyle and Trower, 1979), but there are many cultural variations for most other types of body language (Burton and Dimbleby, 1995).

All signs have significance. Thus verbal and non-verbal communication need to be taken together, and in context, so that the listener considers all possible meanings and does not jump to false conclusions.

In a wider sense, the term 'non-verbal communication' refers to anything that does not require words or which is used alongside words. This can include drawing, painting, music, dance, mime, flag signals and so on in addition to body language. This formal distinction between verbal (word) and non-verbal (non-word) draws attention to the wide range of media available for communication that are not dependent on words. Non-verbal means of communication are more accessible between people of different cultures, do not require an ability to read and write, and are independent of the capacity for speech. Some non-verbal forms, such as dance, mime and the visual arts, are independent of hearing. Other non-verbal forms, such as music and touch, are independent of sight.

Oral communication: using the mouth. The term 'oral' may provide an alternative and more useful term than 'verbal' when referring to spoken communication. For example, instead of asking a person to give a verbal report (which could strictly speaking be written), it would be less ambiguous to ask for an oral report. Better still, there is nothing wrong with asking for a spoken report.

Orientation: the angle or way in which people position their bodies in relation to each other when speaking. It is an aspect of posture that shows how much attention is being paid, what is felt and how conversation should proceed. Observation of interaction (for example, Argyle, 1983) shows that, in friendly conversation, the natural (socially learned) tendency is to sit or stand at a slight angle. Facing too directly feels confrontational; turning further away usually signals lack of interest or a wish to end the conversation. Argyle (1983) and others indicate how relative height is also significant, the higher person having the advantage. The effects can be very subtle, neither person being aware of the situation but nevertheless being influenced by it. In interviews, the interviewer can deliberately signal power by having a higher chair or can inadvertently place the interviewee at a disadvantage by politely offering the only easy chair. Children and people in wheelchairs can be at a disadvantage and be either deliberately or inadvertently made to feel inferior. One solution is for all persons to be seated so their heads are roughly level. In practice, some carers sit on the floor as often as possible when talking with someone in a wheelchair. This reverses the relative heights and can give rise to new experiences. Well-meaning but over-obvious crouching can sometimes be perceived as patronising, particularly if it is too directly face to face.

Paralanguage: use of the voice to convey meaning alongside the words themselves or even in the absence of words. Features include stress, intonation, pitch, tone, quality, loudness, speed of talking, clarity and all the ums, ers, grunts, whistles and gasps. When listening to someone speaking or singing in an unknown foreign language, much of the meaning of the speaker can be inferred from the paralanguage. Absence of this kind of paralanguage in written forms is one reason why written texts need to follow grammatical rules more precisely than speech in order to convey subtleties of meaning accurately and avoid ambiguity.

Phatic communication: a term coined by Jacobson (1960), cited by Fiske (1990: 14), to refer to acts of communication that contain nothing new, no information as such, but that keep existing channels open and available for more emphatic communication later. This might include saying 'Hi' when a colleague passes by, smiling at patients in passing, talking about the weather, sending Christmas cards and so on. In practice, such acts are usually more than just keeping the channels open. Their absence can be a deliberate snub, such as 'cutting someone dead' when passing. In health care, apparently empty or phatic communication can serve the important functions of indicating interest and concern and helping to pass the time in what might otherwise be dull surroundings. It can aid in building a relationship that later makes it easier for someone to talk about emotional concerns.

Process models of communication: The process of communication has traditionally been seen as consisting of three main elements: the sender, the message and the receiver. In early models, only the sender was seen as active, constructing a message that was then transmitted to a passive receiver. The chief purpose of communication was seen as one person seeking to influence another in some way:

sender → message → receiver

There are a number of problems with this basic model. First, it is argued that a message is not something that exists separately from either sender or receiver but that the meaning of the message is something which has to be encoded into signs or signals by the sender and decoded by the receiver. This means that the message received may differ from the intended message. At the time of the Second World War, the basic model was changed to emphasise this point and later refined to include more psychological factors (for example, Shannon and Weaver, 1949; Osgood et al., 1957):

sender (encoder) → signal → (decoder) receiver

Second, it has been recognised that the receiver is not passive but must actively seek out and attend to signals if communication is to be effective. A new model was introduced in the 1970s with a reversed arrow indicating that the receiver must actively attend (Schramm, 1970, 1982):

sender → signal ← receiver

It is even more helpful to think of the transmission consisting of a *text*, following the rules and conventions of language, which is made available for use. The person seeking out and making use of the text is a 'consumer' who is as active and creative as the producer who made the text:

Producer
makes available
↓
Consumer seeks out and makes use of → text

This model (modified from Adams, 1986) is supported by the ideas of de Certeau (1984), who promotes the concept of the 'reader' of a text being as important as the writer. He suggests:

the activity of reading has... all the characteristics of a silent production... A different world (the reader's) slips into the author's place. This mutation makes the text habitable, like a rented apartment. It transforms another person's property into a space borrowed for a moment by a transient. (p. xxi)

While this appears most applicable to literary texts such as novels and plays, or to works of visual art, the model can also apply to all information-seeking and entertainment activities. It is also applicable to intimate interpersonal communication such as conversation and cuddles. A 'consumer' may seek out contact where needs are most likely to be met and interpret what the other is saying or doing in terms of those needs. See also purposes.

This model has been further developed to illustrate the effects of the communication on both producer and consumer (Adams, 1986; Gill and Adams, 1992).

Proximity: the space or distance between people. The study of the way in which space is used in communication is called 'proxemics'. Various writers, including Hall (1969), Morris (1978) and Argyle (1983), have described the patterns used in different circumstances. When these unwritten rules are broken, for example when having to stand close to someone for observations and other procedures, mechanisms such as looking away and moving as little as possible are employed to avoid misinterpretation. Space can be used to create a deliberate impression and bring about the kind of communication that is wanted. For example, in a teaching context, placing the teacher at the front, at a distance from rows of desks, creates an authoritative situation with the teacher in control. This tends to inhibit student-to-student conversation (except perhaps in the back row). Arranging the chairs in a circle or horseshoe so that all participants are equally close and can have eye contact with each other reduces the relative importance of the tutor and encourages open discussion.

Purposes of communication: the term 'purpose' supposes that we can deliberately communicate in order to satisfy requirements or needs. Stevens (1975) identifies eight functions of communication: instrumental, control, information, expression, social contact, alleviation of anxiety, stimulation and role-related function. Argyle (1983) also lists eight motivational sources of social behaviour – biological needs, dependency, affiliation, dominance, sex, aggression, self-esteem and ego-identity – and other social motivations, such as needs for money and achievement. These lists can be condensed into six main categories:

- instrumental
- information and education
- socialisation and control
- social and role-related functioning
- entertainment and leisure (relaxation and stimulation)
- expression or alleviation of emotions.

In all these areas, the processes of sending and receiving (or producing and consuming) are equally important, and it can be interesting to examine the motives or intentions of all parties. For example, the purpose of teaching is generally given as providing information for students, but it should not be forgotten that the teacher has the additional needs of earning a living, social inclusion and personal development. The categories above can be compared with systems for classifying motivation, for example Maslow's (1962) hierarchy of needs, which adds aesthetic and self-actualising needs to the list (see Chapter 7).

Questions: different kinds of question can be identified:

- value-laden
- probing
- leading
- confronting
- closed
- open.

Value-laden questions introduce a note of moral judgement. Burnard (1994) gives the example of 'Does your homosexuality make you feel guilty?'. This makes it difficult for the client to answer either way. Another example is 'Do you think you ought to lose weight?' They may be heard as accusations or condemnations.

Probing questions are 'why?' questions that give an impression of interrogation, for example 'Why do you feel depressed?', 'Why didn't you stick to the diet?' and 'Why did you do that?' They are usually impossible to answer in a way that would lead to a greater understanding of feelings. Like value-laden questions, they can lead to feelings of guilt and blame, and may be responded to with *rationalisations* or *intellectualising*.

Leading questions are those which include a possible answer, with the suggestion that this is the real answer. The respondent is led into agreeing with, for example, 'The car that hit you was blue, wasn't it? or may be trapped between limited options, such as 'Was the car red or blue?' This ignores the possibility of an alternative choice. The respondent would have to contradict the questioner in order to give a different answer. Even if this is managed, the suggestions tend to conjure up mental images that can subsequently interfere with memories and expectations. When a leading question is also value laden, this can put the respondent in an impossible situation. Several writers give the classic example of 'Have you stopped beating your wife?' Whatever the client answers, he will be in the wrong.

Closed questions usually elicit only a short answer such as 'yes' or 'no', or factual information. Examples include 'What is your date of birth?', 'Are you married?' and 'Are you feeling better today?'

Open questions allow a fuller range of answers. No particular answer is expected or predicted. Burnard (1994) gives examples such as 'What did you do then?', 'How did you feel when that happened?', 'How are you feeling right now?' and 'What do you think will happen?'

Value-laden, probing and leading questions have little relevance in person-centred counselling. Probing questions may be used in a psychodynamic context. Value-laden and leading questions have their place in cross-examination in the courtroom. These three approaches are associated with authoritarian styles and may be felt to be bullying.

Closed questions can be used in all contexts when factual information is needed. They need to be used with care in counselling as they do not give opportunity for expression and too many can lead to a feeling of interrogation. They may be used in cognitive therapy or other *didactic* relationships.

Open questions are thought to be useful in many contexts and in most types of therapeutic and educational relationship to explore emotionally charged cognitions and behaviour.

In person-centred art therapy, all questions in relation to images are discouraged. Clients are likely to respond to 'What is that?' as if it were a closed question and provide a short factual answer. There is also a danger that questions will be perceived as probing, leading or value laden, and clients may attempt to provide socially acceptable explanations or rationalisations in terms of popular 'psychobabble' interpretations instead of searching for their own deeper meanings. Open invitations to 'Tell me about that blue bit' may be more productive. Objects should only be named when they are obvious and unambiguous. It can be difficult for a woman to say, 'Actually that isn't a man, it's meant to be me.'

Register: a special variety of language defined according to its use in a particular social setting. These varieties develop to help people communicate about special interests such as occupations, sports and religion. They save time, provide precision and help to develop and maintain group identity. The term 'jargon' is often applied to registers, in a contemptuous way, when a person cannot follow the conversation and feels left out. The differences between registers are mainly ones of vocabulary, but some have their own special grammar. Health-care professionals have to be careful to set aside their professional register and use popular vocabulary when talking to people who are not familiar with medical or social science terms.

Semantics: the study of the way in which meanings are conveyed in language.

Sign language: a specially devised language that can be used by people unable to hear clearly. There are a number of different sign languages in common use, for example British Sign Language, Sign-assisted English, American Sign Language and Macaton. The differences between these systems means that a person proficient in one cannot communicate with someone using a different system. A person from the US using American Sign Language cannot understand someone using British Sign Language, apart from a few signs that they have in common.

Macaton is a simplified language with a limited vocabulary based on those words which are most likely to be needed in a care situation and is used primarily with people with learning difficulties as well as hearing loss.

British Sign Language is an elaborate system, originally developed by people in the Lancashire cotton mills who could not hear each other through the noise of the machinery. It is largely concept based, rather than word based. Each sign is independent of specific English words but represents an idea. For example, the sign for sister involves tapping one's nose in a way that signifies that a sister is 'nosey'. The sign for brother involves rubbing the wrists together, which is derived from the notion that little brothers have dirty cuffs. The connotations, and hence the signs, in American Sign Language are different. For some concepts, a single sign can convey an idea that would take several words. Conversely, a single word like 'birthday' needs two signs: the graphic illustration of a woman giving birth and the sign for book or diary, which indicates 'day'. Sign language has a very different type of grammar from spoken English, since several ideas can be signed simultaneously, giving an indication of how thing appear spatially. Describing events gives a pictorial feel for how things were arranged as the signer uses gestures to indicate where things were. This is very different from spoken English, in which it is necessary to hear the whole of a sentence before the full meaning can be grasped, and which gives a small, but significant, time delay. Spoken English is temporal rather than spacial.

Sign-assisted English is a modified form of British Sign Language. It uses many of the same signs but includes grammatical words from spoken or written English so that the signs are used in sentence form in a temporal rather than spatial way. Words like 'to', which are not really necessary in British Sign Language, can be spelt using the finger alphabet. This is often used with children in order to help them learn to speak and read.

Since sign languages of all types use facial expressions, gestures and postures to convey meanings, there is little of the incongruence or *leakage* that can occur with spoken language where the non-verbal cues may be giving different meanings from the words. People who use sign language often feel it is a more honest and down-to-earth means of communication than speech (for example, Sacks, 1989).

Signs and signals: these words are often interchangeable, but one useful distinction is to think of signs as static (as in road signs) and signals as involving movement or change (as in traffic lights, flag signals or gestures). Common usage usually dictates which is the better term in a particular instance.

In process models of communication, the term 'signal' can be used to refer to anything used for communication that passes between one person and another, that is, spoken words, body language, an essay, book, work of art and so on. Now that the word 'text' has been introduced into communication theory from literary theory, to refer to the content of these items, 'text' can be used as an alternative to 'signal' in most communication contexts. Texts consist of signs.

A sign can be an index, an icon or a symbol. An index is often an unintentional sign, made by a person, or left behind, which gives another person an indication that something is happening or has happened. This would include a crumpled bed, which shows that a person has been there, or a discarded needle, which indicates drug use. The term 'index' also refers to the kind of vocabulary a person uses that gives a clue to social background, education and interests. The terms 'doctor', 'medic', 'consultant' or 'quack' can refer to the same individual; the choice will give some idea of the speaker's attitude.

An icon is a picture that stands for an object and that is intended to look like that object. The signs used in international airports to indicate toilets for men, women and those in wheelchairs are icons that can be understood by everyone, irrespective of their spoken or written language. The signs do not usually look exactly like real people, but they can be seen to represent people. International road signs are also iconic and convey their message quickly in any country. Iconic labels and signs for hazardous materials are used for safety in transport and storage.

A symbol stands for something but does not bear any close resemblance to it. Symbols have to be specially learned and can only be used for communication between people who have agreed on their meanings. Many symbols have more than one agreed meaning, so the context has to be taken into account when deciding which meaning is intended. The decoded meaning will often not be the same as the encoded one, and misunderstandings arise.

Words are symbols. The word 'cat' stands for a small furry creature with sharp teeth and claws, but the sound of the spoken word and the appearance of the letters do not resemble the animal in any way. A few spoken words, such as swoosh and ooze, do sound a bit like what they represent and are slightly iconic; such words are called onomatopoeic.

Silence: many health-care professionals and patients feel uncomfortable when faced with a period of silence. In normal conversation, gaps of silence are usually a sign that one person has finished speaking and is waiting for a response from the other. There are unwritten 'rules' for how long the silence should be allowed to last. French (1994) suggests that each knows when it is someone else's turn to speak. Bradley and Edinberg (1990) found that people who have not had time to build up a relationship or good rapport are uncomfortable with as little as 5–10 seconds of silence. In well-established relationships, silences may be tolerated with more ease and comfort. Those involved can use silence positively as a sign of trust and acceptance or to contemplate and formulate ideas. Conversely, silence may be a sign of anxiety, depression, boredom or preoccupation, or it may be used negatively to convey anger or frustration. The task for the professional carer is to create an atmosphere in which silence can be accepted and used positively and in which different kinds of silence can be accurately identified.

Touch and bodily contact: this can be used as non-verbal communication through physical contact. Touch is one of the most important, and perhaps most subtle, forms of non-verbal communication in health care. It can be used to convey attention, reassurance and friendliness, and express concern and other emotions, as well as being part of the physical care. Attitudes and perceptions of touch are influenced by socialisation, cultural practices, family relationships, gender differences and past experiences, in relation to individual perceptions of personal space and areas of the body that may be touched.

Abraham and Shanley (1992: 125) describe a number of different kinds of touch and their function in caring, making a distinction between instrumental (functional) and expressive (communicative) touch. This has been elaborated by other writers (for example, Barnett, 1972) to give four distinct uses of touch:

- instrumental: deliberate physical contact for some functional purpose, such as taking observations or washing
- expressive: the spontaneous communication of *affect*, such as feelings of warmth and caring
- therapeutic: the transference of energy with intention to heal, such as stroking or holding hands

- systematic: the purposeful manipulation of the soft tissues in order to enhance the well-being of the receiver, as in massage.

Verbal communication: in common usage, the term 'verbal communication' often refers only to speech. It is common in committee meetings, for example, to ask someone to give a 'verbal' report when a written paper is not available. However, more formally, verbal (from the Latin *verbum*) communication is anything using words. Words can be spoken, sung or written. Some people, for example those with learning difficulties or autism, may be able to produce words when singing or in a musical context even when they are unable to speak. Words can also be spelled out using Braille, Morse code or the finger alphabet of British Sign Language. In this sense, a verbal report could be any kind of report that is based on words, whether spoken, sung, written or spelt out on the fingers. Correspondingly, non-verbal means anything without words or used alongside words and includes pictures, mathematical models and many other representations, as well as body language. See also non-verbal communication.

Vocal: making use of the voice, with or without recognisable words.

Voice: a medium for communication that includes speech, singing and non-verbal vocalisations. When working with speech-impaired or deaf adults and children, it is important to realise that, even if speech is virtually non-existent, these people may be able to make considerable use of their voice and communicate a great deal through laughter, humming, grunts and other vocal noises, and can reproduce many aspects of paralanguage. When the voice is used, vibrations can be felt in the throat, in bone cavities in the face and in the chest. Singers may learn to pitch and project notes according to what part of the face or chest is felt to be resonating. Deaf people can learn to identify sounds by feeling parts of a speaker's face and throat. Sometimes, where normal speech is not possible because of damage to the tongue, a voice can be produced by an electronic device that picks up the throat vibrations.

10 Loss and grief therapy

Changes in health status are often referred to in the context of the experience of 'loss'. We can talk about people experiencing loss when there has been: the loss of a relationship through death or separation; failure, removal or alteration of body parts, whether internal or external; or an alteration in physical, psychological or social functioning, such as intellectual capacity, income, role, self-esteem, well-being, security, leisure or sporting activities. Such experiences may be acute or gradual and progressive, temporary or permanent, actual or potential, sudden or anticipated, obvious to others or possible to conceal.

Loss and grief constitute one of the most important areas for concern in professional care, and this book cannot hope to do justice to them. However, a great deal of literature is readily accessible, and it is hoped that readers will be encouraged to look for material that is personally meaningful. This chapter covers some of the main approaches and models that have been developed in the care of dying patients and their families, and in some other situations of loss.

Definitions	
Hindmarch (1993)	Bereavement has come to mean the loss by death of someone close, although it originally referred to the marauding practices of bands of 'reavers' many centuries ago, raiding the livestock of neighbouring clans. Thus to be bereaved implies being robbed or deprived of something or someone of value, so that one is necessarily poorer for the loss. Bereavement is what happens. Grief is what one feels in reaction to the bereavement. Mourning is what one does to express grief.

Approaches, Arguments and Applications

'Loss' may be precipitated in a variety of ways, including disasters (such as earthquakes and massacres), human conflict (war, terrorist action, fights), political and economic changes (redundancy, downgrading), accidents (home, traffic, industrial), congenital conditions, disease, functional irregularity (miscarriage, myalgic encephalitis), medical interventions, self-injury and ageing.

Models and theories developed in connection with bereavement and mourning may be adapted to cope with losses other than those associated with death as similar processes and ways of coping can be identified.

It is generally felt that, following a loss, there is a progression from a position of extreme distress to one of less distress and greater ability to cope. The main debate is whether or not this progression should be viewed as a sequence of stages that finally lead to acceptance of the loss.

There is a common tendency for pioneers who are attempting to analyse a previously uncharted area to look for stages in development. Subsequent research very often shows that this is not the best way to identify elements. Melanie Klein argued that Freud's model of psychosexual stages should be replaced by a way of looking at children's emotional development as the emergence of a child's position with respect to the perceived internal and external world. Piaget's stages of cognitive development have been superseded by descriptions in terms of cognitive styles. The multistage model of memory has been displaced by information-processing approaches. See Chapters 11, 16 and 17.

The word 'stages' in relation to loss and grief is better replaced by phases, components, aspects or positions. These terms indicate that different behaviour might be found on different occasions, but there is no suggestion that they occur in a set sequence. Worden (1991) speaks in terms of tasks, but even these are often numbered in a way suggesting that they may be undertaken in a prescribed order.

A number of models that are based upon the following four approaches can be identified:

- depression
- stress
- stages
- tasks.

Stroebe *et al.* (1993) have classified theories of bereavement as either 'depression models' of grief, which consider grief as an emotional reaction, or 'stress models' of grief, which regard bereavement as a stressful life event.

A number of 'stages' approaches can be found (Hohmann, 1966; Bowlby, 1969, 1973, 1980; Kubler-Ross, 1970; Kerr and Thompson, 1972, Hopson, 1981; Parkes, 1996). These models, particularly the one set out by Elizabeth Kubler-Ross, have contributed to the main debate concerning whether or not the stages should be considered as sequential, one stage following the next (see stages models of the grieving process).

Other models that may be applied to situations of loss include 'coping' strategies, for example Moos (1986) and Danish and d'Augelli (1982). See Chapter 7.

Some changes may bring about positive benefits yet still incur losses. For example, a person with a severe physical problem, used to being surrounded by helpful and caring well-wishers, may lose these relationships if the condition improves and independence is gained. Holmes and Rahe (1967) assign different values to different changes and have suggested that it is the number of changes in a given time, rather than the nature of the changes themselves, that contributes to stress (see Chapter 20).

There may be a range of various conditions that are unusual or do not fit the 'norm', do not involve change for the person concerned and therefore do not lead to any experience of loss, but which are viewed by others as loss, or loss of potential. An example is conditions present at birth, such as a deformity in a limb. This can lead to misunderstandings between the individual and health-care professionals who refer to a person as *suffering* from a particular condition when the individual does not regard the condition as a serious disadvantage.

Glaser and Strauss (1967), using their *grounded theory* approach, identify the following research questions. How can carers:

- recognise and understand psychological reactions of terminally ill people to impending death
- plan the psychological management of distressing emotional, behavioural and physical symptoms in the terminally ill
- introduce psychotherapeutic interventions intended to ease the individual through the dying process
- develop understanding of their own beliefs and fears
- find peer support for stresses involved in caring for the dying?

A focus in their research is on people who have reached a time in their illness when it is realised that they will not recover, particularly those cancer patients for whom dying is a gradual process. They describe this as the 'nothing more to do' phase when the nurse generally takes over from the doctor and changes the emphasis from recovery to comfort. They say, 'A nurse who is able to motivate the patient to die (most nurses we met are not, however) can teach him how to die "gracefully"' (Glaser and Strauss, 1965: 225).

Findings from one area may be adapted in relation to other loss situations. In particular, Kubler-Ross's (1970) conclusions about terminally ill patients are often used in reference to bereavement. There is a wealth of literature, some of it descriptive and anecdotal rather than methodical and replicable.

Key Terms and Concepts

Acceptance: Hinton (1972) uses three main categories of acceptance of impending threat:

- some deny the threat
- others seek as much information as possible
- some move between these extremes.

Schneidman (1978) suggests that it is natural to vary. People experience a wide range of emotions and many never reach acceptance. Saunders (1966) found that levels of acceptance vary from time to time.

Acceptance that involves a coming to terms with impending death when that is imminent, or with loss, so that the quality of the death or continued life is improved, is generally considered to be a good thing. However, it can be argued that acceptance is not always beneficial if it involves a passive 'giving in' that results in a lack of will to live. Eysenck (1985, 1994) believes he has identified a cancer-prone personality type that is co-operative, appeasing and non-expressive of emotions such as anger and hostility (see Chapter 7). Evidence is conflicting, but it is sometimes argued that such people are too accepting and have a lower quality of life than those who refuse to give up their fight.

Anger: this is one of the most commonly found emotional responses to loss and is listed in most 'stages' models of bereavement. Anger may be associated with guilt and blame and directed towards the self. Alternatively, it may be directed towards others. In this case, it is usually regarded as a *defence mechanism*, protecting the person from anxiety, guilt and blame. It is interpreted as involving the displacement or projection of anger towards anyone seen as responsible for the loss, such as family members, health-care professionals, God or the deceased. Some 'stage' models indicate that a person may move from internally directed anger to externally directed anger. See also Chapters 1 and 17.

Anticipatory grief: many losses can be anticipated and therefore the grieving or mourning process can commence before the loss is experienced. Although anticipation can help an individual to prepare for an impending loss, it may also prolong the separation process and intensify the accompanying emotional reactions.

Attachment and bonding: the impact of a loss will be determined in part by the degree of attachment. Bowlby (1988) believes that attachment behaviour stems from the need for safety and security and is intended to maintain bonds. A threat to the bond, such as impending loss through death, may activate attachment behaviours such as crying, clinging, loss of independence and activity.

Bowlby (1951, 1969) asserts that mother love in infancy and childhood is as important for mental health as are vitamins and proteins for physical health and that any kind of psychiatric disorder *always* shows a disturbance in social relationships/affectional bonding, in many cases *caused* by disturbed bonding in childhood. Bonding is defined as 'selective attachment', and although it is now recognised that the mother is not the only person to whom children form attachments, it is considered important for children to have regular contact with a few significant adults. This enables long-term relationships to form and avoids repeated episodes of loss.

Schaffer (1977) gives three stages for the development of attachment in babies:

- Infants' attraction to people rather than things appears at about 6 weeks when babies smile at faces (see also Chapter 14)

- Babies can distinguish between people at about 3 months but still allow themselves to be handled by strangers
- Lasting emotional bonds are noticeable at about 6–7 months when babies miss the mother when absent and show fear of strangers.

Kennell *et al.* (1979) give evidence from the point of view of the caregiver and suggests that skin-to-skin contact is important for a parent soon after birth and needs to occur within a critical period of 6–12 hours after birth for a firm bond to be established. However, Rutter (1979) argues that bonds build up slowly over many months and that 'maternal instinct' is not automatic or immediate.

Different kinds of attachment have been identified, relating to strength and security (Rosenblum and Harlow, 1963; Stayton and Ainsworth, 1973; Tizard and Rees, 1975; Rutter, 1979; Maccoby, 1980). Harlow (1959) is particularly well known for his studies of infant Rhesus monkeys in which he showed that they seek out a soft towelling surface in preference to other surfaces in the absence of the real mother. The 'surrogate' mother can act as a reassurance in new or frightening situations.

Avoidance: social norms dictate that avoidance is an acceptable response to one's own or another person's loss. The loss is not discussed. It is important not to confuse avoidance behaviour, in which the loss is recognised, with denial. Hinton (1980) suggests that dying patients remain quiet to avoid hurting their families: one third did not talk to their partners. Partners tend to avoid the issue in order not to upset the dying person. Avoidance may be important in critical situations where there is a possibility of recovery.

Awareness of death: it is paradoxical that, despite an *entertainment culture* that continuously portrays aggression and death (see Chapter 1), death in an abstract or philosophical sense is a taboo topic. Americans and British alike are reluctant to discuss the process of death or to tell a person that he or she is dying. However, practice in many hospitals is changing. Reluctance among carers to tell a patient whether he or she is dying is proportional to the patient's awareness. The more aware the patient is, the more likely professionals will be to tell the truth.

Glaser and Strauss (1965) identified four levels of awareness that influence the communication patterns between the dying and those with whom they interact:

- closed awareness
- suspicious awareness
- mutual pretence
- open awareness.

They describe five important structural conditions that contribute to the existence and maintenance of the closed awareness context:

- Most patients are not especially experienced at recognising the signs of impending death
- Physicians often find medical justification for not disclosing dying status to their patients, based on beliefs that patients do not want to know and may 'go to pieces'

- Families tend to guard the secret and confirm what the physician has said
- Hospital personnel tend to hide all medical information from patients and couch conversation in medical *jargon*
- A patient has no allies who will tell the truth, as other patients tend to follow ordinary rules of tact and keep quiet.

Crammond (1970) found that 80 per cent of dying patients know that they are dying and wish to talk about it. Kalish and Reynolds (1976) found that 55 per cent thought someone should be told, and 70 per cent said they would personally like to be told. Annas (1974) identified that 90 per cent of patients wanted to know but that 60–90 per cent of physicians were opposed to telling them, and Lasagna (1970) decried how physicians' willingness to tell was proportional to the attractiveness of the patient: greater attractiveness correlates with more willingness to tell. People do not always want to know they are dying, but studies indicate that those who are terminally ill, and people in general, do desire knowledge of their own impending death.

When the doctor decides to tell the patient, this leads to an 'open awareness' context. Conversely, if a patient learns something of the indicators relevant to a terminal condition, this leads to a 'suspicion awareness' context.

In a suspicion awareness context, a contest can develop between patient and carers. The patient may be trying constantly to find out more, but staff are 'carefully and cannily on the defensive'.

When patient and carers all know that the patient is dying but pretend otherwise, a ritual drama may ensue of acting as if the patient is going to live.

In an open awareness context in which all those involved are free to discuss the impending death, there is still no ready answer to problems. The situation is complex and contains ambiguities. These relate to the time and manner of death and to awareness of death itself.

Glaser and Strauss (1965) identified several levels of certainty and uncertainty with regard to death:

- certain death at known time (for example, accident)
- certain death at unknown time (terminal illness)
- uncertain death in known time (critical illness)
- uncertain death in unknown time (chronic illness).

They found that greater problems were associated with higher uncertainty. The problems associated with coming to terms with awareness are discussed under mourning and stages models of the grieving process.

Bargaining for goals: one of the stages in Kubler-Ross's (1970) approach in which she describes patients bargaining with God for extra time. For example, a patient may promise to be a better person if only he or she is allowed to live until a son's wedding.

Creative arts and loss: death and loss are recurrent themes in all forms of art. Powerful imagery can be used therapeutically to bring out into the open thoughts that are normally avoided or repressed. Reproductions of paintings, photographs, films, television drama, poetry and music can be made available for patients with restricted mobility. Taking part in creating paintings, music, drama, poetry, mime, puppetry and sandplay may be possible for those who are mobile.

Art may be used in the context of art therapy (see Chapter 17), with counselling skills as person-centred art therapy, or as a general therapeutic approach (see Chapter 8). Paintings and photographs can be found through galleries and bookshops, some in specially collected anthologies or autobiographies. Music that addresses death can be especially powerful, from Elgar's Dream of Gerontius to tracks by Queen. Several anthologies of poems are available that have been collected especially for people who have been bereaved. Useful sources include *The Long Pale Corridor* (Benson and Falk, 1996), *Stopping for Death* (Duffy, 1996) and the *Oxford Book of Death* (Enright, 1983).

Denial: a defence mechanism sometimes perceived as being used by those who have experienced a loss to protect against anxiety or the implications of the loss. The reality of the loss may be unrecognised or not accepted. It is often considered important not to collude with the denial as this may delay the grieving process. Denial may be exacerbated by some of the language used for death that does not make the finality of the death explicit, for example asleep, gone, departed, passed away, at rest. Carers are advised to use straightforward references to death. Hinton (1984) found that a patient's denial was proportional to carers' attitudes and suggests that carers encourage denial because this is personally less distressing. See also Chapter 17.

Distancing: a process of detachment during which activity may be used to focus attention away from the loss.

Euthanasia: literally a 'good death'; the bringing about of a gentle and easy death, especially for people who have an incurable and painful condition. Retterstol (1990) expresses the common feeling that euthanasia, also known as mercy killing, is a form of suicidal act. The death-bringing act is carried out by someone else on the wishes of a person who is dying or in pain. Pritchard (1995) finds that people who are terminally ill generally do not take their own lives. He cites evidence suggesting that the more serious the prognosis, the less likely people are to contemplate either suicide or euthanasia.

Finding behaviour: this is behaving as if the deceased person is present. It may simply involve a feeling that the lost person is nearby or a sense of a continued presence as if the person is sitting quietly in the same room or walking alongside. Perhaps, even though they are known to be only in imagination, a bereaved person may carry out activities, such as rocking an empty cradle or talking to the dead. Other examples might include making a shrine out of a bedroom or study or continuing to lay the table for two. Such behaviour is often interpreted as evidence of 'denial' but, like *searching*, finding behaviour is observed throughout the animal kingdom. Lorenz (1966) describes how insects continue courting behaviour alone when they cannot find their mate. This suggests that it is a natural response. It may be accompanied by full conscious awareness and acceptance. Such behaviour only becomes a problem when it interferes with normal living.

For Mark

I cradle you back into me
try to feed you with my body
my firstborn that now finds
it so hard to play
you are leaking away from me
I can't stop it
    someone help me

You bear it with the mantle of old age
the sickness   the burning ulcers
I see in your weary face
the muteness of starving children
your quiet acceptance
as you try to make sense of
your frightening world
ajumbleofneedlesandpain
I am helpless
my body hurts
as I stoke your wilting skin
and watch you with a smile
that fronts my tears
at night – away from me –
your cry echoes in my head
    'Mummy make me well'

Judi Thwaite

Dad

I thought you should know
I've planted
your alarm clocks
your mug and razor
and your old Cruikshanks
cycling shoes
between the compost
and the clutter of dead
rhubarb. Somehow
it seemed the proper
thing to do,
rather than just
turning them out
to the bad jokes
of the bin men
without so much
as a thanks
for everything

Stephen Parr

Figure 10.1 Poems of loss and grief

Grief: the emotional experience of those who have been bereaved. Grief is a complex, individualised process that manifests itself in different ways at different times. Following a death, the nature of the reaction is influenced more by how great a part of someone's life the deceased occupied rather than by their emotional involvement (Marris, 1986). Grief may involve physical pain as well as psychological distress, which may precipitate uncharacteristic behaviour in the sufferer. For example, activities such as shopping that previously posed no threat may induce a panic attack after the loss. Feelings can be intense. These include anger, a sense of unfairness, guilt, rage, insecurity, anxiety and isolation. The physical impact of grief may be manifested in apathy, insomnia, loss of weight, palpitations, tightness of the chest or shortness of breath.

If grief is unresolved, it is known as pathological, complicated or *unresolved* grief. In such cases, the grief may be excessive, delayed, absent or prolonged with disruption of the ability to function as usual.

Models focus either on the 'stages' or the 'tasks' of grieving or mourning processes (see below).

Grief therapy: the goal of grief therapy is to help those suffering from complicated or pathological grief to resolve their grief and come to terms with their loss. The mainstream psychological approach is cognitive-behavioural therapy, but any one of more than 400 models, or an integration of any of these, may be chosen (see Chapter 8). The choice will depend on the personal preferences of the client and on availability. The use of creative arts in hospitals, day-care centres and hospices is becoming more widespread, both in a general way for all patients and clients and in unresolved cases.

Guilt and self-blame: in many losses, particularly where there is no apparent reason for death, survivors may feel that they are in some way to blame for the death. This may happen after major disasters like train crashes or in individual cases of loss.

With sudden infant death syndrome, although several theories have been proposed for the cause of death, no definitive explanation has been found. Guilt and blame may be experienced by the parents who seek a reason for the death. See also sudden death.

Miscarriage: the lay term for early accidental termination of pregnancy, usually professionally referred to as spontaneous abortion. The extent of the parents' bereavement and their need to grieve will be determined by what the loss means to them rather than by the gestational age of the baby. Miscarriage in early pregnancy is therefore not necessarily less traumatic than the loss of the baby later in pregnancy.

Mourning: what is done to express grief. This may conform to culturally determined means of expressing grief and bereavement and can include well-established patterns or rituals. Mourning is precipitated by some acknowledgement that the loss has occurred and may be viewed as a means to begin the healing process. Rituals associated with death include viewing the body, the method by which the body is disposed, the withdrawal of the bereaved from social contact and wearing certain colours. Such rituals confirm that the loss exists.

Worden (1991: 10) suggests that there are four tasks of mourning:

- to accept the reality of the loss; this may be indicated by searching behaviour
- to work through the pain of grief
- to adjust to an environment in which the deceased is missing; the deceased may have performed many roles of which the bereaved may not become aware until some time after the death
- to relocate the deceased emotionally and move on with life: releasing the attachment, finding a new place in one's heart or mind for the deceased and continue living.

These tasks may be adapted to cope with losses other than those associated with death. In many health-care situations, the loss can be anticipated so that an additional task that precedes the others may be to prepare for the loss. As with the 'stages' models, these tasks are better viewed as happening in any order, and perhaps concurrently, rather than as an ordered sequence. Many sources assign numbers to them, with the implication that they will be carried out in a prescribed order.

Readjustment: any loss may have physical and emotional consequences to which the bereaved must adapt. For example, a person who has suffered loss of limb function following a cerebral vascular accident or stroke may have to adjust their daily routine to cope with reduced mobility and may also have to come to terms with reduced independence.

Searching: this may be one of the main patterns of behaviour and thought precipitated by loss. Parkes (1996: 43) states that 'the most characteristic feature of grief is not prolonged depression but acute and episodic "pangs"'. The bereaved may seek to be reunited with the deceased to the extent that the presence of the deceased is sought or imagined during everyday activities. The bereaved person may believe that the deceased was spotted in a crowded supermarket or listen for sounds such as the door opening at mealtimes, which might indicate the presence of the deceased. Dreams often include being with the deceased person. Delusions and illusions are common for about one in eight bereaved people. These may be triggered by possessions, smells and music. This can be seen as a universal behaviour demonstrated by many animals. Lorenz (1966) and Bowlby (1961) showed how animals would search for their mate and argued that this is biologically useful. Searching may be accompanied or replaced by *finding* behaviour.

Shock: may be experienced immediately following a loss and last for several days. Characterised by disbelief and denial, the bereaved cannot believe that their loss is real. Numbness may be experienced as a protection against the pain of the loss.

Stages models of the grieving process: many models describe the processes of loss and grieving as consisting of a number of stages. These are helpful to carers in recognising signs and symptoms of distress, but it is important to realise that, for many people, there is no clear sequence from one to the next. The terms 'components' or 'phases' give a better impression of the way in which the different behaviours may vary from time to time. The following models are given in chronological order according to recent publications.

Hohmann (1966, 1975) suggests that a period of mourning is required by people on learning they have a chronic illness or other condition, such as that caused by a spinal injury, and describes four stages of responses:

- denial lasting from 2 weeks to 2 months
- depression, withdrawal, internalised hostility
- aggression, external hostility
- reaction against dependence.

Bowlby (1969) also gives a clear sequence but indicates that responses may appear to indicate coping at first but then a return to distress. This model uses the language of bereavement and is suitable for application to loss of employment, as illustrated below:

- Stage 1   Sense of loss of activity, security
- Stage 2   Searching:
    survival search – for new job, purpose, new earnings
    identity search – for the 'real' me
    fantasy search – what would I like to be
- Stage 3   Finding, period of action, having found some purpose (usually poor and short term)
- Stage 4   Reloss: the vulnerable period, critical stage
    denial of consequences
    escapism into alcoholism, drugs
    depression
    learned helplessness
    hostility
    obsessive behaviour
- Stage 5   Awareness, able to be helped to view situation in a new light
- Stage 6   Burial, closing a chapter, moving forward.

Kubler-Ross's (1970) description of the stages of adjustment to a diagnosis of terminal illness is one of the best-known models:

- denial and isolation
- anger
- bargaining
- depression
- acceptance.

Although she does not describe these experiences as if they always occur in a regular sequence, many interpretations assume that she meant that they do. Kubler-Ross's model relates to her personal experience of caring for dying patients, and she describes how not all the components may be experienced by individuals, many never demonstrating acceptance.

Kerr and Thompson (1972) describe a slightly different set of stages in relation to diagnosis of chronic disability:

- mental shock, fear and anxiety
- grief and mourning
- anger and rebellion.

Hopson (1981) develops this further and describes a transitional process that could apply equally well to good or bad life changes, for example a loss or winning the lottery:

1. immobilisation – shock and numbness
    2.1 reaction – elation or despair
    2.2 reaction – minimisation, making the change seem less important.
3. self-doubt – anxiety, anger, some sadness
4. letting go – accepting the reality of the loss, severing bonds with the past
5. testing – trying out the new self, successes and failures accompanied by mood swings
6. search for meaning – trying to make sense of what has happened
7. integration – between the new lifestyle and the crisis, a disabled person may recognise disability in one area and skills in others

Buckman (1988) gives three simple phases – beginning, illness and final – and suggests ways in which helpers can provide support. He views Kubler-Ross's five aspects of dying not as stages but as reactions that can be seen at any time during the phases of dying.

Parkes (1996) lists grief reactions following a bereavement as if they occur as a succession of phases:

- numbness and denial, experienced soon after the loss, characterised by a sense of unreality lasting from a few days to weeks
- yearning or pining for the deceased to return; the permanence of the loss may not be acknowledged
- despair or depression, the reality of the death is acknowledged, the bereaved person may feel unable to cope with daily living
- recovery or reorganisation.

However, he emphasises (Parkes, 1996: 7) that:

Each of these phases of grieving has it own characteristics and there are considerable differences from one person to another as regards both the duration and the form of each phase. Furthermore people can move back and forth through the phases so that, years after a bereavement, the discovery of a photograph in a drawer or a visit from an old friend can evoke another episode of pining. Nevertheless, there is a common pattern whose features can be regarded as a distinct psychological process.

Hindmarch (1993) describes a whirlpool model of grief, a pictorial representation developed by Dr Richard Wilson at Kingston Hospital out of his experiences of working with bereaved parents after the death of a child. This is not supported by research, but it indicates more clearly than the stages models how an individual can be caught up in many different emotions at once.

Sudden death: Worden (1991) suggests that the following features are likely to be pronounced where death is sudden:

- the absence of anticipatory grief work
- shock
- nightmares and intrusive images
- an inability to take the initiative in seeking help
- an inability to 'actualise' the death
- fantasies, which are likely to be worse than reality
- guilt and self-blame
- scapegoating
- displacement
- involvement of the legal and medical authorities
- personal death awareness, heightened, for example, when the partner was of the same age
- feelings of unfinished business
- a search for meaning.

Wright (1996) focuses on the particular problems faced after a sudden death and stresses that special care is needed in breaking bad news. In particular, euphemisms such as 'lost', 'passed on' and 'slipped away' are open to misinterpretation if a person is not expecting the news. Wright gives the example of one man telling them:

When the doctor came in and said 'I am afraid we have lost her', I thought what a damned fool. How could they allow a woman who is so sick to leave the hospital? You see, my wife was always a bit wayward and if someone said something she did not want to hear she would just walk out. I remember saying, 'What do you mean? How could you just let her walk out?' He looked embarrassed, and said 'She is dead'. I remember being angry and saying, 'Well why didn't you say so?'

Suicide: special care may be needed after a suicide, especially if the death was sudden and unexpected. Taboos surrounding suicide are even greater than for other forms of death. Family and friends may be preoccupied with apportioning or avoiding blame and be unresponsive to offers of help. Wright (1996: 45) cites Henley (1983), who found that 'death by suicide results in a bereavement more devastating than any other form of death'. Her study revealed a lack of emotional support and a strong avoidance of communication. Reactions may be influenced by particular schools of thought, for example awareness of psychodynamic approaches that explain destructive behaviour in terms of a 'death-wish' or by the stigma attached to mental disorders. A knowledge of socioeconomic patterns and the incidence of suicide can help to dispel myths.

Unresolved grief: grief can become a problem and require special counselling if it is:

- chronic
- exaggerated, for example depression, anxiety or post-traumatic stress disorder
- masked by other symptoms or drugs, or not expressed because of discouragement from family.

11 Memory and Response to Memory Changes

Memory is a concept that refers to a variety of behaviours, in particular the three interrelated processes of registration, storage and retrieval of information. That is, how information gets into our memories, where and how it is stored, and how to find it when we want it. Memories appear to depend on cognitive processes similar to perception and include search for meaning and gap-filling. There are many different kinds of skills and information that can be remembered, and it is accepted that memory is not a single process.

Definitions	
Hunter (1957)	an abstraction, a shorthand way of referring to certain kinds of activities... [and] ambiguous in the sense that the word is used to refer to very different kinds of activities.
Miller (1962)	the retention of acquired skills or information.
Drever (1964)	that characteristic which underlies all learning, the essential feature of which is retention.
Gregory (1981)	memories are hypotheses of the past [in the same way as] perceptions are hypotheses of the present and immediate future. Like perception, memory depends upon gap-filling, and guessing from inadequate (stored) data.
Baddeley (1982)	the capacity for storing and retrieving information.
Blakemore (1988)	learning is the acquisition of knowledge and memory is the storage of an internal representation of that knowledge.

Approaches, Arguments and Applications

Theoretical approaches centre around the different kinds of memory that can be distinguished and whether these can be related to distinct physiological processes or areas in the brain. There is strong evidence (for example, Gregory, 1981) that most memories are not accurate reconstructions but that memory, like perception, involves the mental processing of limited information, and in order to make sense of what has happened, the gaps are filled with whatever makes most sense, depending on other available information, personal needs and interests. At the present time, there is no single integrated theory of memory; the predominant psychological perspective lies within cognitive psychology, but each school of thought makes important contributions.

Issues for health psychology include awareness of changes in memory as a result of ageing or damage or deterioration of the brain and nervous system, effects on memory of the physiological and psychological state, such as mood, context and style of questioning, and implications for effective communication. There are implications for health-care professionals both as teachers and learners, and in particular for those working with people with learning disabilities.

Brain damage may result in memory changes such as amnesia, confabulation and confusion. Psychometric tests for assessing memory changes may make use of simple tasks such as free or ordered recall, span, backward span and duration. Work with elderly or confused patients may include reminiscence and reality orientation. The serial probe technique and similar tests may be used in the diagnosis and monitoring of dyslexic conditions.

A number of strategies exist for helping consolidation of memory and avoiding unhelpful or negative interference. These include: pausing, repeating and questioning when giving information; giving concrete examples; encouraging visual imagery; putting material to immediate practical use; practising overlearning; associating new information with something that is already familiar; encouraging recognition when recall appears difficult; reducing similar material that can interfere; avoiding or reducing anxiety; and providing written reminders.

Biopsychological approaches: these include studies of the relationship between physiological processes and psychological experience, such as the following:

- electrical stimulation of specific areas of the brain to evoke memories, for example Penfield (1958)
- the study of people who have brain damage due to illness, accident or stroke, for example Milner *et al.* (1968), Blakemore (1988) and Baddeley (1990)
- the study of maturational changes throughout the lifespan, for example Stuart-Hamilton (1994), the effects of ageing and hormonal changes, for example during the menstrual cycle and in pregnancy and the menopause
- studies of the ways in which synaptic processes and interconnections between neurones and different areas of the brain are modified by memory, and the different areas that are associated with different kinds of memory
- the effects of drugs and diet.

Cognitive, behavioural and social approaches: these look at the ways in which individuals develop strategies and processes of memorising, remembering and forgetting.

Four fundamental measurable effects are identified – recall, recognition, reconstruction and relearning – normally measured in terms of the number of trials needed to achieve accuracy, from Ebbinghaus (1885).

Early behavioural models (for example, James, 1890; Hebb, 1949; Broadbent, 1958; Waugh and Norman, 1965) distinguished only between short-term (STM) and long-term memory (LTM) and suggested that memories go into a long-term memory store (LTS) from the short-term memory store (STS) after a process of rehearsal. Sensory memory was then added to this as a preliminary stage (for example, Atkinson and Shiffrin, 1971). Models based on these simple ideas are known as multistore, gateway or dual-process models. Diagrams imply that memory resembles a set of boxes and that there is a simple progression through the stages of storage. This idea was based on experimental data involving regulated tasks of memorising. Alternative views of memory are given by the levels of processing approach of Craik and Lockhart (1972) and Neisser (1976), and the dynamic memory theory of Schank (1982). Newer, information-processing approaches have led to short-term and long-term processes being viewed as much more complicated than behavioural experiments could reveal. As with other 'stages' models (see Chapter 10), the pioneering ideas have been superseded.

LTM can be subdivided into episodic or autobiographical, and semantic. This separates things remembered in the context in which they were first encountered and those remembered independently of how they were learned. Procedural and remote memories can also be regarded as distinct systems. Baddeley and Hitch (1974) propose that there is transfer in both directions between short-term and long-term memory. STM may act as a working memory with a central executive and a number of subsidiary slave systems such as the phonological loop and visuospatial sketchpad. Memories that have been stored long term can be brought into short-term awareness in order for ideas to be worked on.

When applying theories of memory in health care, it is important to note the dates of publication of various approaches and the sources used. Even recent publications may be relying on early multistore or 'box' theories. Observations in health care may need to be reinterpreted in the light of newer ideas. For example, difficulties in LTM, which have previously been explained in terms of interference with transfer from short-term to long-term storage, may be due to problems of retrieval from LTM into working memory as a result of a faulty executive system.

Other cognitive approaches to memory and forgetting include the Gestalt theory of forgetting, interference theory, cue-dependence, memory as reconstruction, and eye witness testimony.

Psychodynamic approaches: theories of the unconscious workings of the mind include the idea of motivated forgetting, which suggests that we deliberately repress memories which are disturbing. See Chapter 17.

Key Terms and Concepts

Accessibility: whether or not the stored information can be retrieved. That is, whether one can actually 'find' something in memory that is believed to have been learned. It depends on the way in which information has been encoded and is to be distinguished from availability, which depends on whether the information has been stored at all.

Acoustic, auditory or echoic store: the short-lived memory store of perceptions of sounds. Some writers use this term for the sensory store, implying that storage takes place before the sounds have been interpreted and processed by the cortex. Other writers suggest that even the simplest storage involves cortical organisation.

Acoustic code: the coding of sounds in the appropriate sensory store (echoic store or acoustic store), which makes them available for interpretation and processing.

Acronym: the use of initial letters (either of a title or a list of items to be memorised) to form a pronounceable word. Acronym titles are common in all walks of life, for example **TENS** (**t**ranscutaneous **e**lectrical **n**erve **s**timulation). Acronyms for lists are commonly used in education: **PAIL** (**p**uncture, **a**brasion, **i**ncision, **l**aceration – for types of wounds) and **DICE** for the main theories of forgetting – **d**ecay, **i**nterference, **c**ue dependence and **e**motion.

Activity trace: reverberating activity in the receptor and effector cells involved in a sensation, related to sensory and short-term memory.

Amnesia: the inability, either total or partial, to remember. Anterograde amnesia refers to inability or difficulty in recalling or recognising events that have occurred *since* the onset of illness, that is, forwards in time from the illness. Retrograde amnesia is impairment in recalling events that occurred *before* the onset of illness, that is, backwards in time. Both conditions may appear together. Brain damage may result in severe effects on long-term memory. It is now established that there are a number of critical lesion sites that give rise to a global amnesic effect, all of which are structures in the *limbic system*. Other evidence suggests an alteration in the active processes of retrieval rather than in passive reminiscence. Analysis of the amnesic syndrome has contributed to current theories of memory, and to a move away from the simplistic view of memory as a set of boxes towards active information-processing models. People with Alzheimer's disease differ from other amnesic patients in showing a clear deficit in working memory, both verbal and spatial memory span being impaired. They appear to show a combination of the amnesic syndrome with disturbance in the central executive system.

Analogue: used in theories of memory to refer to information stored in the brain that corresponds to a representation or image of the thing to be remembered.

Availability: whether or not the information has been stored and is available for retrieval. Early assumptions that all experiences are available somewhere in the brain (supported by the findings from electrical stimulation) led to beliefs that hypnosis would facilitate accurate recall.

Backward span: a test procedure in which a participant is required to repeat a list of items in reverse order.

Capacity: a more general term than 'span' for the number of items or amount of information that can be retained and reproduced following a single presentation.

Central executive system: this is a subsystem suggested by Baddeley and Hitch (1974) as being used for processing short-term memory tasks. When concurrent processing is required (that is, maintaining a memory and doing another attention-demanding task at the same time), the central executive helps to co-ordinate these tasks in the slave systems. If there are too many items for the slave systems to cope with, some items can be transferred to long-term memory, which acts as a back-up. See working memory.

Chunking: a mnemonic process or strategy of remembering a long list of items in a series of groups or chunks, such as remembering a telephone or credit card number in chunks of three (Miller, 1956). It is most helpful if the number of chunks is within the person's span, and a hierarchy of chunking is sometimes used, in which each set of subdivisions is within the span. Miller (1956) produced the most well-known account of the limitations of memory span to the 'magic' number of seven, plus or minus two.

Confabulation: the disorder of confabulation is distinguished from classical amnesia in that the patient may produce 'memories' that have no basis in actual events or occurrences and may arise in patients whose performance on standard tests of anterograde memory and learning is within the normal range. Confabulation can be considered a 'paramnesic' disorder, that is, alongside amnesia, a bit like it but not the same. In some cases, such as in alcohol or drug-induced states, or in non-pathological situations, confabulation may be a deliberate ploy.

Context dependence: an example of cue dependence in which recreating or imagining the context (place, time and physical conditions) in which the material was first learned can assist recall.

Control processes: transient processes such as rehearsal, which, according to the multistore model, transfer information from one structural component of memory to another.

Cue dependence: recall is sometimes enhanced if the participant recreates or imagines the physiological state or the context in which material was learned. This is sometimes noticed in everyday life when one forgets what one went to fetch but can remember it by returning to where the idea first occurred.

Curve of forgetting: graph showing the rate of forgetting or the amount forgotten during time.

Decay (trace decay): gradual disappearance of neural activity.

Duration: investigations of the duration of short-term memory have focused on the rate at which material is forgotten in the absence of conscious attention and rehearsal.

Dynamic memory theory: the approach of Schank (1982) that suggests a flexible model allowing for the changing dynamic aspects of memory. The model includes notions of memory organisation packets (MOPs), which define a way in which some items in memories are organised into plans, scenes and schemas (or scripts), and thematic organisation points (TOPs), which define a way in which some memories are organised into themes.

Efforts after meaning: a term used by Bartlett (1932) to indicate how people strive to make sense of what has happened, which involves making inferences or deductions about what could or should have happened, and may involve altering the content in order to make more sense.

Eidetic image: traditionally, an image that revives an optical impression with hallucinatory or near-hallucinatory quality. It is common in children but rare in adults. People with this facility were referred to as Eidetic or as an Eidetiker (from the German). The term is nowadays sometimes used for visual memories with a special clarity, also called photographic memory.

Electrical stimulation: studies by Wilder Penfield (for example, Penfield, 1958) seemed to provide evidence that memories were located in particular regions of the brain. Patients at times reported experiencing vivid visual or auditory memories during stimulation of points in the temporal lobes, the hippocampus and the amygdala. However, excision of these areas did not seem to erase memories. It is likely that most memory impairment after brain damage results from an interference with the processes of memory rather than with localised memories as such. It is not possible to identify one specific area in the brain responsible for memories: different types of memory (for words, pictures and physical skills) are stored or processed in anatomically different sections of the brain.

Encoding: a term used to denote the way in which information is coded in suitable ways either in the appropriate sensory modality (visual, auditory, kinaesthetic, and so on) or according to personal schemas for storage and retrieval. This can be contrasted with use of the term 'encoding' in communication (see Chapter 9).

Episodic or autobiographical memory: this refers to memories of personal experiences and events. This memory is difficult to research as it is rarely possible to check its accuracy. Some studies indicate that young and old produce equal numbers of such memories and that early spontaneous reminiscences may be dimmer than recent memories but can become stronger if often rehearsed. Elderly people are generally slower to produce reminiscences (Rabbitt and Winthorpe, 1988). There is little clinical evidence to support the cliché that elderly people live in the past (but see also reminiscence). When considered alongside other aspects of long-term memory, this provides a more complex approach to memory than does the early multistore model.

Eye witness testimony: an area of research (for example, Wells and Loftus, 1984) that involves laboratory studies, recall of details of films, simulations or real situations in a variety of conditions.

False memory syndrome (recovered memories): terms usually used to refer to memories that arise under hypnosis but which are subsequently suspected of being false. Early beliefs included the assumption that hypnosis can free individuals from normal conscious constraints and facilitate accurate recall. This came from experiments with electrical stimulation that suggested that all experiences were possibly stored somewhere in the brain in photographic fashion. It was also supported by psychodynamic theories of repression. Although some hypnotists hold strong beliefs that such memories are genuine, most cognitive researchers argue that such memories are as vulnerable to distortion, search after meaning, inferences and reconstruction as any others, if not more so because of the necessary element of suggestibility in hypnosis. In contexts other than hypnosis, the term 'pseudomemories' may be used. See also hypnosis in Chapter 12.

Flashbulb memory: this refers to a type of episodic memory in which people recall vivid details of when and where they were and what they were doing when they heard some particularly important news. As with other memories, the details may not be accurate even though they appear vivid.

Forgetting: failure at any time to recall or recognise an experience or item when attempting to do so, or to perform any action previously learned. There are several broad categories of the theories of forgetting: decay theory, interference theory, cue dependence, inadequate processing during encoding or storage, Gestalt theory and motivated forgetting (repression).

Free recall: in a free recall task, the order of recall does not matter.

Fugue: a period of loss of memory, when the individual withdraws for a time from the normal lifestyle.

Gestalt theory of forgetting: this suggests that memories change with time in a qualitative way, losing irregular and unexplained detail, filling in gaps and tending towards regular patterns.

Hierarchical network model: a model by Collins and Quillian (1969, 1972) of semantic memory, which shows how some information is processed according to meaningful hierarchies similar in some ways to scientific classification systems. However, unlike scientific systems, the hierarchical schemas are often highly individual and are not always readily articulated without prompting from others.

Hippocampus: the area of the brain most closely associated with specific memories for information, particularly the learning of new information. See Figure 5.2.

Iconic store: the term 'iconic' may be used for any memory, mode of representation or cognitive process using visual or other images that resemble the actual object (for example, Bruner, 1964). This may refer to imagining an apple being cut in half, in which the sound, appearance, smell, taste and feel of the apple and the act of cutting can be imagined. However, iconic store usually refers only to short-term sensory storage of visual stimuli in terms of physical features such as size, shape, colour and location but not meaning (Sperling, 1960, 1963).

Imagery: the term is usually restricted to visual images but can include memories or imaginings of touch, taste, smell, sound and autokinetic sensation. Bruner uses the term 'iconic' to refer to thinking in visual images. The key word technique uses visual image links to aid memory. Imagery is often used to help in problem-solving. See also Chapters 9, 14 and 16.

Immediate memory: a term sometimes used for short-term memory.

Inferences or deductions: finding additional meaning for an event beyond the actual information available.

Initial letter sentences: learning a list of items in the correct order by taking the initial letters of the items and making an easily remembered sentence or saying. For example: **P**ortsmouth **F**ootball **C**lub **v**ersus **M**illwall **R**overs could be used to memorise the nutritional groups of **p**roteins, **f**ats, **c**arbohydrates, **v**itamins, **m**inerals, **w**ater and **r**oughage.

Interference or inhibition: any intervening activity that affects the retention of learned material. Retroaction (retroactive interference or inhibition) is the effect of recent activity on previously learned material. 'Proaction' ('proactive' interference or inhibition) is the effect of past activity on future learning. Interference can be either positive (improving retention) or negative (hindering), but common usage may often refer only to forgetting. The term 'inhibition' is usually reserved for negative effects.

Key word technique: a mnemonic using visual image links between familiar key words and the unfamiliar foreign or technical terms to be learned. For example, someone learning about intrinsic and extrinsic knowledge may visualise the interior of a room to remind them that intrinsic means inside and an EXIT sign to remind them extrinsic means outside.

Leading questions and memory: a form of question used in interviewing that suggests the answer that should be given. Apart from trapping people into giving certain answers, it is thought that some leading questions can actually affect how a person interprets and thus remembers an event (Loftus and Palmer, 1974). For example asking a witness of an accident whether one of the cars involved was blue may lead the witness to visualise a blue car and subsequently confuse the imagined car with the memory of the accident.

Levels of processing (LOP): a model proposed by Craik and Lockhart (1972) in which the durability of memory is seen as a direct function of the depth of processing rather than of the structures of short- and long-term memory. Items that have been more deeply processed will be retained for a longer period of time. Two types of rehearsal are identified: maintenance rehearsal, which simply repeats items in the form in which they were presented and which probably restricts them to short-term memory; and elaborative rehearsal, which includes additional associations and meanings and which can serve to transfer items into long-term memory. Three levels are suggested: the structural or shallow level, associated with visual physical appearance (with words this corresponds to the visual appearance of the word); the phonetic or phonemic level, associated with sounds (with words this corresponds to the sound of the word); and the semantic level, associated with meanings. See also semantics in Chapter 9.

Long-term memory (LTM): any memories that last for more than a few seconds can be described as long term. According to trace decay theories, memory seems to depend on how strongly a structural trace is developed in the brain and thus how likely it is to be reactivated at a later date, either spontaneously or when required. According to the levels of processing theory, retention depends on how the information is processed rather than on different kinds of storage.

Long-term memory can be subdivided into *episodic* (or autobiographical) memory and *semantic* memory (after Tulving, 1972). *Procedural* and *remote* memories are also long term. Much long-term memory seems to be material specific and processed in associated areas of the brain. Changes to

LTM can give rise to several identifiable types of memory loss. Whereas there is little ageing effect on short-term memory, there is a pronounced effect on LTM. This may be due to problems in *encoding* or with retrieval from LTM owing to a faulty *executive system*. This is particularly noticed with remote memories for non-autobiographical items or events that have taken place within the person's lifetime, such as the names of famous people. Memories for recent famous names are better than for distant ones, and in controlled test conditions, fresh memory inputs are more likely to displace remote or distant memories than recent ones (Stuart-Hamilton, 1994). Older people may also have more difficulty distinguishing between things they have actually done and those they have only thought about. This may lead to difficulties in recalling whether they have posted letters, turned off the gas or locked the door.

Malleability (suggestibility): the idea that eye-witness testimony may inadvertently be distorted in response to certain kinds of questioning such as leading questions. Some people may be more prone to this than others, and factors such as vividness of imagination may be as important as compliance.

Material-specific memories: names of things or places, and appearances of people, particularly faces, places, views, routes and so on are handled by different areas of the brain.

Mediators: according to behaviourist theory, mediators come between a stimulus and a response. In interference theory, they refer to activities that affect whether recall will be hindered or enhanced.

Memory as reconstruction: the idea that misremembering may result from memories being transformed or distorted at the time of retrieval owing to leading questions, subsequent information, emotions or other interference effects (for example, Loftus and Palmer, 1974). See also redintegration.

Metamemory: knowledge about one's own memory: what its capacity is, how best to remember things, awareness of one's own memory abilities and limitations. Although there seems to be no age difference in accuracy, it is reported that elderly people think that their semantic memory has declined and have low confidence in their memories.

Mnemonic (pronounced nem on´ ic): any device or strategy intended to aid the memory. Examples include acronyms, chunking, rhymes, associations, key word technique and initial letter sentences.

First letters are often used to make easily remembered items. A distinction is made between acronyms (pronounceable words) and sentences. Abbreviations of titles into initials, such as NHS, are not normally referred to as mnemonics.

Modality-specific: a term used either for storage that occurs in the sensory system that received the information, which does not appear to be processed by some other location or central processing system (for example, Baddeley, 1990), or for storage in the *cortex*, which is still closely related to the relevant sensory mode.

Multistore (dual process) model: this postulates two separate processes for short-term and long-term memory and suggests that memory is transferred from a short-term to a long-term store by rehearsal (for example, James, 1890; Atkinson and Shiffrin, 1968, 1971). This early behavioural model has been superseded by more complex information-processing models such as working memory.

Ordered recall or serial learning: in tests, the participant is to be marked correct only if all items are repeated in their exact order of presentation.

Overlearning: material is regarded as underlearned when it has not been learned sufficiently for one perfect repetition and overlearned when the participant is required to go on with the learning trial after one perfect repletion has been achieved. Early studies, for example Kreuger (1929), showed that the greater the original overlearning, the slower the rate of forgetting.

Paired-associate learning: the participant is presented with items in pairs, the task being to learn the second item of the pair as a response to the first. On subsequent trials, the participant is presented with the first stimulus and required to produce the response item. Learning a language often uses this method.

Partial reports: incomplete memories or reports of memories that can be deliberate or inadvertent due to interference and other effects.

Pattern recognition: an idea from the multistore model that information will be transferred from sensory to short-term memory accompanied by a verbal label from long-term memory if a match occurs between a pattern in long-term memory and the incoming sensory data.

Perseveration: continuation in time of neural processes set up by incoming stimuli, regardless of the duration of those stimuli. An example of this is the involuntary, persistent repetition of a word or phrase (by people with brain damage, organic mental disorders or schizophrenia) in response to different questions.

Phonological (articulatory) loop: this is the name given to the process that deals with the sounds of words, and is one of the slave systems suggested by Baddeley and Hitch (1974). Memory traces of the sounds of words in the phonological store are assumed to fade and become unretrievable after 1.5–2.0 seconds but can be refreshed by subvocal rehearsal or inner speech, which feeds back into the store. The memory span will be determined by how many items can be refreshed before they fade away. This plays an important role in learning to read.

Phonological (articulatory) suppression: an experimental task used to lend support to the working model of memory. A participant repeats meaningless data out loud at the same time as trying to carry out another task. The meaningless data use up the resources of the phonological loop so that it cannot perform other functions.

Primary and secondary memory: alternative terms for short-term and long-term memory respectively, associated with the early work of James (1890).

Procedural memory (PM): defined by Tulving (1985), Anderson (1985) and others as information from long-term memory that cannot be readily articulated. It includes memories of activities that we know how to do but cannot readily describe and corresponds to muscle memory or Bruner's (1964) enactive mode of representation. This kind of memory seems to be handled in the *cerebellum* of the brain and can remain intact even if other kinds of memory are lost through brain damage (for an example, see the description of Clive Wearing, in Blakemore, 1988; Baddeley, 1990; Gross, 1996). Activities such as playing a musical instrument, juggling, riding a bicycle and driving seem to involve this kind of memory.

Prospective memory: the use of memory to remember to do something in the future.

Reality orientation: For people with dementia or who are disorientated, the strategy of reality orientation is sometimes used. This involves helping the person to orientate to time, place and person by the use of clocks, calendars, signs and labels for rooms and so on. This can, however, appear confrontational and upsetting if the person is contradicted, and needs to be used with sensitivity.

Recall: demonstration of retention and retrieval in which the participant reproduces (in words or in concrete images, pictures, sounds and so on) what has previously been learned; the external evidence that an item or list of items has been learned.

Recognition: perceiving (or recalling) an object accompanied by a feeling of familiarity, or the conviction that the same object has been perceived before. The recognition method requires the participant to learn certain items (the targets) and then point out those items in a given list, which may include items which were not in the original list (the distracters). This kind of test may be adapted to distinguish between items a participant has actually handled and those only thought about.

Redintegration: the word 'redintegration', now rare in common usage, means restoring or re-establishing in a united or perfect state. According to the *Shorter Oxford English Dictionary* (1983), it was first used in psychology by Sir William Hamilton in 1836, in his Law of Redintegration or Totality, to indicate that thoughts which had previously been part of the same total act of cognition later suggest each other. It is now used to indicate a search of memory, started by a few cues, leading to some kind of coherent whole. Since processes of interpretation, interference, confabulation, suggestibility and so on also have to be taken into account, the integrated wholeness that is perceived may be substantially different from the original perception.

Rehearsal (or repetition): repeating to oneself the items that are to be recalled. This is a common tactic for memorising a telephone number long enough to dial it.

Relearning: it is often easier to relearn something even if the original material seems to have been forgotten, as in relearning a foreign language. Ebbinghaus (1885) identified relearning as one of the four measurable types of memory, alongside recall, recognition and reconstruction. Even severely brain-damaged patients who show little awareness of learning new information sometimes show relearning abilities and improved relearning savings.

Relearning savings: in laboratory tasks, the number of trials needed to relearn material is compared with the original number of trials and the saving is expressed as a percentage:

$$\text{Savings score} = \frac{\text{original trials} - \text{relearning trials}}{\text{original trials}} \times 100\%$$

Reminiscence: recall that is passive rather than active, that is, appearing spontaneously and without effort, often after a period of rest. Reminiscence can have a therapeutic effect, and some writers believe that 'reminiscence therapy' should be encouraged with elderly people to enable them to come to terms with experiences towards the end of their lives (Kermis, 1983). However, this is inadvisable in some cases, particularly where there is confusion, as people may be unnecessarily reminded of losses. Reminiscence can also be a response to boredom, particularly where the present life is uneventful (Rabbitt and Winthorpe, 1988), or where deafness leads to difficulty in conversation and monologues of reminiscences are a way of coping with visitors.

Remote memory: is sometimes used to refer to memories of non-autobiographical events that have occurred within a person's lifetime.

Repression (motivated forgetting): this is an example of a defence mechanism and is a psychodynamic term used to describe memories that are unconsciously hidden because they are disturbing. According to Freud, much forgetting is unconsciously motivated in some way. Some memories can be difficult to uncover, but psychodynamic therapies encourage a client to bring them to light, in the belief that such recovery will eventually lead to improved mental health. Repression may be a beneficial coping mechanism, and unless there are problems, too much pressure to seek out recent hidden memories may not be helpful. See also Chapters 8 and 17.

Retention: the persisting trace left behind as an after-effect by an experience; the neurological indication that an item has been learned.

Retrieval: reproduction of a retained memory or location of items in the memory; one's own knowledge or experience that an item has been learned.

Schema (plural schemas or schemata): a term used by Piaget in the 1920s to refer to cognitive frameworks built up from past experience for organising, interpreting and recalling information. A schema is personal and individualistic, not always readily articulated and thus less definite than a *concept*, which can be verbally expressed. See Chapter 16.

Semantic memory: a term used for items independent of personal experiences, such as use of language, general knowledge and academic learning. Some semantic memory may require significant effort in encoding information so that it can be retrieved at will, but it can usually be retrieved independently of when and where the information was originally acquired. Semantic memory seems to survive ageing and can be related to *crystallised intelligence*. Older people are usually as good as or better than younger people at recalling meaningful facts and information.

Sensory memory: according to Baddeley (1990), this is the initial registration of information in the senses, lasting up to 100 milliseconds and representing a stage of memory before information is processed by the brain, for example the *persistence of vision*. Other writers may use the term 'sensory memory' for storage in the *cortex* that is short lived and associated with the related sensory modality. See also Chapter 14.

Serial probe technique: an experimental task in which a sequence of digits is presented and one of the digits is selected as the probe, the participant then being asked to recall the digit that follows the probe (for example, Waugh and Norman, 1965).

Serial reproduction: developed by Bartlett (1932) for investigating reconstruction, this early technique examines the way in which a message may be progressively altered when an account is reproduced from memory on a number of successive occasions. It can be compared with the Gestalt theory of forgetting.

Short-term memory (STM): usually refers to storage of a few seconds, involving higher mental processes in the cortex of the brain, such as remembering a telephone number long enough to dial it. Changes in STM are very varied. Studies of STM loss distinguish between capacity and duration. It is found that there can be significant changes in some tasks with no noticeable difference in others. For example, a person may have difficulty recalling words presented aurally but no difficulty with visual presentations. This can be explained in terms of Baddeley and Hitch's (1974) concept of working memory. The subsystems appear to be independent and are assumed to be processed in different parts of the brain. Investigations also show that a person may have no trouble recalling single items, presented either aurally or visually, but will make errors with two or more items. Or there may be severe difficulty in recalling more than one item presented as either an aural or a visual stimulus, but less difficulty when both types of presentation are given simultaneously for each item (Warrington and Shallice, 1969). Simple STM span shows little or no decline with age. However, when extra demands are placed on participants, the age effects generally become apparent. Backward span procedure and concurrent processing indicate that elderly people are significantly worse at these tasks. Baddeley (1982) suggests that the central executive is the prime cause of this age-related decline.

Slave systems: According to the working memory model of Baddeley and Hitch (1974) and their later work, short-term memory consists of a central executive system and subsidiary slave systems that handle modality-specific information. Two such slave systems are the phonological loop and the visuospatial sketchpad or scratchpad.

Span (span of apprehension): the longest list of to-be-remembered items the participant can reliably repeat back, usually after a single brief presentation. 'Digit span' denotes memory for numbers, 'word span' for word lists and so on. Most people can remember about seven random digits (Miller, 1956) but only about four or five random words or letters (McCarthy and Warrington, 1990).

State dependence: empirical evidence is mixed, but memory may be affected by the level of emotional arousal associated with the item to be remembered or the context in which the remembering is required. State dependence is an example of cue dependence in which a person recreates or imagines the physiological state or mood in which material was originally learned in order to assist recall. Examples include using alcohol or drugs, or thinking of tiredness or happiness.

Structural change or trace: changes in the form of synaptic or dendritic growth that (possibly) facilitate neural connections and therefore the firing of a particular sequence on a later occasion, related to long-term memory.

Theories of memory based on this notion used to rely more on supposition than on physiological evidence. However, there is increasing evidence that denser growth corresponds to areas connected with repeated physical activity such as learning to play the violin.

Structural components: Sensory memory, short-term store (STS) and long-term store (LTS) are referred to as structural components in the multistore model. Control processes such as rehearsal serve to transfer memories from one structure to another.

Subspan and supraspan: Lists or material less than the participant's normal span is described as subspan, anything beyond this span being supraspan.

Transfer: the (positive or negative) effect of learning one task upon the learning of another.

Triggers: items that act as cues that set off a train of memories. In everyday experience, snatches of songs or certain smells can trigger vivid memories. See also reconstruction, cue dependence and redintegration.

Verbal memory: this term was traditionally used only for memory for individual words, and much early research focused on the memorisation of lists of real words compared with nonsense syllables. This showed that nonsense items were more easily remembered if associated with real words and images. More recently, it has come to include symbolic representation, which uses meaningful phrases and sentences to code information and memory for speech and written material. Random lists of words are processed less well than meaningful prose.

Visuospatial sketchpad (scratchpad): this refers to the rehearsing of items as visual images in terms of how and where they would occur in the normal visual field. An example would be imagining a football game while listening to a radio broadcast. This is one of the subsidiary slave systems suggested by Baddeley and Hitch (1974).

Working memory: Baddeley and Hitch (1974) and Baddeley (1990) suggest that short-term memory functions as a set of subsystems acting as temporary working memory systems and enabling us to perform a range of cognitive tasks. Baddeley and Hitch conceive the working memory as consisting of a controlling central executive system and a number of subsidiary slave systems. Two such slave systems are the phonological (sound) loop and the visuospatial sketchpad. When someone is trying to solve a problem, visual and sound memories are brought into consciousness or short-term working memory, where they can be continuously rehearsed via the sketchpad or sound loop. Other sensory memories may also be involved in different slave systems. These processes are organised by the central executive system until the problem is solved and the solution committed to either paper or long-term memory. See also Chapter 16.

12 Mind and Altered States of Consciousness

The concept of consciousness is one which has occupied and puzzled philosophers and scientists throughout history.

It is very difficult to relate our perceptions of awareness of ourselves and our mental processes to what is known about the functioning of the central nervous system. This chapter explores some ideas about the relationship between brain functioning and mental experience and what is known or believed about different or altered states of awareness, in particular sleep, dreaming, hypnosis, hallucinations, dementia and the effects of psychoactive or psychotropic drugs. Those aspects of conditions such as epilepsy, schizophrenia and autism that can in some ways be interpreted as an altered state of consciousness are also included here.

Definitions	
Ayer (1963)	[Descartes'] view is that a person is a combination of two separate entities, a body and a mind or soul. Only the mind is conscious; the physical properties which a person has are properties of his body. The two entities are separate in the sense that there is no logical connection between them....
Gregory (1981)	we would expect theories of consciousness to be related to theories of perception... then we may suspect that our knowledge of ourselves is a construction: perhaps very much as perceptions are hypotheses of the physical world.
Dennet (1991)	We must abandon the dualism of mind and body that is our legacy from Descartes and the idea that there is some part of the brain that is the seat of consciousness.

Definitions (cont'd)	
McGinn (1993)	Neural transmissions just seem like the wrong kind of materials with which to bring consciousness into the world, but it appears that in some way they perform this mysterious feat. The mind–body problem is the problem of understanding how the miracle is wrought, thus removing the sense of deep mystery.
Chalmers (1995)	distinguishes between what he calls the 'easy problems' and the 'hard problem' of consciousness. The easy problems are those to do with how a person integrates information and responds appropriately, including talking about what is happening; the hard problem concerns what we actually mean by subjective experience. Chalmers suggests that some philosophers are addressing only the easy problems and that consciousness may be a fundamental in itself, not reducible to anything more basic, and requiring new principles to explain it.
Ornstein (1973)	An ASC [altered state of consciousness] may be defined… as a qualitative alteration in the over-all pattern of mental functioning, such that the experiencer feels his consciousness is radically different from the way it functions ordinarily. An SoC [state of consciousness] is thus defined not in terms of any particular content of consciousness, or specific behaviour or physiological change, but in terms of the over-all patterning of psychological functioning'. Ornstein lists as ASCs: dreaming, hypnogogic and hypnopompic states, alcohol intoxication, effects of marijuana and LSD, meditative states, so-called possession states and autohypnotic states.
Rogers (1980)	studies appear to reveal that people in an altered state of consciousness feel they are in touch with, and can grasp, the 'evolutionary flow' of the development of consciousness in the human species.

Approaches, Arguments and Applications

The study of consciousness is an area of psychology very much interrelated with and dependent on philosophy and physics. A sense of the history of these disciplines can be helpful in considering what it makes sense to say in the light of our current knowledge of the nature of matter and the way in which things work in the physical world.

The language used in the definitions from philosophical enquiry may seem difficult and unfamiliar, but it can be seen that the terms 'conscious' and 'unconscious' do not simply refer, as they might in the accident and emergency department, to whether a person is awake or not but to what we mean when we talk about our awareness of ourselves and the world and how this may change. This has important implications for professional care, particularly for people with conditions that are viewed as abnormalities or mental disorders. The implications of the study and discussion of consciousness involve ethical and moral considerations of the effects of drugs, brain surgery, 'brain death', the use of hypnosis and so on, and also practical ways of caring for people with altered sleep patterns, under anaesthetic, in a coma or with mental health disorders.

Philosophical approaches: psychology, philosophy and physics are struggling with the puzzle concerning the interrelationship between mental processes and physiological processes in order to try to understand what causes what. There is a need to know whether our mental experiences bring about changes in our brain functioning, whether changes in brain functioning bring about certain experiences, whether there is always a mixture of both, or whether both are created by something else, at present unknown.

The main philosophical debate appears to be whether the Cartesian mind–body dualism is still an appropriate way of talking about consciousness, and if not, what *paradigm* should now replace it. The Cartesian *dualists* talk in terms of the mind being quite separate from the body, others, the *reductionists*, in terms of mental activity arising from (or capable of being reduced to) the biological activity, and still others, *monists* or *identity theorists*, that mind and brain are not separate at all but identical, the concepts of mind and brain being simply two rather different descriptions of the same thing. So-called *mysterians* (Chalmers, 1995) assert that we will never understand consciousness at all. Gregory (1981) gives a useful review of some of the different approaches.

Biopsychological approaches: studies include the measurement of brain activity using EEG, CAT, PET and MRI scans corresponding to different states of consciousness. Theories try to provide neurological explanations for: how and why we sleep and dream; what happens in the brain and nervous system during hypnosis; the effects of drugs on the nervous system and how and why hallucinations occur; and alterations in brain functioning in conditions such as schizophrenia, autism and dementia. The motor nervous system, but not the autonomic nervous system (ANS), is regarded as being under voluntary conscious control. There are exceptions to this as voluntary control can be gained over the ANS through hypnosis, yoga and biofeedback and lost in the motor system owing to damage in the CNS.

Behavioural and social learning approaches: behaviourists are not concerned with a concept of mind but view it only as a black box, unknowable and not amenable to scientific study. This perspective considers only observable behaviour without concern for what is going on inside the individual or any conscious awareness of this. All behaviour is regarded as conditioned or learned from others. Free will and intentions are regarded as illusory. Experimenters look for learning experiences whereby patterns of sleep, expectations of hypnosis, drugs and altered perceptions are conditioned through association and observation of others when certain behaviour is selectively reinforced by tangible or social rewards.

Social psychology approaches: these look at the ways in which we communicate our ideas and feelings and how we influence each other. This includes study of the language that we use to try to convey our inner experiences and by which we infer what another person is experiencing. This language-based awareness seems to be at least part of what we mean by consciousness.

Cognitive approaches: in this century has come the realisation that much, perhaps nearly all, of our mental activity takes place without awareness, and that we engage in very sophisticated *information-processing* without being able to give any account of what we are doing. We can think and solve problems while functioning on a sort of 'autopilot', but we do not know how we do this. Gregory (1981) describes consciousness as a kind of moving beam of light searching and illuminating facets of the mind. Current consciousness consists of whatever is being lit by the patch of light of the beam, and there is a great deal more around it which is not lit for the moment, some never being lit. We are also aware that we can shift from one state of consciousness to another and that our experience of ourselves and of the world varies according to mood, drowsiness, sleep, hypnosis and the effects of drugs. Increased awareness of what to look for and an awareness of our own processes (metacognition, metamemory, and metacommunication) can lead to greater access to processes that otherwise remain under autopilot.

Psychodynamic approaches: these have indicated that our emotional experience also seems to be influenced, or even governed, by deliberately hidden or *repressed* unconscious activity. Freud talked as if the mind were structured in terms of three distinct layers: the conscious, the preconscious and the unconscious. The unconscious part contains the deliberately repressed material, kept hidden through defence mechanisms. Some of this may leak accidentally into consciousness in a symbolic way through dreams, but the symbolic coding usually prevents total awareness so that the dreamer remains protected from disturbing thoughts and memories. Therapies address this hidden or repressed unconscious mental activity. The symbolism is believed to be decodable through inferences concerning which defence mechanisms are operating and a systematised analysis of the reasons behind them. Analysis of dreams may assist with understanding and may lead to more effective coping mechanisms. Comparisons may be made with symbolism found throughout the visual arts.

Humanistic approaches: all behaviour is viewed as meaningful and language as symbolic. Visual art forms and music can be more powerful expressions of meaning than words, but these symbols need not be viewed as obscure or requiring specialist interpretation. All symbols that an individual finds in dreams and art arise as part of that individual's personal experience. An individual will bring whatever meaning he or she thinks of, and the meaning for each individual comes from within that individual, whether looking at his or her own *text* or something from another person. Meanings will be due in part to the individual's knowledge of cultural products and other people's interpretations of them. The true or real meaning is whatever makes most sense to the individual.

Creative arts therapies: these explore different means of communicating about emotions and experiences, including dreams and altered states of consciousness, using methods that are not dependent on words or which use words in special ways.

Key Terms and Concepts

Anaesthesia: the aim of anaesthesia is to depress the functions of the central nervous system while maintaining the functions of other vital body organs (Sear, 1992; Carrie *et al.*, 1996). The main implication for psychological care is the realisation that, from time to time, reports are given that a patient has been conscious during an operation, has felt pain and has been able to hear without being able to communicate this. In all cases, hearing is the last sense to be lost and the first to be regained.

Helpers are now advised not to say anything in the presence of a patient under anaesthetic that they would not want the patient to hear. There is a need for more information about the minute signs that might indicate some degree of consciousness.

Apparitions: an immaterial appearance of something as if it were really there. This can involve any one of the senses or a combination of senses. Most apparitions that are reported are described solely as visual, but this is likely to be because vision is normally the prominent sense and other sensory experience is ignored. Green and McCreery (1989: 1) suggest that we think of an apparition as a figure of a person who 'isn't really there' superimposed on the normal environment. Green and McCreery distinguish between apparitions and waking dreams in which the whole environment is perceived as different from normal and there is a temporary loss of awareness of the normal physical surroundings. Note that the word 'hallucination' refers to the perceptual *experience* and the term 'apparition' to the *object* which is perceived.

Autism: Anthony Clare and Lawrence Bartak (in Williams, 1992) describe how people with autism have difficulty in understanding other people's facial expressions, emotional reactions and conversational tones, and find it hard to process information dealing with people and relationships. Bartak asserts that this is not caused by bad parenting, as was once thought, but by an abnormality of brain development; there may be a link with vitamin B12 metabolism.

Baron-Cohen (for example, 1989) has attempted to isolate some of the variables and test hypotheses systematically. He describes how many autistic children have difficulty appreciating what someone else might be thinking and cannot see that someone else might have a point of view different from their own.

Hobson (1993) describes autism as a profound disturbance in interpersonal relatedness and gives examples of people with autism who cannot grasp what is meant by friendship or what it means to have a friend. Both Hobson and Baron-Cohen are exploring autism in the context of a child's development of mind and are looking for better ways to trace and describe normal and abnormal development.

Autohypnotic: inducing a hypnotic state in oneself. As with other hypnosis, this may refer to any state that is believed to be hypnotic, from relaxation to trance or sleep. Autohypnosis can be practised by most people who are susceptible to hypnosis and may be induced by saying a code word or repeating a sequence of words or numbers that has been learned.

Autophany: seeing an apparition of oneself.

Autoscopy: seeing oneself from a distance, as in an out-of-body experience.

Clairvoyance: popularly defined as foreseeing the future. Green and McCreery (1989) argue that clairvoyance can be regarded as particularly vivid hallucinatory perceptions in which details are 'seen' or known which would not be perceived under normal visual conditions.

Coma: early beliefs about coma are exemplified by Glaser and Strauss (1965: 29):

> As an interactant, the comatose person is what Goffman has called a 'nonperson'. Two nurses caring for him can speak in his presence without fear that, overhearing them, he will suspect or understand what they are saying about him. Neither they nor the physicians need to engage in tactics to protect him from any dread knowledge.

However, it is now realised that, as with anaesthetic, some people in a coma are responsive to the environment. Families may bring in favourite music or read out loud in the hope that such stimuli will help the patient to regain consciousness. Helpers are advised, as with anaesthetised patients, not to discuss patients in their presence.

Confusional state: a general term for any condition in which there is a loss of orientation or difficulty in scoring on simple psychometric tests of memory, attention span or other cognitive function.

Delirium: an acute confusional state caused by disturbance of the central nervous system metabolism. This may happen as a result of fever, drugs or inadequate diet. It may be confused with dementia, but the onset is usually very rapid. Children and elderly people are most vulnerable. Behaviour tends to be either extremely apathetic or hyperactive. Memory, attention span and other cognitive skills are poor. Unlike those with dementias, delirious patients are particularly subject to illusions. Recovery can be spontaneous.

Dementias: Stuart-Hamilton (1991) defines dementia as the 'global deterioration of intellectual function resulting from atrophy of the central nervous system (CNS)'. He states that dementia can occur at any age, and although the probability of becoming demented increases with age, it should not be considered to be a disease of older people. The psychological abilities of patients with dementia are quite different from those of unaffected elderly people, and dementia is not a natural part of the normal ageing process. By definition, the label 'dementia' is only given where there is no other known cause, such as a tumour, in which there is a clear relationship between mental functioning and the state of the brain. However, it is only possible to confirm this through autopsy, and most diagnosis therefore takes place on the basis of what is apparent to an observer. Haase (1977), cited by Stuart-

Hamilton (1991), has identified about 50 different causes of dementia, the more common ones being classified according to five main types: Alzheimer's disease, multi-infarct dementia, Pick's disease, Creutzfeldt–Jacob disease (CJD) and Huntington's disease. The progression of the disease is different in each type, depending on the order in which different parts of the brain are affected. Parkinson's disease and syphilis can also cause dementia or dementia-like symptoms. There are a number of other illnesses that are easily confused with dementia, such as pseudodementia, delirium and depression.

Diurnal/circadian rhythms: these are the daily biological rhythms that become established over roughly a regular 24-hour period. Diurnal refers specifically to the daytime period, the opposite of nocturnal or night-time. Circadian, from the Latin *circa*, round about, and *dies*, day, refers to approximately 24-hour cycles and is a recently introduced term, dating from 1959. When daily routine is altered, for example by travelling to a different time zone, starting shift work or going into hospital, the rhythms are disrupted. With long-term change, there is usually an adjustment period of between 5 days and 2 weeks during which new rhythms are established.

Dreaming: most people believe they dream for a few minutes most nights; others will say they never dream. Sleep research shows that dreaming or *REM* sleep generally occurs as part of a personal cyclical pattern of sleep, occupying roughly 10 minutes in each period of an hour and a half. Most dreams are forgotten unless the person is awakened at the time. Dreams with emotional content that waken the sleeper are thus likely to be remembered best, as are those which occur at times when the sleeper is disturbed by a loud noise or by pain or indigestion. The adage that cheese at bedtime causes dreams may have some truth if it causes indigestion.

Most people describe their dreams in terms of their visual images, but dreams can create fantasy situations with imagery in all the usual sensory modes: seeing, hearing, smelling, tasting, touching and proprioception (Oswald, 1966, 1984). People with sensory loss recreate in their dreams what is normal for them or what has been available in their past. Thus someone blind from birth is unlikely to have visual dreams, but someone blinded later in life may well continue to have visual imagery. Dream imagery is probably largely built on memories of anything that has been encountered, or heard or read about, but with fantastic elaborations.

As it is not always possible for people to trace the memories that could account for the stuff of their fantasies, some theories of dreaming incorporate explanations that go beyond real-life experience. There are biological, behavioural, social, cognitive and psychodynamic explanations. Fanciful, or non-scientific, descriptions include reincarnation, communication with other worlds and so on.

Biological explanations include the notion that brain activity during REM sleep is purely random, but if roused, a person will try to make sense of the various snippets of thought and turn them into meaningful stories. Oswald (1966, 1984) believes that the dreaming period is allocated to the growth and repair of the tissue of the brain. This fits with the observation that babies sleep and seem to dream a great deal while their brains are growing rapidly. This is disputed by others, for example Horne (1988), who believes that deep stage IV sleep is also used for brain recovery.

In the 1960s Christopher Evans, cited by Aldiss (1970) and Peter Evans (1991), believed that the main purpose of sleep was to allow us to dream, not to consciously explore ideas but to enable the brain to sort out its new experiences and to put its files in order. He compared the brain with a computer. At the time he was writing, in order to update information in a computer, it had to be taken off-line, that is, disconnected from the task it was controlling, to run through the programs and make modifications where necessary. If it was not taken off-line, all the stages of the reprogramming would get confused with the task. Thus Evans saw the purpose of sleep as taking the brain off-line, to prepare for revising and clearing the brain's programs concerning recent events and experiences.

Dreams, by this analogy, are the running through of the programs and their reclassification. Yet we are not normally aware of this clearance of experiences. Only when the process is interrupted, because of some external or internal disturbance of the sleeper, will consciousness interact with the clearance activity, and we experience a dream. A dream is thus an experience (important or not) that is in the process of being sorted and classified. Evans believed that the content is mostly trivial and that we are aware only of the few sequences that are sufficiently emotional to wake us up. Similarly, if we are restless for some reason, we might become aware of the irrational 'rubbish' that accounts for most of our REM activity and possibly inject new meaning into this rubbish as we become aware of it.

This theory, together with what is known of the switching mechanisms, provides an interesting explanation of hallucinations: that the brain becomes muddled and confused because of some interference with the procedure for going off-line, and sorting occurs while the person is awake. It also suggests that sleep is essential and not just a wasted period of our lives – that we should not try to stay awake, sleep-learn or take sleeping pills such as barbiturates that allow stage IV but suppress REM sleep. Also, LSD might be activating the dream mechanism at unsuitable times when the brain is not off-line, and could well have permanent effects.

Psychoanalysis, and other psychodynamic approaches, assume that dreaming is a symbolic encoding of painful and disturbing unconscious material. Explanations vary according to which school of thought they originate from. The most well-known ones are the Freudian and the Jungian. Therapeutic intervention, and the interpretation of dreams, may enable the person to become aware of repressed thoughts and memories and confront them.

Epilepsy: Sander and Thompson (1989: 7) gives the medical definition of epilepsy as 'the occurrence of transient paroxysms of uncontrolled discharges of the nerve tissue of the brain, leading to epileptic attacks'. Seizures range from momentary 'absences' or blankness to a generalised convulsive attack. The causes are not clear, and in about 60 per cent of cases no cause is identified. The experience of seizures or fits varies from person to person: there may be a warning such as a peculiar sensation of a smell, or an 'aura'. Often there is little awareness either of having a fit or of momentary absences.

False awakening: there seem to be two types of false awakening. In one type, people believe they have woken up normally but then begin to doubt whether they are really awake and look around them trying to work out whether they are awake or not. Sometimes they realise they are not awake and then have a *lucid dream*. Some people experience repeated false awakenings and may imagine themselves to have dressed and set out for work, only to 'wake' again a little later and find themselves still in bed. This can be repeated several times before the sleeper truly wakes. In the second type, sleepers may believe that they have woken normally but then have a sense of foreboding or excitement and may experience what appear to be hallucinations, before fully waking.

Hallucinations: the experience of an apparent perception of an object that is not present and that is not related in any obvious way to sensory stimulation. This can occur in any of the sensory modes, vision, hearing, touch, taste, smell, *proprioception* or *interoception*. Visions and voices are the most commonly described experiences. These are traditionally regarded as mysterious or frightening and contribute to folklore and views of insanity. In contrast, it is not usual to talk about the experience of the existence of a limb that has been amputated as an hallucination, presumably because the experience can be reasonably explained in terms of the neural activity and can be seen to be imagined. It may be that there is no justification for regarding a schizophrenic person's voices as physiologically different from the amputee's itchy foot. It is perhaps one person's realisation that the sensation must have been imagined, and another's conviction that it was real, that distinguishes between different mental states. Rankin and O'Carroll (1995) report that non-psychotic individuals disposed towards hallucination obtain lower scores on tests of the cognitive skills involved in discriminating between memories of words imagined or heard.

Hypnobate: a sleepwalker.

Hypnogogic: usually used to denote experiences while falling asleep. Originally from the Greek for inducing sleep.

Hypnopompic: a term used for the state between sleep and waking, or experiences while waking, before being fully awake.

Hypnosis: the term 'hypnosis' can be used in several ways. First, it may be used to refer to sleep that has been induced by an hypnotic or sleep-promoting drug. Second, it may refer to a state of semi-coma induced by deliberate mild poisoning or intoxication, such as 'barbiturate hypnosis'. The term is mostly used to refer to a condition in which one individual complies to an unusual extent with the suggestions of another, usually accompanied by the feeling that the experience is not quite the same as the normal state of consciousness and that the compliance is involuntary (Naish, 1986). This condition is sometimes described as a trance.

In 'trait' approaches, it is argued that some people are more susceptible to hypnosis than others, and this is the generally held belief. Many people also believe that hypnosis can be imposed against one's will. However, 'skills training' approaches, described by Naish (1986), argue that responses to hypnosis can be learned. Learned responses may include the willingness to comply and the ability to imagine vividly what is being suggested, which can improve with practice. The experience will depend to a large extent on what the individual expects to experience. If the individual expects hypnosis to feel trance-like or different in some way from normal consciousness and complies with suggestions, this is what will be experienced. Similarly, if the individual complies with suggestions while expecting his or her responses to feel involuntary, this is what it will seem like. On the other hand, a person who expects things simply to happen, without any effort or willingness to comply, will resist or not experience hypnosis. Someone who does not expect anything to happen and who makes no effort to comply is also unlikely to experience anything. These skills training approaches argue that hypnosis requires effort on the part of the hypnosee rather than the hypnotist and that those people who believe themselves to be good subjects will experience more of the expected effects than those who believe they are not susceptible, say that hypnosis is a fraud or hold other negative attitudes towards it. Research into hypnosis continues, and reliable scales have been developed that can measure a person's suggestibility (Fellows, 1988). See also Chapter 11.

A popular use of hypnosis is in entertainment, in which the stage hypnotist selects susceptible people from the audience and then induces what is normally viewed as a trance-like state during which suggestions are made that the volunteers will carry out bizarre behaviours without any memory of the suggestion and without voluntary control. This is usually judged as harmless fun, but from time to time reports are made of people who believe that they have suffered permanent ill-effects. Reputable stage hypnotists have a voluntary code of conduct that discourages extreme suggestions and includes screening people for known heart defects or epilepsy or other conditions making them vulnerable.

Hypnotherapy: the use of suggestion to help someone make changes to their lifestyle or state of being. In most cases, it involves suggesting that the client is in a state of deep relaxation and of talking through the client's beliefs, perhaps worries or fears, and about aspects of self-concept or lifestyle. Suggestions about improvements in habits or lifestyle may be made, and the client may form an intention to carry out the suggested changes. Hypnotherapy may be used in attempts to treat eating disorders or stress or to give up smoking. Most hypnotherapists refer to the hypnotic state as deep relaxation rather than trance-like (see also hypnosis).

Hypnotic: this term can be used to refer either to something sleep-inducing or soporific, or to someone who is susceptible to hypnotism.

Hypnotics: drugs used for treating insomnia. The main categories are barbiturates and benzodiazepines. Barbiturates are only used with severe intractable insomnia, if at all. They produce tolerance, have toxic effects and reduce the proportion of dreaming sleep. Benzodiazepines are believed to act on specific receptors close to the GABA receptors (see Chapter 5). Rebound insomnia is common. Cyclopyrrolene is also thought to bind to GABA receptors but at a different site from the other benzodiazepines. Quality of sleep is better, and studies suggest it may be superior to other hypnotics with regard to undesired effects. Other hypnotics include chloral hydrate and chlormethiazole. Promethazine and diphenhydramine are antihistamines whose sedative effects may be used to help induce sleep.

Hypnotic state: this refers to whatever state is achieved when a person believes him or herself to have been hypnotised. It may be a state of calm relaxation, such as that used in some forms of hypnotherapy, it may be trance-like or it may be sleep. It might be perceived as a regression to childhood or past life.

Insomnia: the inability to sleep or the perception that one is not getting enough sleep. For some, particularly older people, this may only be in comparison with what is thought to be normal or the 'right' amount of sleep (see sleep duration). For older people, who probably do not need as much continuous sleep as they have been used to, and who may be 'napping' during the day, help with planning a new routine or finding things to do when awake during the night may be helpful. However, where insomnia is caused by illness, pain, stress or medication and is interfering with rest and daily activities, pain and stress management advice and hypnotics may be needed. See also sleep deprivation.

Lucid dream: a dream in which the dreamer is aware that he or she is dreaming.

Metachoric experiences: experiences in which the normal field of perception is completely replaced by an hallucinatory one. Green and McCreery (1989) give waking dreams, lucid dreams and ordinary dreams as examples and point out that the hallucinatory environment may be an exact, or nearly exact, replica of a real one, as in a false awakening or an out-of-body experience.

Multiple personality: an extremely rare condition, sometimes known as *grande hysterie*, in which a person apparently has the experience of being a different person on different occasions, sometimes with, sometimes without, awareness of this change. Schreiber (1974) describes Sybil, who would suddenly find herself in strange surroundings without any understanding of how she came to be there, and who gradually came to realise that she was living part of her life as one person, part as another. During her treatment, various other personalities emerged, some of whom were aware of the other 'selves'. Dual personality is dramatised in stories such as *Dr Jekyll and Mr Hyde* by Robert Louis Stevenson, in which a doctor, experimenting with drugs and the occult, succeeds in separating himself into two alternating characters, one good, the other evil. This can be related to Jung's beliefs about an *alter ego* and the *principle of opposites*. Multiple or dual personality is often confused with schizophrenia in everyday language, but the conditions are quite different.

Myoclonic jerk: the most common type is a sudden spasm that may occur in the early stages of falling asleep, resulting from a tiny burst of activity in the brain. This may be linked to a missed heartbeat. It is sometimes associated with a brief dream image such as tripping over a step. It may be particularly noticeable in situations in which a person is trying to stay awake, or appear as if awake, such as in lectures. See sleep cycle. Other kinds of myoclonic jerk may occur in conditions such as epilepsy.

Narcolepsy: a condition characterised by irresistible, usually brief, attacks of sleep or uncontrollable drowsiness, possibly with mumbled speech, double vision and stumbling. Attacks may be precipitated by boredom or when carrying out a monotonous or repetitive task. People with this disorder pass quickly into dreaming sleep without going through the usual stages and tend to report vivid dreams (Oswald, 1966).

Negative hallucination: a sensory experience in which a person fails to perceive something in the environment, such as not seeing an object being looked for, only to find a moment later that it was there all the time. Such experiences are common and are probably responsible for belief in poltergeists, which are said to hide objects playfully. Under hypnosis, a person may respond to suggestion that an object is not present or not visible.

Orthodox sleep: the early name for ordinary deep sleep with big slow EEG wave traces, so named to distinguish it from paradoxical sleep, which was not understood at the time.

Out-of-body or ecsomatic experiences: experiences in which the person continues to act normally but seems to be perceiving what is going on from a position that is not the same as where the actual body is, such as feeling as if one is walking a few paces behind oneself or watching oneself in bed from beside or above the bed.

Paranormal: outside the normal range of scientific investigation.

Pseudodementia: severe depression in elderly people may result in low motivation and poor scores on psychometric tests of memory and other cognitive functions. This may be confused with dementia. However, these people are usually well orientated. Their level of activity tends to vary through the day, and they are usually well aware of their poor performance.

Psychotropic (psychoactive) drugs: drugs that affect mood or other psychological states or experiences: mind-altering substances ('tropic' as a suffix meaning bending or altering). This group includes everything from food to legal and illegal substances that have an effect on the central nervous system and affect mental processes. Psychoactive drugs interfere in three main ways with the processes by which brain cells pass messages across the synapses: by mimicking natural neurotransmitters, by increasing endogenous neurotransmitter release or by blocking natural neurotransmitters, or a combination of these.

Moon and Karb (1993) list psychotropic medications as antipsychotic, antianxiety, antidepressant and antimanic agents. Messer and Meldrum (1995) suggest that it is helpful to make a rough classification according to whether the drugs are predominantly depressant or stimulant:

Depressant	**Stimulant**
Anticonvulsants	Cerebral stimulants
Anaesthetics	Hallucinogens
Anxiolytics	Antidepressants
Hypnotics	
Neuroleptics	
Analgesics	
Alcohol	

According to the Parliamentary Office of Science and Technology (1996), the most common drugs to be used illegally are cannabis, Ecstasy, amphetamines and lysergic acid diethylamide (LSD). Some of the effects are well documented; others can only be guessed at.

REM sleep: rapid eye movement sleep. It was called 'paradoxical' sleep early on in research because it was obviously deep sleep but the brain patterns were like those of waking. The term 'paradoxical sleep' was first used with study of cats before the association with dreaming was understood. It is not absolutely proved, of course, but most experimenters believe that we do most of our dreaming during REM sleep and that everybody dreams. We only recall dreams after being awakened or disturbed.

Schizophrenia: the word is derived from the Greek words for 'split' and 'brain'. The common misperception is that schizophrenia means split personality as in the story of *Dr Jekyll and Mr Hyde*. However, that kind of dual or *multiple personality* is an extremely rare disorder quite different from schizophrenia. Schizophrenia is fairly common, affecting one in every hundred or so people at some time in their lives, and the name comes from the perception that people seem split off from reality or that there is a split between thoughts and feelings. The term was first introduced in 1912, gradually replacing the term dementia praecox, which dates from 1891 and was used to label young people who developed symptoms. The latter name may still be used by relatives of people now in their late 70s or 80s.

As Howe (1990) describes, the diagnosis of schizophrenia covers a variety of conditions with a number of characteristic symptoms. These can include feelings of paranoia, suffering from delusions, hearing voices that torment and persecute, believing that their own thoughts can be heard by others and feeling that other people are 'out to get them' and are manipulating them into unpleasant situations. Behaviour ranges from explosive anger and aggressiveness to extreme withdrawal and unresponsive states of immobility. Causes are not known, although there does appear to be a genetic component, sometimes linked with high creativity (Hoffer, 1983, cited by Howe, 1990).

Evidence suggests that delusions and hallucinations may occur because the person's brain is overwhelmed by sensory information, perhaps because the brain is unable to filter out unnecessary information and allow for selective attention processes. Srivastava (1995) indicates that there is a lack of the protein PSA-NCAM, which gives healthy people's brains the flexibility needed to filter large amounts of sensory information. The brain of a developing fetus contains large quantities of the protein, which assists nerve cells to grow towards their targets and controls the formation of synapses. Soon after birth, the protein disappears from most of the brain but remains in those areas where synapses are continually being reorganised, such as the hippocampus, which is concerned with learning, remembering and processing new information.

There also appear to be high levels of dopamine associated with schizophrenic symptoms, and it is known that disruption of the hippocampus can stimulate the overproduction of dopamine. An alternative opinion is that the levels of dopamine may be within normal limits but cannot be tolerated.

It is not clear whether the altered brain chemistry is a cause or an effect of symptoms. Moreover the levels of protein can only be determined through post-mortem analysis. It is hoped that current knowledge will lead to new ways of diagnosing schizophrenia and maybe find ways of increasing the level of PSA-NCAM in relevant areas.

Carol North (1987) describes her experiences of childhood and adolescence dominated by visual and auditory hallucinations and voices, which she believed to be real. She suffered a lack of understanding and empathy from some professionals (but kindness from others) through a variety of unsuccessful psychotherapeutic interventions, until she was suddenly helped by kidney dialysis. This is thought to have filtered out toxins in her blood. She experienced a dramatic reduction in hallucinations, which can be ascribed to reduction of 'noise' in her central nervous system.

Earlier approaches to schizophrenia indicated that patterns of communication within families might exacerbate the condition. R.D. Laing (1967) describes a 'double-bind' situation, which he believes contributes to the cause. This takes place when a parent or other significant person imposes conflicting demands on a child so that, whatever the child does, he or she will be judged to be wrong. See also value-laden and leading questions in Chapter 9. It is now more widely held that awkward or faulty patterns of communication are likely to arise either because the person with schizophrenic tendencies responds in non-standard ways or because other members of the family also have some schizophrenic tendencies, these not being marked enough to have been diagnosed as such.

Sleep: a recurrent healthy state of inertia and unresponsiveness (Oswald, 1966). We usually find that we have to sleep. We cannot (and usually do not want to) do anything to prevent ourselves sleeping, but it is not fully understood why we sleep. It appears most probable that sleep is needed for brain repair and recovery but not for other physiological processes (Horne, 1988).

Calder (1970) cites studies reporting that, during sleep, a hormone is released that is responsible for growth: human growth hormone (hGH). Cell division (mitosis) and synthesis of somatomedin (a protein that stimulates the growth of cartilage) occur at night and are inhibited by cortisol, glycogen and catecholamines produced during the day. Adam and Oswald (1983) concluded that much of healing takes place at night, or during resting and sleeping, and this remains a widely held view. However, Horne (1988) argues that the conditions of night-time, resting and sleeping need to be considered separately. Cell repair takes place most efficiently during wakeful resting and can be shown to be reduced during sleep. Human growth hormone is released at night, but this continues to occur during sleep deprivation and is likely to be associated with circadian rhythms rather than sleep as such; its function in adults is not understood.

Sleep is commonly subdivided into REM sleep, during which dreaming occurs, and non-REM or slow wave sleep (SWS). Horne (1988) suggests that a further useful division is into essential or core sleep and optional or behaviourally learned sleep. He suggests that core sleep takes place during the first part of sleeping and that about 5 hours (three cycles, see below) are necessary for most people on a long-term basis.

188 PSYCHOLOGY FOR HEALTH CARE

Awake: small irregular beta waves, eyes open, thinking

Threshold: alpha rhythm, relaxed wakefulness, drifting, eyes closed

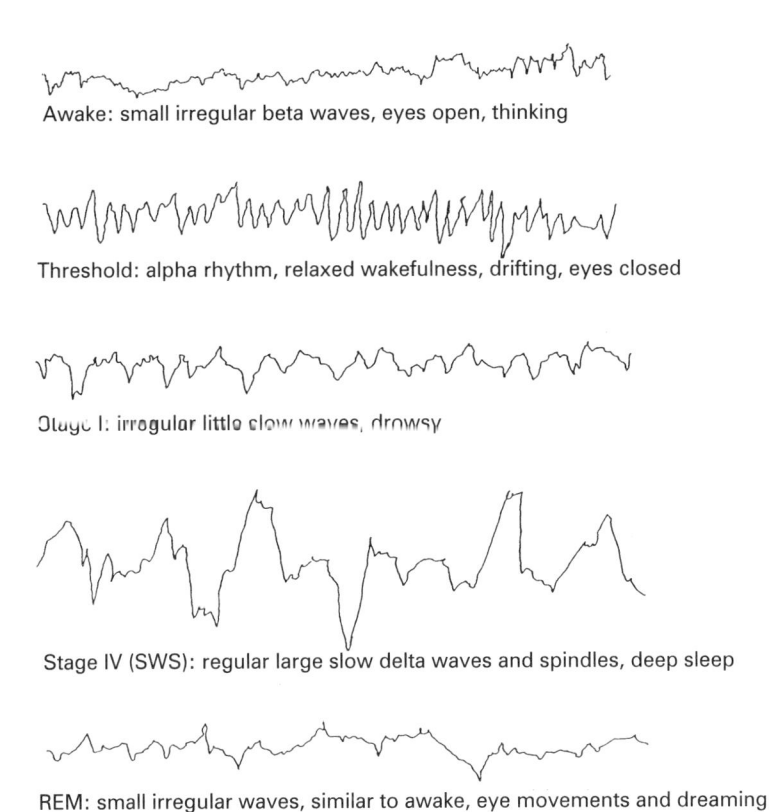

Stage I: irregular little slow waves, drowsy

Stage IV (SWS): regular large slow delta waves and spindles, deep sleep

REM: small irregular waves, similar to awake, eye movements and dreaming

Figure 12.1 EEG wave traces in sleep

Sleep cycles: sleep occurs in a series of cycles throughout the night, on average four or five cycles of about an hour and a half each. Different stages of sleep can be identified through the observation of visible signs, difficulty of waking and characteristic EEG traces (Table 12.1) (see also Chapter 5). The waves when awake (beta waves) are similar to those of REM sleep. These are small irregular traces. During 'orthodox' sleep, the waves gradually become slower and bigger from threshold (alpha waves) to stage I and on to stage IV (delta waves) (see Figure 12.1). Each person has a unique style and timing, so much so that experimenters watching the EEG recorder can predict what is about to happen. Typically, each cycle consists of a gradual descent through stage I, stage II and stage III to stage IV, which is deep or delta sleep, followed by dreaming or REM sleep. After about 10 minutes of dreaming, the first REM period ceases. The person may turn over in bed, and begin the cycle again, down through stage II to stage IV, slowly rising again for another REM dream. The entire cycle is repeated four or five times. Towards morning, the person no longer sinks to the bottom in delta sleep, and REM periods are longer. Sleep becomes lighter, the body temperature

Table 12.1 Stages of a normal sleep cycle

Stage	Brain waves	Behaviour and sensations	Depth of sleep	Physiological changes	Dreams
awake	**beta**: small irregular waves	concentrated thought, activity			coherent thoughts
threshold	**alpha**: small, even rhythm 9–13 per second	serene relaxation, no concentrated thought	relaxed wakefulness		fragments of thought
myoclonic jerk	tiny burst	sudden spasm	momentary arousal		
I	small, pinched, irregular, changing	floating, drifting sensation, idle thoughts	can still be woken easily	muscles relaxing, pulse even, breathing regular, temp. falling	little fragments of images and thoughts
II	growing larger, quick bursts	if eyes are open, will not see	needs modest sound to awaken	eyes roll slowly from side to side	low-intensity dreams, rarely recalled
III	large, slow waves, one per second	removed from the waking world	needs louder noises to awaken	muscles relaxed, breathing even, heart rate slow, temp. and blood pressure down	as stage II
IV	**delta**: very large slow waves	period of bed-wetting, sleep-walking or oblivion	most difficult to wake	temp. and blood pressure at lowest	poor recall, apparent oblivion
REM	irregular, small, similar to when awake	rapid eye movements as if watching	hard to bring to surface and reality	low muscle tone, rising pulse, blood pressure, breathing and temp., twitching	very vivid dreams, 85% of the time

The entire cycle is repeated roughly every 90 minutes, or about four or five times in a night.

begins to rise and body chemistry changes, ready for waking. On awakening, a fragment of dream may be recalled, a moment of awakening or nothing at all. It is extremely rare for anyone to recall enough to account for all the time spent in REM sleep, although some people can if wakened at the time.

Sleep deprivation: under experimental conditions, deprivation of slow wave, deep or delta sleep (SWS) tends to lead to physical symptoms, aches and pains, depression and apathy. Deprivation of REM sleep may lead to mood changes, hostility, irritation, anxiety and behaviour changes, which may be perceived as changes in personality. When deprived of all sleep, it is the delta sleep that is made up first. When deprived only of REM sleep, volunteers tend to lapse into REM sleep almost as soon as they are allowed to close their eyes (Oswald, 1966). No physiological effects of sleep deprivation have been reliably found, and psychological effects are felt to be due more to levels of motivation rather than to impairment up to about 3 days of deprivation. After this time, there are measurable changes in cognitive function, and this suggests that sleep is essential for brain repair and restoration.

Sleep duration: most people have an idea of what they consider to be the right amount of sleep – and do their best to make their children conform to that norm. The usual figure given is 7–8 hours a night, more for young children, and considerably more for babies. There are some, particularly older people, who go to the doctor complaining of insomnia because they are not having a regular 8 hours sleep, even if they do not have any other symptoms. 'Good' sleepers generally fill in questionnaires to the effect that they take about 7 minutes to get to sleep and have about 7 or 8 hours of sleep a night. 'Poor' sleepers think they take an hour to fall asleep, wake at least three times in the night and only have a few hours sleep (McGhie and Russell, 1962). Perceptions can be listed as follows:

- 8%   less than 5 hours
- 15% 5–6 hours
- 62% 7–8 hours
- 13% 9–10 hours
- 2%   more than 10 hours.

Laboratory findings suggest that, for those in the first group, people's beliefs about how long they sleep can be widely inaccurate: they often sleep for as long as the others but perhaps at a higher level, and with a different sort of pattern.

Horne's (1988) division into essential and optional sleep suggests that the majority of people could thrive on 5 hours of sleep but that extra sleep is used to conform to social patterns, occupy the dark hours of the night and provide a surplus that allows for coping readily with short-term deprivation.

Sleep paralysis: unpleasant dreams in which the dreamer struggles to escape some impending danger but is unable to move. EEG records show that the main muscles are indeed paralysed, as during all dreaming sleep, but there may be facial twitching and strangled cries.

Sleep switching mechanisms: various parts of the brain are interconnected and responsible for controlling sleeping and waking. The pineal body (or pineal gland), deep inside the brain at the top of the brain stem, is the part of the brain that controls the biological clock – the diurnal rhythms. One of its functions is to receive information indirectly from the eyes, and it responds to darkness by producing melatonin. The melatonin affects those brain cells that produce serotonin, and this in turn affects the switching mechanisms.

Pineal body → melatonin→ serotonin → switches

In the brain stem, there are three distinct 'switches': for waking (reticular activating system), deep sleep (raphe system) and dreaming sleep (locus coerulus):

- The switch for normal, deep (stages I–IV), sleep is called the raphe system. If this is destroyed, the owner becomes incapable of sleep, however tired
- At the same time as the raphe system is switching on to permit sleep, the activating system switches off. The full name for this is the *reticular activating system*, and it is probably active when noradrenaline is present. When it is switched off, information from the sense organs and other parts of the brain do not reach the higher centres of the cortex
- A third switch, the locus coerulus (from the Latin, meaning blue region), is important in dreaming sleep: it prevents the dreamer getting up and acting out the dream.

Serotonin is also implicated in control of mood. A lack of serotonin, perhaps because of a lack of sunlight, may be responsible for seasonal affective disorder (SAD) (see Chapter 2).

Sleepwalking: it is well known that most people move quite a bit during sleep and that some talk or sleepwalk. These bodily movements tend to occur during periods of deep, stage IV, delta sleep and, surprisingly, are rarely associated with dreaming or the recall of dreams.

Sleepy sickness: Oliver Sacks (1991), in *Awakenings*, describes patients who are among the few survivors of an epidemic (encephalitis lethargica) that occurred in the 1920s. (The term 'sleepy sickness' is usually used to distinguish between this condition and the sleeping sickness transmitted by the tsetse fly in Africa.) Sacks describes in detail what the experience was like for the people as he tries out various treatments, in particular high doses of L-dopa, which 'woke' the patients and brought them back to a state of consciousness.

13 Pain and Pain Management

Pain is an unpleasant subjective experience generally associated with tissue damage. Some of the definitions given below could apply to all sorts of unpleasant experience, and there is little in the words themselves to make it clear quite what is involved. It is only by talking with others about experiences and finding that same word – 'pain' – is used to refer to certain kinds of feeling that one can come to have some kind of shared meaning for the word. There is disagreement on the exact range of experiences correctly identified by the word 'pain'.

Definitions	
C.S. Lewis (1940)	A particular kind of sensation... recognised by the patient as that kind of sensation, whether he dislikes it or not... or any experience, whether physical or mental, which the patient dislikes ... synonymous with suffering, anguish, tribulation, adversity or trouble.
Sternbach (1968)	an abstract concept which refers to (a) 'a personal private sensation of hurt', (b) 'a harmful stimulus which signals current or impending tissue damage', and (c) 'a pattern of responses which operate to protect the organism from harm.
McCaffery (1968)	what the experiencing person says it is, existing when he says it does...
McCaffery (1983)	an unpleasant sensation interwoven with a reactive or emotional component, and the emotional component itself may intensify the perception and expression of the pain encountered.
Merskey (1979)	An unpleasant sensory and emotional experience associated with actual or potential tissue damage or described in terms of such damage.

Definitions (cont'd)	
Wall and Melzack (1984)	a need state, just like hunger and thirst... the purpose of pain is to signal to the body impending injury or that it needs to rest.

Approaches, Arguments and Applications

Some writers, like Sternbach, Wall and Melzack, quoted above, believe that pain may represent a threat and result in some kind of reaction or response, but this seems to apply only to acute pain for which the cause is known and which does seem to be acting as a warning signal. With chronic pain, the cause is often not known, and it no longer seems to serve any purpose. C.S. Lewis (1940) includes mental suffering and anguish, which need not be associated with a physical sensation. He also suggests that there might be some kinds of sensation of pain that are not disliked. This suggests that it is the meaning of the pain for a person and not just the sensation that has significance. Skevington (1995) disagrees and argues that the definition by Merskey (1979) is particularly useful in the context of health care as it makes it clear that experiences resembling pain but which are not unpleasant, and unpleasant emotional experiences that are not connected with sensory qualities, should not be regarded as pain. McCaffery's (1968) definition is favoured by many health professionals as it suggests that an open approach is necessary, but it does little to explain what pain actually is or why we feel it.

Most modern approaches take the view that the perception of pain is psychologically determined. In contrast, early theories of pain assumed that all sensations of pain were due only to tissue damage.

Two early theories of pain are the specificity theory and the pattern theory. The specificity theory was based on the assumption that there are specific nerve fibres that, when damaged, carry pain messages directly to the brain. The pattern theory added to this the belief that other fibres that normally carry messages of warmth, cold and pressure can also convey pain if stimulated in a particular way. Both these theories lead to a linear model of pain indicating that tissue damage leads to stimulation of the pain-carrying nerves, which in turn leads to a sensation of pain and then to pain behaviour. When these theories were first developed, it was not understood how they interrelated, and there was much argument over which one was 'right'. It can now be seen that there are elements of truth in both approaches, and also that neither is wholly adequate.

If these are the only theories used, and all pain is explained in terms of the linear model, certain assumptions automatically follow. Medical treatment of pain was, until recently, conducted primarily according to these assumptions:

- If the amount of pain is seen as proportional to the amount of damage, it would follow that the dose of analgesics needed is proportional to amount of damage, irrespective of individual differences

- If pain behaviour is seen as proportional to pain, it would follow that if no pain behaviour is being exhibited, no pain is being felt. This would mean that babies and other people who do not express pain behaviour feel no pain and do not need analgesics
- If pain behaviour is seen as proportional to damage, it would follow that if there is no detectable damage, pain behaviour is inappropriate. If pain behaviour is exhibited, this would indicate that the pain is imagined and is not deserving of analgesics or other medical treatment.

Pain is now viewed as a much more complex process. Some talk about the puzzle or paradox of pain whenever it is difficult to explain why pain is felt or not felt or an individual's experience seems to contradict all expectations (Melzack, 1973). Although specific nerve pathways have been identified, there are various instances of the 'presence of pain in the absence of damage' and the 'absence of pain in the presence of damage', and the specificity theory is not sufficient for the following reasons:

- Not all specialised nerves are specific only to pain; for example, naked nerve endings in the ear that carry pain messages also carry messages of touch, hot, cold and so on
- Internal organs are poorly innervated and generalised; pain can be felt which is not related to specific pathways
- Damage in one part of the body can give rise to pain sensations elsewhere – *referred pain* – which does not always follow specific paths
- Similar damage gives rise to very different reports of pain, depending on circumstances and the past history of patient
- Because of congenital and acquired insensitivity, despite an intact nervous system
- As a result of phantom pain after amputation.

To try to provide explanations for these phenomena, the gate control theory was developed (Melzack and Wall, 1965, 1982; Melzack and Dennis, 1978; Wall and Melzack, 1984). This is based on evidence that pain messages carried by certain nerve fibres can be interrupted before reaching the brain. Specific pain-carrying nerves have been identified. Examples of these are the A-delta fibres, which convey immediate or sharp pain, and C fibres, which carry dull and aching pain. These specific nerve fibres are in the peripheral nervous system. This system can only connect with the central nervous system by means of the synapses in the spinal column. If the chemical action at each synapse can be altered, the pain messages will not be able to cross the gap. This can happen in response to physical or psychological stimuli. The pain messages can be interrupted by physical counterirritants, such as rubbing or applying warmth or cold. They can be affected psychologically as a result of the action of endorphins, which can be produced in the brain in response to cortical activity. It is found that our memories, the way in which we coped with previous experiences, our beliefs and expectations, all processed within the cortex, are somehow able to alter the levels of endorphins, so that we can, in effect, have control over how much pain we feel.

This 'control' is largely unconscious and not easily conjured up by sheer willpower but is responsive to our lifelong experiences and can be affected by counselling and support. Analgesics are no longer given solely in proportion to the visible damage but in response to how the patient perceives his or her pain. Where possible, a variety of psychological interventions are also used. Acute pain may be treated primarily with analgesics with supporting short-term counselling to encourage positive attitudes. Earlier 'no pain, no gain' attitudes have been replaced by 'less pain, more gain' approaches (Allis, 1992), and analgesics may be administered before pain is likely to be felt. The suggestion is that if the patient never experiences pain beyond manageable levels, he or she will not anticipate pain and will, therefore, become proficient in 'keeping the gate closed' (see gate control theory).

For chronic pain, more structured approaches are needed, and many pain clinics employ a multimodal regime. Relaxation, massage, exercise, group counselling, individual and family pain management counselling and even faith healing may be combined with the administration of pain-relieving drugs or TENS. Counselling may be focused on encouraging positive confronting attitudes, learning from past experiences, fostering self-efficacy and diminishing learned helplessness or sick-role behaviour.

Biopsychological approaches: these include the linear model based on specificity theory and pattern theory, and the gate control theory, which help to relate our experience of pain to physiological processes and explain the action of biological, physical and psychological interventions. Related interventions include medication, exercise, relaxation, slapping, rubbing or massage, warmth, infra-red lamps or heat rubs, cold from ice packs, menthol or camphor, and TENS.

Behavioural approaches: these consider how pain behaviours may be learned and maintained or strengthened through conditioning. Interventions involve changing pain thresholds and pain tolerance, and altering learned helplessness and sick-role behaviour, either individually or by involving the family.

Social approaches: these are based on social learning theory, communication theory and a knowledge of groups and social support systems. Interventions include developing improved pain assessment techniques, paying attention to subtle cues from body language, providing appropriate role models and setting up group therapy sessions and support groups.

Cognitive approaches: these are based on health belief models and include models of confronting and avoiding attitudes to pain. Interventions are aimed at helping people to examine their beliefs, memories and expectations about their pain and their ability to manage it. Strategies include the use of distraction, imagery, information-giving and the facilitation of self-efficacy.

Psychodynamic approaches: these encourage exploration of repressed memories and conflict, relating to early experiences and the way in which defensive behaviour may have developed. The aim is to improve insight and work towards more effective management of pain.

Humanistic and integrative approaches: these aim to empower the patient, giving the patient control over the amount of analgesic to be given, and involvement in care and planning. Any approach which interrupts a habitual cycle of pain and distress can help the patient towards a more positive pain management. Multimodal pain management may include complementary therapies such as *Alexander technique* to teach beneficial posture and movement, hypnosis, exercise, relaxation, acupuncture, massage, aromatherapy, shiatsu, yoga and similar techniques to improve muscle tone and reduce tension and pain, chiropractic and osteopathy to realign bones and muscles. Faith healing may be used.

Key Terms and Concepts

A-beta (Aβ) fibres: large-diameter nerve fibres in the peripheral nervous system that can carry messages of warmth, cold and pressure to the central nervous system.

Acupuncture: a technique based on ideas suggesting that life or ch'i energy flows along meridians. It is carried out by inserting needles or exerting pressure at key points on the body. Some of the meridians connect with the organs they are thought to influence, but it is believed to work by boosting the production of natural endorphins and 'closing the gate' (see gate control theory). It has been found to raise the *pain threshold* in about 25 per cent of participants. Although used mainly as a method of pain relief, it can also be used to treat a variety of physical and psychological problems.

Acute and chronic pain: Loeser and Fordyce (1983) consider that chronic and acute pain have nothing in common. It is helpful to make the following distinctions between acute and chronic pain.

acute	chronic (3–6 months or more)
short lived	long lived
reversible	seemingly incurable
often localised	often diffuse
seen as a warning	no longer a warning
cause usually identified	cause may be unknown
associated with anxiety	depression and exhaustion
short-term psychological intervention helps.	long-term psychological adjustment is needed.

Turk *et al.* (1983) identify three kinds of chronic pain:

- chronic/recurrent: repeated intense episodes of pain from a benign cause, for example migraine headaches
- chronic/intractable: constant discomfort with varying levels of intensity from a benign cause, for example back pain
- chronic/progressive: continuous, increasing in intensity as the underlying cause worsens, for example associated with malignant conditions.

A-Delta (Aδ) fibres: myelinated nerve fibres in the peripheral nervous system that carry messages of immediate or sharp pain to the central nervous system.

Adjuvants: helpful or auxiliary items not related directly to the patient's illness, such as relieving the physical discomfort caused by a loaded bowel.

Analgesics: pain-relieving medicines or drugs (painkillers). Pain can be reduced by interfering in some way with the nervous pathways between the brain and the site of injury in the periphery. This can be achieved locally or systemically by administering analgesics that act at appropriate points in the pathway. Opioids such as codeine, morphine and cocaine affect the transmission of pain messages in the spinal cord and their reception in the brain. Non-opioid drugs, such as paracetamol, and non-steroidal anti-inflammatory drugs (NSAIDs), such as aspirin and ibuprofen, reduce the strength of impulses in the peripheral nervous system or in the brain stem. The injection or topical application of local anaesthetic produces a transient, reversible blockade of nerve function and numbs the area.

Aspirin: an analgesic with anti-inflammatory and antipyretic activity, which, when it enters the bloodstream, acts at the site of injury by blocking the release of prostaglandins, which cause the firing of nociceptors. This reduces the frequency of nerve impulses or action potentials in the pain-carrying nerves.

Assessment of pain: the treatment of pain relies on a thorough assessment, the aim of which is to discover the causes, intensity, location, duration, antecedents and consequences of the pain. Information about the following should also be sought: factors that ease or worsen the pain; coping strategies that have been used and their effects; the coping resource available; related or concurrent symptoms; and the meaning and significance of the pain to the sufferer.

Methods of pain assessment include the direct observation of behaviour, structured interviews, a patient's diary (for example, Fordyce, 1976); and the use of *assessment scales, pain questionnaires* and the *multiple-baseline approach*.

Assessment scales: a pain assessment or rating scale can be used to indicate a person's perception of the intensity of their pain. Scales are not useful for setting standards or comparing patients but are helpful in monitoring a particular patient's changes in experience, perception and tolerance. Three kinds of scales are most commonly used: visual analogue, numerical rating and verbal descriptor.

A visual analogue scale consists of a straight line with one end marked 'no pain at all' and the other marked 'worst possible pain'. The patient is asked to mark the point on the line that represents the present pain level. If subdivision lines are included on an analogue scale, the sensitivity of the pain measure may be reduced as the user may have a tendency to mark the scale near or on those lines. Numerical rating scales (for example, Linton and Gotestam, 1983) consist of a continuum from 0 to 10, 0 signifying no pain and 10 unbearable pain. Verbal descriptor scales (for example, Tursky, 1976; Houde, 1982) use words such as 'none', 'slight', 'moderate', 'severe' and 'unbearable' to try to convey differences in pain level but are often unable to convey subtle changes. Although the words are placed at equal intervals along a line, the intervals do not necessarily signify consistent changes in pain intensity. Some assessment tools (for example, Bourbonnais, 1981) combine numerical and verbal descriptor scales.

Special scales based on pictures of facial expressions are available for use with children. Horgan and Choonara (1996) have devised the Liverpool

Infant Distress Scale, which is designed to assist nurses in assessing pain in neonates by close examination of their behaviour and facial expressions.

C fibres: unmyelinated nerve fibres that carry messages of dull or aching pain from the body to the central nervous system.

Children and pain: Allis (1992) discusses the way in which doctors have assumed that babies under 6 months of age do not feel pain and that 'society is hysterical about making a four-year old a heroin addict'. Allis reviews technological and psychological advances in assessing and managing pain. Collier *et al.* (1993) cite research by Burr (1987, 1993), Devine (1990) and Eland (1985) in relation to the myths associated with pain and distress in children. They list the following 12 common inconsistencies or myths that are repeatedly discussed in the literature:

- Active children cannot be in pain
- Children will always tell you when they are in pain
- It is often being restrained during procedures, rather than any pain involved, that children find distressing
- Parents know the best way to manage their children's pain
- Children cannot accurately tell you where it hurts
- There is generally a 'usual' amount of pain associated with any procedure
- Children feel less pain than adults
- Children forget pain more quickly than adults
- It is unsafe to administer narcotics to children because they become addicted
- Narcotics always depress respiration in children
- The best way to administer analgesia is by injection
- The less analgesia administered to children, the better it is for them.

Cognitive appraisal: sorting out the beliefs, knowledge and understanding that persons may have about their situation and the pain they are experiencing, the value they place on the experience and their expectations. See also Chapter 6.

Congenital insensitivity to pain: a rare genetic variation in which the person feels no pain despite having an intact nervous system. As the warning function of pain does not operate, injuries and illnesses can go unnoticed and may deteriorate.

Context: intuitive experience and research indicate that the context in which an injury or potential pain-producing event occurs can greatly affect the amount of pain experienced. Toothache is less noticeable when one is busy. Injury during sport, particularly matches, may be ignored. Rough horseplay with children is not seen as painful, whereas similar treatment in another context would be. Injuries sustained in war appear less painful than similar civilian injuries (Beecher, 1956, 1959). Pain-reducing relaxation techniques practised prenatally may be effective in normal childbirth but not in a late miscarriage, when the baby is known to be dead.

Counterirritants: these act by stimulating sensory A-beta nerves, which compete with pain signals from the affected area. Counterirritants can include warmth, for example from a hot water bottle, infra-red lamp or rubefacient embrocations (heat rubs); cold, for example from an ice pack, menthol or camphor; rubbing, slapping or massage; and electrical stimulation (TENS). See also gate control theory.

Culture: cross-cultural studies reveal differences in patterns of behaviour, but it is not clear whether these are related to different experiences of pain or to different coping mechanisms. For example, Zborowski (1969) reported that third-generation Americans and Irish immigrants were more stoic, admitting less pain than Jewish immigrants, who tended to avoid pain situations but give immediate expression if in pain.

Distraction (attention diversion): a common-sense technique used to help people when anticipating or experiencing pain, for example, from injections or the removal of stitches. It is most effective with brief, localised peripheral pain in which the pain threshold is raised; that is, the intervention may be noticed but not perceived as painful. In acute and chronic pain situations in which the pain may be 'attended to' by the sufferer, distraction can help to refocus attention elsewhere. Tan (1982) identifies three categories of techniques of distraction:

- attention diversion to external events, which involves focusing on aspects of the environment, such as counting the slats in the blinds or stripes on the wallpaper, watching television, listening to music (portable CD or cassette players are useful in hospital settings), playing board games, painting, talking to others or any activity that is enjoyed.
- attention diversion to internal events, such as doing mental arithmetic, composing a poem or listening to one's own heartbeat
- somatisation, which involves focusing on pain in a detached manner, for example analysing the pain as if preparing to write an article about it for a magazine.

Dorsal horns: the region of the spinal cord where incoming *afferent* (sensory) nerves make connections with the central nervous system.

Empathic pain: recognition and entering into the feelings of pain of another person. Examples are sometimes quoted of twins feeling each other's pain, of fathers-to-be feeling labour pains and of the carers or friends of a patient experiencing pain in the same part or the body, although usually only for an instant.

Endorphins: morphine-like substances produced within the organism. The word is a contraction of endomorphine. See opioid peptides.

Enkephalins: see opioid peptides.

Exercise: thought to stimulate the production of endorphins, enkephalins and serotonin so that the input of stimuli via the 'gate' is altered and pain tolerance increases. Those with chronic pain may need advice on whether activity despite pain is worthwhile. See also Chapter 7.

Faith healing: like acupuncture and hypnosis, faith healing has been found to raise the pain threshold and tolerance in suggestible and imaginative people, although there is no evidence that it alters the production of endorphins. It is offered in some pain management clinics.

Gate control theory: Melzack and Wall (1965, 1982), Melzack and Dennis (1978) and Wall and Melzack (1984) developed the gate control theory in which they consider that pain messages carried by the specific nerve fibres (A-delta and C fibres) can be interrupted before reaching the brain by the action of other nerve fibres.

The model suggests the action of a gate in the dorsal horns of the spinal column where nerve fibres meet. Pain messages may be carried through the *substantia gelatinosa* of the dorsal horns to special *T-cells* in the spinal column, which relay pain messages to the brain. However, messages of heat, cold and pressure carried by large-diameter A-beta fibres may activate intervening nerves in the substantia gelatinosa, preventing the pain messages reaching the T-cells and thus closing the gate. This may explain why applying warmth or cold to a painful area, simple massage or *TENS* can act as counterirritants and reduce, mask or even replace pain.

In addition, messages descending the spinal column from the brain can also close the gate. It appears that this process involves the production of natural pain-suppressing substances in the brain stem and spinal cord such as the endorphins, enkephalins and dynorphins (opioid peptides), which act in a similar way to morphine. This can be activated by memories of previous painful experiences that have been managed well, the perception of supportive surroundings and a positive meaning of pain, which lead to expectations that coping will occur again. In contrast, memories and expectations about poor pain control and factors such as boredom and anxiety can lead to opening the gate.

This theory can account for many of the psychological, anthropological and sociological data concerning individual and cultural differences in pain experience and behaviour.

As it stands, the gate control theory does not examine the relationships between the sizes of fibres and pain sensation, nor does it explain individual differences in pain avoidance behaviour in relation to high pain sensation, that is, when pain messages are still getting through the gate.

Gender: there is considerable debate, but little research evidence, surrounding the issue of whether men or women have a greater tolerance of pain. There do seem to be differences. Women appear to report more emotional distress, but it is not clear whether this is related to the amount of pain felt. Levine and de Simone (1991) found that the amount of pain reported depended on the gender of the person reported to: males reported less pain when reporting to females in a clinical setting and took fewer analgesics when looked after by a female nurse, perhaps wishing to preserve a macho image. No differences were revealed with female patients.

Group counselling: used in multimodal pain clinics, where the guided sharing of experience helps to reduce anxiety and feelings of isolation, and can help to focus attention on positive attributes and the development of coping strategies. Sessions may be led by a psychologist or trained nurse.

Hypnotism: as a method of inducing deep relaxation or distraction by focusing attention on suggested specific emotional or physical experiences, hypnotism has been found to be effective in raising the pain threshold by as much as 85 per cent. A trance-like state is not necessary. It is not clear whether hypnotism can directly affect the production of natural opioid peptides. See also Chapter 12.

Ibuprofen: a non-steroidal, anti-inflammatory, non-narcotic analgesic, available for oral administration as tablets, sustained-release capsules or syrup. It is also available as a gel for direct application to an affected area. The main action, as for aspirin, is at the site of injury.

Imagery: this may be used in a number of different ways to help a person to develop new perceptions in order to alter cognitions or act as a distraction from the pain. Tan (1982) lists three main types:

- imaginative transformation of the pain, which involves the interpretation of pain sensations as something other than pain, for example transforming it into other sensory qualities such as warmth or tingling, or minimising the sensations as being trivial or unreal
- imaginative inattention, which involves evoking imagery that is incompatible with pain and that distracts from it, for example conjuring up images of an enjoyable holiday
- imaginative transformation of the context in which the person is encouraged to acknowledge the pain and to think of a situation or context in which it would not be troublesome, such as being a hero who has been wounded while rescuing someone from the enemy.

Linear models of pain: models of the process of the pain experience that are based on early specificity theories.

Sternbach (1968) identifies a three-part linear process, in which each stage leads to the next and there is direct proportionality between the stages:

$$\text{noxious stimulus} \rightarrow \text{sensation} \rightarrow \text{response}$$

The response may be behavioural (lifting a hand away from the flame or screaming), emotional (feeling anxious or upset) or physiological (autonomic nervous system arousal).

This linear process can be outlined in more detail, incorporating stages suggested by von Frey at the end of the nineteenth century:

$$\text{noxious stimulus received by nociceptors}$$
$$\downarrow$$
$$\text{tissue injury}$$
$$\downarrow$$
$$\text{impulse in pain pathway}$$
$$\downarrow$$
$$\text{activation of pain centre in brain}$$
$$\downarrow$$
$$\text{pain sensation}$$
$$\downarrow$$
$$\text{pain behaviour}$$

These linear models give rise to certain assumptions that, until recently, influenced pain treatment (see Approaches, Arguments and Applications above).

Local anaesthetics: these prevent the generation and propagation of action potentials at any point along a nerve. Since the pain-carrying fibres are of smaller diameter than other nerves, the action on these is greater, and the experience is of a reduction in pain without the loss of other sensations or motor control.

Massage: pain relief can be gained by massage at or near the affected site. It is probable that the relief is gained either through distraction, through the release of endorphins or because massage interferes with pain messages. See gate control theory. Blood flow is also increased to the area, and this can give a sense of warmth and relaxation.

Morphine: an analgesic and narcotic drug obtained from opium and used medicinally to relieve pain. It acts by binding to specific pain receptors in the brain (particularly the brain stem) and the dorsal horns of the spinal cord. It depresses the activity of T-cells and affects the ways in which pain messages are transmitted and received in the brain. When misused, morphine may produce respiratory depression and a state of euphoria, which can lead to addiction.

Multimodal pain management programmes: some pain control clinics offer a variety of therapies and treatments. Not only do some approaches suit some people better than others, but it is believed that the combination is far more effective for everyone than are single treatments. See *pain management*.

Multiple-baseline approach: a cognitive approach that includes observation of specific pain behaviours; see, for example, Lefebvre (1981), Rosenteil and Keefe (1983), Kerns *et al.* (1985), the Pain Experience Questionnaire (PEQ) and the Multidimensional Pain Inventory (MPI). The questionnaires are used to help patients and carers to identify patients' beliefs about their pain.

Nociceptors: these are specialised receptors in the skin and elsewhere that respond to noxious (harmful) stimuli such as excess heat, cold, pressure and chemical substances. When stimulated, messages (action potentials) are carried along specific nerve fibres to the central nervous system.

Non-opioids: analgesics that do not contain opium or opium derivatives.

Non-steroidal anti-inflammatory drugs (NSAIDs): these inhibit prostaglandin synthesis. The group includes aspirin and ibuprofen.

Opiate: a narcotic drug containing opium, or generally a substance that soothes or stupefies.

Opioid: a substance containing derivatives of opium such as morphine, cocaine, codeine, and related chemicals, for example natural opioid peptides.

Opioid peptides: a group of neurotransmitters (enkephalins, endorphins and dynorphins) that can be released from neurones and seem to work in similar ways to morphine by binding to specific receptors in the central nervous system. They act mainly in the brain stem and the dorsal horns of the spinal cord. Enkephalins and endorphins have important functions in influencing behavioural responses to painful stimuli by depressing the activity of T-cells and affecting the ways in which pain messages (action potentials) are transmitted and received in the brain.

Opium: the impure narcotic and addictive drug obtained from the opium poppy.

Pain behaviour: behavioural responses to pain vary widely from one person to another and are determined by many different physical, psychological and sociocultural factors. Examples of these include the nature of the disease or injury suffered, the emotional state of the person in pain, the pain threshold and tolerance, the beliefs and expectations that the person holds about pain and social norms, which dictate appropriate ways of behaving.

Turk *et al.* (1985) suggest that pain behaviour can be classified into four types:

- facial/audible expressions of distress, such as grimacing, moaning and clenched teeth
- distorted ambulation or posture and behaviour that is self-protective, such as moving in a guarded way, stooping or holding the painful area
- negative affect, for example irritability
- avoidance of activity, such as social withdrawal or the avoidance of housework, activities, hobbies, exercise or any sort of stimulation.

It can be helpful to distinguish between two contrasting kinds of pain behaviour: confronting and avoiding. Confronting involves facing up to painful situations and taking part in recommended activities in the belief that this will eventually lead to reduced pain. Avoiding behaviour includes withdrawal and the avoidance of painful activities, which people believe will reduce pain. Although pain avoidance may be seen as appropriate for acute pain or as an effective coping mechanism in the short term, it may not be so for chronic pain, when it may be necessary for people to confront their pain and learn new behaviours that, while initially painful or difficult, may lead to better long-term outcomes.

Experience in practice suggests that people use a mixture of these coping strategies, varying from occasion to occasion. Some writers believe that they are related to personality characteristics and identify people as confronters or avoiders according to their typical characteristics. Philips and Jahanshahi (1986) suggest that chronic pain headache sufferers may be either confronters or avoiders. They believe that chronic pain may be sustained by pain avoidance behaviour, which is influenced by the following three types of cognition:

- the balance of expectations about the effects of engaging in events: expectations that there will be an increase of pain on exposure and a decrease with avoidance
- self-efficacy beliefs: the beliefs about the individual's capacity to cope with the pain produced
- memories of past experiences.

Woodgate and Kristjanson (1995) describe three types of behaviour in children: confronting, avoidance or withdrawal, and 'making it good'.

Pain-carrying fibres: these include A-delta and C fibres.

Pain management: pharmacological or other approaches may be used to treat the cause of pain or alter perception or sensation. This may reduce pain or, where pain cannot be eliminated, help people learn to live with and cope with their pain in a constructive way. Strategies are designed to empower the person by confronting learned helplessness and may generate a sense of optimism. Non-drug measures include radiotherapy, surgery, nerve blocks,

TENS, traction, acupuncture, physiotherapy, occupational therapy, relaxation, massage and aromatherapy, and talking.

Lazarus (1981) uses the acronym BASIC ID for a multi-modal approach to the treatment of pain:

- B behaviour
- A affect
- S sensation
- I imagery
- C cognitions
- I interpersonal fractors
- D drugs

Behaviour-focused interventions include the use of operant conditioning techniques to alter or extinguish pain behaviour and to reinforce attempts to cope (for example, Fordyce, 1976). Anticipatory pain can be linked to classical conditioning. Gains from displaying pain behaviour, such as avoidance of disliked activities or obtaining attention from others, can be explained in terms of reinforcement. See Chapter 4.

The affect or mood may need to be the target of interventions if the person in pain also experiences associated depression or anxiety. See Chapters 2 and 6.

Pain sensations can be altered directly by using counterirritant techniques such as massage, manipulation, the application of heat or cold, acupuncture or TENS. Surgical interventions may be used in severe cases to remove or disconnect part of the peripheral nervous system in order to prevent the pain signals from reaching the brain. Indirect strategies to alter pain sensation include exercise. See Chapters 6 and 7.

Imagery can be used for attention diversion and cognitive restructuring. See above and Chapter 6.

Strategies addressing cognitions include giving information, cognitive restructuring, using coping statements to emphasise the ability to tolerate pain, self-efficacy beliefs and distraction. See Chapters 6 and 7. Hayward (1975) identifies two kinds of information:

- procedural: how, when, where and who will carry out surgery
- sensory: the nature, severity, location and duration of pain expected after surgery.

Interventions that have an interpersonal focus include the development of language used for communication, the interpretation of body language and other signs, responses to pain behaviour and the use of role-models. See Chapters 4 and 9.

There are several useful ways of classifying the main types of drug that are used to treat pain. These can be classed as opioid or non-opioid, centrally acting or peripherally acting, systemic or local, and direct or indirect. See analgesics.

Pain questionnaires: can be used to obtain a range of information about a person's pain. An example is the McGill Pain Questionnaire devised by Melzack (1975). This contains four parts:

- the location of pain on the body, including whether it is internal or external
- a description of the pain in relation to three components:
  – emotional-motivational, such as terrifying, vicious, tiring
  – sensory-perceptual, such as pounding, stabbing, burning
  – cognitive-evaluative, such as unbearable, troublesome
- how the pain changes with time
- the present pain intensity.

Pain threshold: the level of stimulus that is just noticeable as painful. This can be lowered by discomfort, insomnia, fatigue, anxiety, fear, anger, sadness, depression, boredom, introversion, mental isolation and social abandonment (Twycross, 1975). It can be raised by distraction, counterirritants, acupuncture, hypnosis and counselling or therapy.

Pain tolerance: technically, the level of stimulus at which the sensation or experience of pain is perceived as just on the borderline of unbearable. Hence, raising pain tolerance (strictly speaking) means raising the level of pain that is just bearable. However, in practice the term is used to refer to pain that is readily bearable, and increasing tolerance usually means bringing perceptions of pain within a reasonably comfortable range rather than having them at the top limit. There are big differences between what can be tolerated in the short term and in the long term, so tolerance usually refers to both level and duration.

Paracetamol: an analgesic with antipyretic activity similar to aspirin but without anti-inflammatory activity. It inhibits prostaglandin synthesis more in the brain or brain stem than in the peripheral nervous system.

Paradoxical pain: pain is sometimes increased by measures that would normally be expected to reduce pain. For some people, morphine can actually increase pain.

Patient-controlled analgesia (PCA): a strategy for dealing with acute pain, particularly following surgical intervention (Ferrant *et al.*, 1990). The patient can control the amount and rate at which an analgesic drug is administered within preset safety limits, usually by means of a digital pump connected to a catheter. It is found that many people experience less anxiety, and subsequently less pain, when they are in control of this timing and do not have to rely on routine drug administration, attracting someone's attention, or being otherwise constrained. However, it has also been noted that a few people may feel more anxious when having to take responsibility.

Pattern theory: pattern theories relate pain to the patterns (frequency and strength) of impulses in the nervous system rather than to specific pathways. Thus any excessive stimulus (heat, cold, pressure and so on), rather than just those affecting specialised nociceptors and A-delta or C fibres, can produce pain. Livingstone (1943) proposed that small stimuli can sometimes set off reverberating circuits that send volleys of impulses to the brain and are interpreted as pain. These theories are better able than specificity theory to account for differences in pain perception, but none of these early theories explains individual differences as satisfactorily as does the gate theory.

Phantom pain: any unpleasant sensation that is felt in a part of the body which has been removed by disease, accident or surgery. The person may complain of sensations that are not usually regarded as being painful, for example, itching, tingling or sweating. Explanations include persistent spinal cord and brain activity without input from the periphery, persistent peripheral activity in the severed nerves, and neuromas in the stump. There is some evidence that people who are fully informed before an operation about the existence of this phenomenon, and the explanations for it, are less likely to experience it.

Placebo medication: *placebo* is from the Latin meaning 'I shall be acceptable or pleasing.' There are two types of placebo:

- Inert placebos are those which contain pharmacologically inactive substances and are knowingly used as placebos
- Active placebos are those which contain some compound with pharmacological activity and which are prescribed in the knowledge that their pharmacological activity is not appropriate, in the mistaken belief that it is, or is at a level below the recommended dose for clinical effectiveness.

Melzack and Wall (1982) state that placebos can be effective in treating pain. The pain-relieving effects of placebos are thought to stem from the belief of the receiver that they will work. Fields and Levine (1984) suggest that positive expectations trigger the release of natural opoids. As the administration of placebo medication can involve deception, health-care professionals need carefully to consider the ethical issues involved in their use. See also Chapter 18.

Post-herpetic pain: chronic pain which may arise from permanent nerve damage even after healing has apparently occurred.

Psychogenic pain: pain that does not appear to have any organic or neural origin, such as *empathic* pain. The assumption is that the pain is somehow psychologically generated, perhaps as a result of a vivid imagination or suggestion. See also Chapters 12 and 20.

Referred pain: sometimes known as transferred pain, this is pain felt not where the damage actually occurs but somewhere else in the body. For example, it is common for someone who has toothache to feel pain in the ear and for people to feel pain across the shoulders after abdominal operations in which the abdomen has been distended with gas. With angina, the pain usually radiates down the inner aspect of the left arm and is often accompanied by a feeling of suffocation.

Van Wynsberghe *et al.* (1995) offer two explanations for referred pain:

- Sensory impulses from the organs and skin share the same pathways
- The real source of the pain develops from the same embryological structure as the area of the body to which the pain is referred, the structures thus being supplied by branches of the same peripheral nerve.

Specificity theory: early approaches (originating with Descartes in the seventeenth century, and developed by von Frey at the end of the nineteenth century) identified naked or free nerve endings (nociceptors) in the skin that respond to noxious (harmful) stimuli and send impulses along pain pathways to a specific area of the brain (the pain centre). Lyn (1984) identifies two groups of pain-carrying nerve fibres: thin, myelinated A-delta fibres (immediate or sharp pain), and unmyelinated C fibres (dull or aching pain). Early specificity theories contributed to the development of linear models of pain. Current anatomical details of the nervous system are incorporated into the gate control theory.

Substantia gelatinosa: the complex arrangement of intervening neurones in the dorsal horns of the spinal column which, when activated, interfere with the transmission of pain messages from the peripheral nervous system to the central nervous system.

Transcutaneous electrical nerve stimulation (TENS): the transmission of tiny electrical impulses across the skin. Small flexible electrodes connected to a control box are placed at or near a painful area. The level of stimulation is usually controlled by the patient after instruction. The sensation is one of a slight tingling. This stimulation affects many nerve endings in the skin and seems to interfere with pain messages as a counterirritant, similarly to rubbing (see gate control theory). If resources allow, people may use this at home once they have mastered the technique. Like patient-controlled analgesia, this method of pain control can give the patient confidence in managing pain and reduce anxiety.

14 PERCEPTION AND RESPONSE TO PERCEPTUAL CHANGES

The study of perception is the study of how meaning is brought to the information received by the senses, the way in which we make sense of our world, both external and internal. Our senses are continuously receiving data about ourselves and the environment and sending signals in the form of action potentials *to the brain. Most of this incoming information is monitored unconsciously so that much of our behaviour and all of our physiological processes are automatic. However, we pay conscious attention to some of it and can talk about what we identify and make conscious decisions about what we do.*

It is often said that we see what we want to see or what we expect to see, and it is realised that these processes are not just a passive 'picking up' of sensory messages but involve a great deal of 'gap-filling' and hypothesising from incomplete data.

Definitions	
Drever (1964)	the process of becoming immediately aware of something; usually employed of sense perception, when the thing of which we become immediately aware is the object affecting a sense organ; when that object is recognised or identified in any way perception passes into apperception. [Note – this distinction between perception and apperception is no longer used: the terms sensation and perception are preferred.]
Gregory (1971)	a matter of reading non-sensed characteristics of objects from available sensory data... [the] senses monitor characteristics immediately important for survival... Their information is useful before objects are identified. [Sense] responses are primitive – pre-perceptual

Definitions (cont'd)	
	reactions, not to objects but to physical conditions (for example, the reflex action of withdrawing the hand from a hot object). Recognising objects, and behaving appropriately to their hidden aspects, comes later.
Stratton and Hayes (1993)	the process by which we analyse and make sense out of incoming sensory information.

Approaches, Arguments and Applications

Understanding the processes of perception helps in appreciating the similarities and differences between people. In one way, the individual's interpretation of surroundings is unique, depending on individual past experiences, needs and interests. This can be particularly important in hospitals and other care settings where the new patient perceives the sights, sounds and smells quite differently from the experienced professional. On the other hand, there are recognisable patterns of perception that can help us to anticipate people's responses and plan accordingly. For example, the colour scheme of a room can influence mood. Background sounds of monitors can invoke fear or reassurance depending on how they are organised and explained. Choosing materials and activities for long-stay patients can be influenced by a knowledge of visual, auditory and tactile perception processes.

If something cold and wet touches your back while you are sunbathing, you are likely to react with a primitive response, either leaping up and away in a startled fashion or 'freezing' until the danger passes. The sense receptors in the middle of your back cannot tell you whether you have been attacked by a monster from the deep sea, a friendly dog, a bunch of seaweed or a friend's hand. If you were brave enough to put your hand round behind your back without looking, the sense of *haptic* touch in your fingers could give more detailed information. Vision provides a much more comprehensive picture. Vision and hearing can give advance warning of an event that is about to happen and the opportunity for evasive action if necessary.

Vision seems instantaneous. We do not appear to have to 'feel round' an object with our eyes in the same way as we would with our hands: it seems as if we simply look and know. However, evidence seems to indicate that we do have to go through a similar process of sorting out the outline, distinguishing an object from its background, assessing texture, colour, distance, patterns or special features and matching these up with previous experience. We pay attention to things that have importance for us individually, depending on our needs and interests. One of the current debates in cognitive psychology is whether perception involves mainly top-down or bottom-up information processing (see Chapter 6). It does not always make sense to separate the different psychological approaches, but the following distinctions may be helpful.

Biopsychological approaches: these provide detailed information of how the senses function: how they receive data about external and internal conditions and transmit messages to the central nervous system. The structure and function of the specialised areas of the central nervous system can be described. Special studies have provided information on, for example, colour perception, visual perception of lines at different orientations, the development of vision in visually restricted fields, visual neglect, the loss of perception for faces, movement, the effects of drugs and strokes and brain damage, split brains and the reflex arc. Information is provided on how information is transmitted between the different areas of the brain and how it is co-ordinated and established as memory traces. The foundation is laid for *reductionist* approaches to the discussion on the nature of consciousness and how this is related to the nervous system (see also Chapter 12).

Cognitive approaches: these form the main perspective for the study of perception, which covers all the mental process, both conscious and unconscious, involved in paying attention and in recognition and interpretation. Studies of particular note include those on inverting goggles, impossible and ambiguous figures, illusions, perspective, constancy, depth perception, selective attention and perceptual *set*. Debates centre on the type of information processing involved in perception and the comparison of these processes with memory.

Social psychology approaches: Cross-cultural studies indicate how perception is affected by background and upbringing and group studies show how perception is susceptible to group or peer pressure. Studies of language and interaction show how the words we use determine the meanings we attach to perceptions and how we communicate with each other.

Psychodynamic and humanistic approaches: these help people to articulate the emotional processes and personal experiences that influence perception.

Key Terms and Concepts

After-image: there are two kinds of after-image: positive and negative. Images, particularly bright ones, tend to persist as a positive after-image after the source is removed. This is also known as persistence of vision. This may be noticed dramatically when waving a 'sparkler' or fluorescent strip around in the darkness: it is possible to write one's name in the air.

A ghostly, negative after-image may be seen by many people when they have been staring for a few moments at a stationary image and then look away to a blank surface, although not everyone readily achieves this effect. After staring at a black square on a white background, the after-image is a white square on a dark background. With coloured images, the *complementary colours* are seen. Bright images, such as on a television screen, can give noticeable after-images, particularly if the set is turned off suddenly. These effects can interfere with vision, so that mistakes can be made in interpreting monitors.

Auditory location: picking out the direction from which a sound is coming. The ability to do this accurately depends on having similar hearing in both ears as the perception of direction depends on an evaluation of the differences in timing and loudness of the sound arriving at each ear.

An interesting illusion is often noted where a sound is directly behind or in front of the listener. Since the signal arrives at both ears simultaneously, it may not be possible to tell whether the sound is coming from front or back. This has implications for calling to a person from behind as there may be momentary confusion about where the voice is coming from. This is particularly true of people with Alzheimer's disease who have difficulty processing information, in whom confusion may lead to frustration and aggression. Helpers are advised never to approach a person from behind or speak abruptly while out of sight (Rau, 1993).

Where there is some long-term loss in one ear relative to the other, normal daily experience will usually lead to a relearning of auditory location. Following a sudden loss, it can be helpful if practice is arranged under supervision so that the person can be given accurate feedback on which to build relearning.

Where a person has totally lost the hearing in one ear, auditory location is very difficult, and the person may have to rely on constantly looking around in order to tell where sounds are coming from. Hearing aids that bypass one ear and send sounds arriving at the deaf side to the better ear cannot help with auditory location and may cause some confusion.

Binocular disparity: the differences in the images registered on the retinae of the left and right eye. These differences are processed in the brain to allow the perception of depth and distance.

Colour constancy: this is the tendency to see objects as unchanging in colour even though the light source changes, provided that the change is not too great. As we move from sunlight into artificial light, we do not usually perceive a change in colour, but photographers have to adjust their cameras because the light is actually rather different. We only notice changes when the light source is dramatically different, such as sodium or mercury street lighting – and even then some people can adjust and perceive objects and clothing nearly as well as in sunlight. However, as mentioned above, the light source does affect how we see colours in a room and can affect our mood and our ability to detect small changes in colour, even if we are not aware of it.

Coloured lights: the colour of an object depends on the frequencies (or wavelengths) of the light that is reflected from the object into our eyes. Artificial light contains a restricted range of frequencies and will alter the way in which objects are perceived. When designing a room in terms of colour, the lighting must also be taken into account. It is also possible that nurses or other carers may miss vital signs of a change in a person's condition if the lighting prevents the accurate perception of changes in skin colour. Lighting can also affect the way in which colour test strips, such as for glucose in the urine, are interpreted. Street lighting, with sodium or mercury lamps, gives very limited colour perception; red will tend to look black, and it is possible that blood at the scene of an accident will be missed. See also colour constancy.

Colour of surroundings: colour in our surroundings is very important to us, even if we are only vaguely aware of it. Certain colours, usually bright or zingy combinations, are found to invigorate us; quiet colours, such as pale green, are soothing; dull colours can be enervating, sapping us of energy. Rooms with a specialist use, such as for counselling after rape or intensive care, and children's wards, can be carefully designed to provide the optimum conditions to promote a feeling of well-being.

Colour vision: the retina of the eye contains cells called cones that respond to the different frequencies (or wavelengths) of light.

It has traditionally been believed that there are three main types of cone, and it is sometimes convenient to refer to these as red-sensitive, green-sensitive and blue-sensitive respectively, since red, green and blue are regarded as primary colours. However the cones are not sensitive only to one colour each but to a range of frequencies (Figure 14.1). The addition of the discovery of a fourth cone (Mollon, 1990) may shed new light on colour vision and help to explain some of the discrepancies between men and women, such as in the description of blue, green and turquoise. See also colour vision variations.

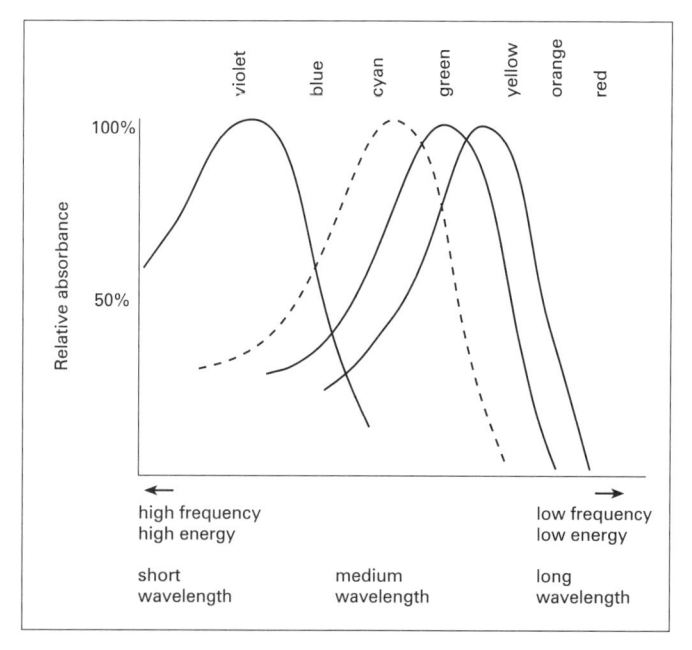

The solid curves are for the cones, the dotted line for the rods. Note that the so-called red-sensitive and blue-sensitive cones have their peak sensitivities in the yellow-green and violet respectively.

Figure 14.1 The colours of the spectrum and the relative sensitivity curves believed to be typical of the three main types of cone found in the human retina (*adapted from Dartnall and Bowmaker, cited in Barlow and Mollon, 1982*)

Sunlight (white light) is the range of frequencies that can stimulate all types of cones simultaneously. Coloured objects do not present all these frequencies to the eye. A red object reflects the red components but absorbs the others, and stimulates mainly the red-sensitive cones. In the same way, a green object reflects only the green components and so on (Figure 14.2).

White light can be passed through a filter to remove, for example, the red component. This makes the light appear blue-green or cyan (minus-red) (see complementary colours). If this illuminates a red object, it contains no red light to be reflected, and the object appears black. The same effect is noticed with mercury street lighting, which contains no red component.

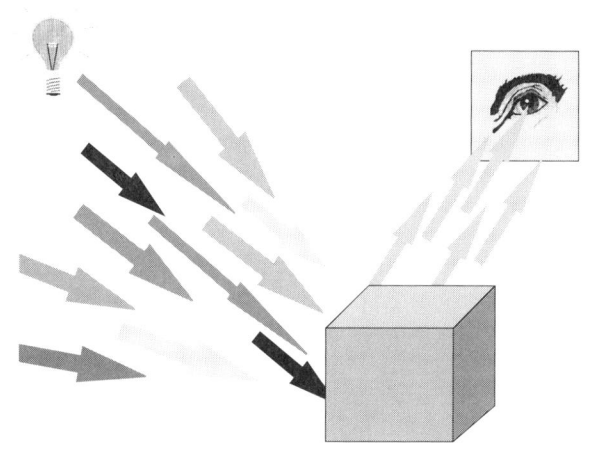

The colour that an object appears to be depends on the components of the light that are reflected into the eye. Thus a red object reflects only the red components, a green object only the green and so on

Figure 14.2   Colour vision: colour of objects

Colour vision variations: we tend to talk about 'normal' colour vision and 'colour blindness', but no-one is really blind to colour: there are just differences in the ways in which colours are perceived. There are a number of commonly occurring variations.

In the most common kind, the person does not distinguish clearly between red and green. This is hereditary and involves a gene carried on one of the X chromosomes, being therefore sex-linked, occurring in 8 per cent of males but only 0.4 per cent of females (although 16 per cent of women are carriers) (Barlow and Mollon, 1982). These people have only two kinds of cone (**di**chromacy). All have the high-frequency (blue-sensitive) cones. Some then have *either* the low frequency (red) *or* the middle frequency cones (green) but not both, whereas others have a type of cone with a range of sensitivity somewhere between the usual low and middle ranges. In other rarer types of dichromacy, the blue-sensitive cones are missing; these people can distinguish between red and green but make 'mistakes' with blues.

In other kinds of variation, there may be three types of cone (**tri**chromacy) but with ranges of sensitivity different from the majority. These people see slightly differently and make different choices in controlled tests. In recent research (Mollon, 1990), it appears that some people may have four types of cones and be able to discriminate more finely than usual, particularly in the green and blue regions of the spectrum. Moreover, women who have these four kinds of cone, and vision superior to 'normal' men, may be carriers of other types, and their sons may inherit a deficiency.

Complementary colours: when the word complementary is spelt with an e instead of an i, it means adding whatever is needed to make the full complement, that is, a complete or whole set (as in complementary therapies). When applied to coloured lights, this means adding complementary pairs of colours to make white light.

The three primary colours for lights are deep red, green and blue. When a filter of one of these colours is held up in front of a spectrum, it lets through only a small part of the spectrum, about one third, and is known as a 'narrow-band' colour. Each primary colour then has a complementary colour representing the remaining two-thirds of the spectrum in each case and is thus a broad-band colour.

Cyan (minus-red) is complementary to red. See also colour vision. Magenta (minus-green) is complementary to green and yellow (minus-blue) complementary to blue. Blue and yellow spotlights shone together make a white spot and so on. In each case, a narrow-band colour (one third of the spectrum) is being added to a broad-band colour (the other two-thirds of the spectrum) that makes up the whole of the spectrum.

With paints, pigments, printing inks and dyes, the broad-band colours of magenta, yellow and cyan (or the nearest available) are the three best primaries as they make the most useful mixes. Mixing paints is known as 'subtractive' mixing and is the exact reverse of the 'additive' mixing of lights. The complementary pairs are regarded as opposites on a colour wheel or circle. When painted next to each other they give a dazzling effect as a result of after-images forming round the edges. See also Adams (1989).

Dark adaptation: as a person moves between areas of dim and bright light, the eye has to adapt to the varying conditions. This happens by the iris expanding or contracting to let in varying amounts of light and by the retina responding to the different levels of illumination. The human retina consists of a mosaic of rods and cones, each receptor having its own separate nerve. The rod nerves encode information in dim light; the cone nerves encode bright light and colour. Rod signals and cone signals co-exist all the time and are combined in varying degrees depending on conditions. Dark adaptation is needed when going from a bright area into a dark one. At first, the eye is insensitive so that hardly anything at all can be seen, but improvement begins rapidly for most people. It can take half an hour to reach full dark-adapted sensitivity. The iris responds quickly to the change and the pupils enlarge, but the pigments in the retina take time to recover: the pigments are bleached by strong light and need time to be naturally restored. People working in an environment that requires frequent changes may learn to compensate, and they need to be aware that a newcomer will take longer to adjust.

Depth perception: the seeing of objects and the space around them in three dimensions. This occurs with solid objects even though the retinal image is only two-dimensional. The term is commonly used to refer to vertical depth, the most well-known experimental work being that of Gibson and Walk and the 'visual cliff' apparatus (see any introductory psychology text, for example Bee and Mitchell, 1984; Cardwell *et al.*, 1996; Gross, 1996). Clues to depth perception are given by relative size, texture, the partial hiding of further by nearer objects, geometrical perspective, accommodation of the lens, *motion parallax* and the difference between the two images received by the two eyes. It is not yet known exactly to what extent depth perception is inborn or learned. Babies have many months of visual experience before they can move independently, so it is not possible to test them before they have had time to learn.

Dichotic listening: listening to two different messages simultaneously, one relayed to each ear. Experiments of this kind contribute to understanding of attentional processes and levels of processing.

Disorders of perception: specific disorders may occur owing to illness or following a stroke. Examples are actual sensory loss leading to reduced perception, visual neglect, visual interference patterns (such as spots, wavy lines or blank spaces in the visual field, sometimes found during a migraine or when under stress), auditory interference patterns (such as the ringing due to tinnitus) and exaggerated illusions or hallucinations that may occur where there is sensory loss, understimulation or overload. Perceptual changes may cause anxiety where the cause is not known to the individual as they may be interpreted as being a mental disorder. Many disorders can, however, be linked to alterations in the senses, to biochemical changes in the brain and nervous system or to damage to the brain.

Distortions: a type of visual illusion in which we judge something as a different length or shape from what it actually is. We genuinely make a mistake, usually because there are distracting surroundings. Examples of standardised distortions used to illustrate this are Muller–Lyer lines and the Ponzo effect (for example, Cardwell *et al.*, 1996; Gross, 1996). In day-to-day situations, this kind of distortion is common, although it rarely causes major problems. Most people learn the hard way that if they wish to move a heavy piece of furniture from one corner of the room to another to fit it into a convenient space, it is wise to measure the space first!

Faces: the perception of faces seems to be a special area of perception. Babies appear to have some recognition of faces very early in development. It is possible to have a loss of recognition of faces following brain damage even when other perceptual process appear to be intact. Illusions involving faces tend to be very strong.

Fantz (1961) believes that newborn babies pay more attention to pictures of faces than to other complex figures. Hershenson *et al.* (1965), however, did not find this difference, if alternative figures of very similar complexity were used, until about 4 months of age. Kleiner (1987) and others have found that newborn babies prefer abstract patterns, while older babies prefer face-like patterns. These studies tend to suggest that face recognition is learned rather than innate, but all seem to agree that, to a baby several months old, faces are extremely interesting. See also Sternberg (1995: 416) and Fontana (1990: 82).

Fictions (embedded figures): a type of illusion in which we see something that is not there, usually created out of a 'space' with apparent boundaries formed by other parts of the figure. A widely cited example is the Kanizsa triangle, in which the illusion is not a simple space but cuts across other parts of the figure (for example, Gross, 1996: 206). Art students are trained to look at negative spaces in order to help with the relative positioning of lines and angles, and much art is created with special attention to these spaces.

Figure–ground reversal: a number of drawings have been produced that illustrate how perception involves the processing of what constitutes the figure and background. The best-known example is of Rubin's vase/two faces (for example, Gregory, 1971: 16, 1990: 322; Gross, 1996: 218). In this, two interpretations are possible, depending on what is selected as the figure and what as the background. This illustrates that we make a mental decision about what we are seeing rather than simply passively receiving a stimulus.

An intriguing example is given in Figure 14.3. If the black blocks are regarded as the figure against a white background, the arrangement looks simply like a pile of children's building blocks. If, however, a mental switch is made so that the black area is regarded as the background, a very different perception results!

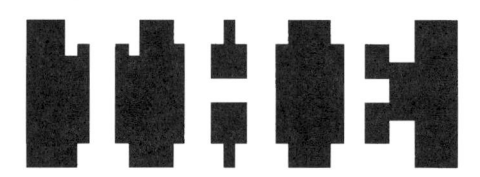

Figure 14.3   Figure–ground reversal

Gestalt theory: a school of thought in psychology that introduced to the study of perception the notion that 'the whole is greater than the sum of its parts'. The German word *Gestalt* means an organised whole or pattern. This approach argues that, in order to make sense of something, we have to pay attention to the parts and then integrate this information into a whole. The key elements identified are similarity, proximity, continuity, closure and figure–ground and part–whole relationships. This means that when we look at a picture or diagram, we pay attention to marks that are similar to each other, we notice where things are close together, and we look to see whether there are any continuous flowing lines or shapes, even if these have gaps or spaces in them. In this way, we can pick out a figure from its background, identify familiar shapes and see how each part relates to the whole picture.

These processes are automatic and unconscious, and perception is spontaneous. Although the Gestalt principles do not provide the whole story, they provide some basic ideas for understanding perception.

Habituation: becoming accustomed to a repeated stimulus so that it no longer registers and we cease to pay attention to it. This happens chiefly because the nervous system is 'programmed' to register a change in stimulus more strongly than continued stimulation. This is noticeable with the ticking of a clock. After continuous exposure to the ticking, we are no longer aware of it, although we can bring our attention back to it if we wish. However, if the clock suddenly stops, we immediately notice the change. This effect is necessary to protect us from information overload: we can safely ignore anything which is not changing and use our resources to deal with new data that might be important. There is some suggestion that habituation (together with other selective attentional processes) does not function well in some people suffering symptoms of schizophrenia or autism (see Chapter 12). Habituation at the level of the nervous system can be compared with the more complex processes of desensitisation (Chapters 1 and 4) and stress inoculation (Chapter 20).

Hearing (auditory sense): this can be described as an *exteroceptor, telereceptor* or *mechanoreceptor* sense (see senses). The ears enable information to be picked up from a distance by the successive action of sound waves or pressure changes on the eardrum, small bones in the ear and small hairs (auditory receptors) in the cochlea. Movement of the auditory receptors creates *action potentials* that travel to the auditory areas of the cortex on both sides of the brain (see Chapter 5). Hearing enables discrimination of the following variables:

- pitch
- loudness
- emphasis
- timbre or quality
- location (see auditory location).

Hearing can be very important in the interpretation of *paralanguage* (see Chapter 9), and people with hearing loss may be insensitive to nuances of meaning conveyed by tone of voice.

Identity constancy: being able to recognise an object as the same object even when viewed from a different angle or distance or under different lighting conditions. For example, a cup can still be recognised as being the same even when someone is moving it around the room, despite the fact that the retinal image is continuously changing. This may be lost if an object is viewed from an unusual angle or only a tiny part of it can be seen, an effect that is exploited in the party game using close-up photographs of bits of familiar objects.

Illusions: the perception of something that does not actually exist but which, unlike an *apparition*, is clearly related to specific visual stimuli. Gross (1996: 206) cites Gregory (1983) and classifies illusions as distortions, ambiguous figures, paradoxical figures and fictions. A detailed account of illusions is given in Robinson (1972).

Gregory (1990: 329) points out that perception and conception are not the same thing, so we can be seeing an illusion but knowing we are seeing it. We are not conceptually deluded, even though we are, as Gregory says, 'perceptually illuded'. This notion poses interesting questions for theories of perception. Most theories describe perception as interpretation in the light of previous experience, but if this were so, we would not be able to identify something unless we had seen it before, and we would never be able to see anything new. Gregory argues that perhaps perceptual processes have to happen very fast to warn of danger and cannot access all of the knowledge stored in our memories, so that a great deal of perception involves gap-filling and hypothesising. In contrast, conceptual processes of understanding our experience and organising ideas for planning and using language for communicating ideas takes a long time and continues to develop throughout life.

Impossible figures: specially contrived drawings that break the rules of perspective or 'play games' with visual perception. Perhaps the best known example is Penrose's 'impossible triangle'. Robinson (1972: 176) cites Penrose (1958), Schuster (1964) and Fisher (1968) as having produced a whole range of such figures. The artist M.C. Escher has incorporated many of these figures into his paintings. William Hogarth (for example, in an engraving in 1754) has also played extensively with the rules of perspective. See Gregory (1971: 51–3) and Escher (1967).

Kinaesthesia: the sense of movement and position felt through the sense receptors in the muscles. It is this sense that provides information about where all the parts of the body are and what they are doing at any particular moment without having to look, and creates a kind of 'mental map' of the body. If you close you eyes, put both hands up in front of you, about a metre apart, the fists loosely clenched and the forefingers extended, and attempt to touch your forefingers together, you may find that your kinaesthetic sense is not particularly accurate! People who have brain damage that upsets this internal sense lose their 'body maps' and cannot tell what their body is doing. Sacks (1985) describes a few people who have learned to compensate for this by watching themselves in mirrors all the time. See also *proprioception*. Note that in neurolinguistic programming, the name 'kinesthetic' (K) is used for a combination of sensation and emotion that is expressed in terms of how a person 'feels'.

Motion parallax: the apparent relative motion of objects owing to the motion of the observer. The simplest way to observe this is to line up two vertical objects, for example two coffee mugs, at different distances away, close one eye and move one's head from side to side. The nearer mug will appear to move from side to side relative to the distant one. When travelling (by car, train and so on), nearer objects flash past more rapidly that distant ones. This relative movement gives clues to the distance of objects and contributes to depth perception. In the cinema, a landscape filmed from a moving vehicle is seen as more 'solid' than a static picture. When two objects are at the same distance, they will appear to move together and are said to be in a position of 'no parallax'. Instruments with a graded scale can give rise to parallax errors if the markings on the scale are at a slightly different distance from the eye than the item being measured. To avoid this error, instruments should be held exactly in line and not viewed at an angle.

Müller–Lyer illusion: this is one of the most commonly known visual illusions, in which lines of equal length appear different because of the presence of different arrowheads. A line with outward facing arrowheads appears shorter and a line with inward-facing arrowheads appears longer than a comparison line with no arrowheads. The extent of this illusion appears constant within Western society, most people seeing the same size difference. There have been many attempts to explain this illusion, but none is conclusive or universally accepted (see Gregory, 1971; Robinson, 1972).

Necker cube: a two-dimensional drawing of a cube will normally be perceived as three-dimensional. Continuous staring at the drawing usually results in the perspective suddenly jumping or switching spontaneously from one interpretation to another, the front face becoming the back one. The after-image will also reverse spontaneously, indicating that the switching must occur in the brain rather than in the retina. If a fluorescent wire cube is used in a darkened room, it can be a strange experience trying to touch the edges of the cube if the perception is reversed as the brain is receiving conflicting information from the different senses of vision and touch. Some strange *motion parallax* effects can also be seen. People who gain sight after having been blind may experience similar confusion.

Neglect: a lack of attention or perception of parts of the body or of the surrounding environment. Visual neglect is an inability to perceive objects in part of the visual field. The term 'hemianopia' is used where half of the visual field appears to be lost. This may occur together with paralysis of one side of the body (hemiplegia) which can occur after a stroke. Hemianopia may be a temporary symptom of migraine. Sacks (1984) gives a vivid description of how he 'lost' one side of the visual field during a migraine following an accident. The most striking effect is that the sufferer usually has no awareness that there is anything missing. This may also be associated with a change in spatial awareness, which can be revealed by observation of behaviour and of drawings made by the person. The person may be seen to continually move the head to one side and may end up continually lying on one side, staring at the wall, unaware that there is anything else to look at or that there is any point in turning the other way. Drawings may show information that the person knows about all heaped up on one side of the drawing, for example the numbers of a clock all placed around a half circle or all the features of a face on one side. Curiously, the drawings do not necessarily look wrong to the person who drew them, although it is possible, with hard work and feedback, for an individual to learn to produce near 'normal' drawings.

Perceptual constancy: the tendency to judge things as the same even though the retinal image has altered as a result of different conditions. The main examples are identity, size, shape, location, brightness and colour constancy.

Perceptual set: a tendency to notice certain aspects of what is around rather than others. This is part of the selection and interpretation process, which directs attention to things of importance and protects one from overload. In familiar terms, this refers to the judgement that we see what we expect to see or what we want to see. This may be strongly influenced by the language we use to refer to things or people, as in diagnostic labelling. See also set in problem-solving in Chapter 16 and labelling in Chapter 3.

Proprioception: a general term that can be used for the combination of all internal body senses which give information about the body's position and movement. It includes both the muscle sense (kinaesthesia) of where all the parts of the body are and the sense of balance in the inner ear (vestibular sense), which tells about movement in relation to the horizontal and vertical. Proprioception gives complete information about position and motion in the external world. It depends on the basic physical principles of gravity and inertia and allows a person to know how much and how rapidly to move in order to reposition or move one part of the body without disturbing other parts or losing balance. For example, proprioception enables the source of an itch to be located and scratched without falling over. Anyone watching babies or toddlers will appreciate that proprioception is often learned the hard way! See also kinaesthesia.

Saccadic eye movements (saccades): perpetual, apparently random, rapid and relatively large movements of the eye that are essential in the process of centralising a target on the fovea, the most sensitive part of the retina. Centralising in this way provides the greatest acuity, but Cornsweet (1970) showed that if there were no movement, images would tend to stay in exactly the same place on the retina. Inability to renew the chemicals needed for vision, and natural *habituation* of the receptors, would then result in a lack of visual sensitivity.

The movement is most clearly noticeable in a darkened room in which a spot of light is projected onto a wall. The spot appears to move, jumping about irregularly. The effect is termed 'autokinetic'. The amount of movement varies from person to person but can also be influenced by suggestion and by a tendency to conform to group norms. See also autokinetic effect in Chapter 19.

Selective attention: one of the problems for theories of attention and perception is working out how the brain and nervous system process incoming stimuli and make decisions about which bits to pay attention to. Conscious attention can be deliberately directed towards any of the senses (apart from interceptors) at any time, but the greatest part of the selectivity takes place automatically at an unconscious level of processing. Habituation plays a part in this as the nervous system stops responding to repeated stimuli after a while, but this still leaves a great deal of other incoming information to sort. One suggestion (known as the filter model) is that all the information is taken in and then filtered by some process that identifies and selects only those items of interest and importance. Another suggestion is that it would be impossible to monitor all incoming information, even at an unconscious level, so the processing must involve a kind of sampling procedure in which a regular sample of the incoming data is taken in turn from each of the senses and examined for importance. The *thalamus* in the centre of the brain acts as the chief interchange of neurones in the brain, routing information from the senses and passing it on to the relevant areas of the brain, and may play a part in the selection of material in response to signals from the cortex. All approaches indicate how the conscious awareness of incoming information is limited to a tiny fraction of what is available in the world (both externally and internally) and that limits are essential in order to protect from 'information overload'.

Sensation: the term used in physiology and psychology to refer to information received by the senses. It is linked to the notion of irritability, used in biology, which indicates how parts of the body are responsive to the environment and can provide information about the surroundings. Irritability and sensation are defined as essential differences between living and non-living organisations of matter and energy, and the need for sensory input appears to be fundamental to living creatures. Although rarely mentioned specifically, it it is helpful to include it in Maslow's (1962) hierarchy of needs, alongside the other basic physiological needs such as nutrition and respiration (see Chapter 7). See also sensory deprivation.

Senses: it is usually taught that there are five 'special senses' – seeing, hearing, touching, tasting and smelling – which have been recognised from the time of Aristotle and provide information about the outside world. In the early 1800s, Bell added a sixth sense, muscle or kinaesthetic sensation, to Aristotle's original five. This tells us where all the parts of the body are and how they are moving in relation to the outside world. It is now also recognised that the balance organ in the inner ear provides information about the body's orientation and movement; this is referred to as the vestibular sense. The kinaesthetic and vestibular senses are usually known collectively as proprioception. It is now common to refer to six senses – seeing, hearing, touching, tasting, smelling and proprioception – which can be classified in different ways.

Gross (1996) cites Sherrington (1906), who names three groups of senses:

- exteroceptors
- interoceptors
- proprioceptors.

In this classification system, the exteroceptors are the five 'special senses' that give information about the external environment. Interoceptors pass information to the brain about the internal physiological state of the body, for example of blood glucose levels. Proprioceptors include the kinaesthetic and vestibular senses (although in some texts, proprioception refers only to the muscle or kinaesthetic sense).

An alternative classification is given by Messenger (1979), who argues that the location of the stimulus is a key distinction. He limits exteroceptors to receptors that pick up data at the surface of the body (such as hairs that respond to touch), interoceptors being inside the body with some proprioceptors at the joints. He adds a fourth group – telereceptors (sound, sight and smell) – which can pick up signals distant from the body.

Messenger makes a further classification according to the kind of signal that can be processed:

- mechanoreceptors (pressure, tension, vibration and sound, involved in touch, balance and hearing)
- chemoreceptors (chemicals involved in smell and taste)
- thermoreceptors (warmth, cold and changes in temperature)
- electroreceptors (not specialised in humans, but there is a generalised response to electrical stimulation, such as in TENS, and electric shock)
- photoreceptors (sensitivity to light, mainly vision, but also thought to occur in other ways that affect the pineal gland and responses to daylight).

Through all these senses, a complete mental map is built up in relation to the environment. The only information about oneself and the world that the brain receives is through these senses. To this is then added rational thought and imagination, such that understanding can be brought to the incoming information. Damage to any of these senses, to the nervous system that carries messages to the brain or to the brain itself results in limited or faulty information. This may need to be compensated for through the greater use of other senses, new ways of interpreting data or other complex individual strategies.

Sensory deprivation/overload: too much or too little incoming information from the senses can disturb the smooth organisation of perception and lead to symptoms of stress and even to hallucinations and confusional states. The early work of Heron (1957) dramatically demonstrated the effects of boredom on individuals who were deprived of normal sensory stimulation. Volunteers wore masks that allowed through only diffuse light, earmuffs that prevented distinct sounds, and cuffs on the hands and feet that prevented any discrimination of touch. This did not cause a complete loss of sensory input but a reduction in patterns and recognisable input.

Many of the volunteers reported having hallucinations after only a short period in this state. Cognitive skills were severely impaired, many were confused and unsteady after the experience, perceptions were distorted with a marked loss of constancy for size, and some were measurably more susceptible to persuasive arguments. This has important implications for the care of people with marked sensory loss, older people in whom all the senses provide reduced discrimination, and those in whom daily routines are repetitive and boring. There may also be implications for people with severe learning difficulties, whose perceptual processes are not well developed and who have difficulty making fine discriminations between different types of input.

Similar disturbances are found where there is an overload of sensory stimulation with bright lights, loud sounds and excessive touch or handling. The overload interferes with the normal perceptual processes of fine discrimination.

This combination of sensory monotony and sensory overload is believed to be at least partly responsible for what has come to be known as the *ITU syndrome* or 'post-pump psychosis'. Patients in intensive care are subjected to much stressful stimulation and continuous background noise and are isolated for long periods. They are found to be prone to perceptual disturbances, visual and auditory hallucinations, disorientation and paranoia (Isaacson *et al.*, 1982; MacKellaig, 1987). Their situation is further exacerbated by sleep deprivation, feelings of helplessness and an inability to communicate.

Shape constancy: like other forms of constancy, this refers to the perceptual interpretation remaining constant even when the viewer and object move relative to each other. For example, a round plate continues to be seen as a circle even when placed at an angle to the viewer so that the retinal image is not circular but oval (elliptical).

Size constancy: this refers to our perception that objects and people remain the same size when we are moving towards or away from them, or when they have moved. The image on the retina is changing, so the judgement about lack of change is a mental one. It is thought that babies have to learn this constancy but that it is present by 18 weeks (for example, Slater, 1989).

It is found by most people that size constancy has not been learned in a vertical direction (as most visual experience takes place in a horizontal plane) and the view from a tall building or an aeroplane often gives the impression of toy cars and people below. Things no longer look the right size. It seems that aeroplane pilots soon lose this effect as they develop new size constancy in the vertical direction.

Smell (olfaction): this is defined by Messenger (1979) as a distant chemical sense. The receptors in the nose and nasal passages respond to airborne and water-borne stimuli even in very low concentrations. In Western cultures, smell is a neglected area of study, and little has been known about it until recently. For most people, the perception of smell is largely unconscious except in response to strong smells. It is often found that smell plays a significant part in the detection of certain conditions and that many nurses and doctors are alerted to changes in a patient's state of health by a change in smell, even if they cannot name the change or describe to an observer what they are noticing.

Subliminal perception: a perception of a stimulus that is below the normally measured limit or threshold of perception. This is said to occur when a stimulus is very brief or at very low intensity. It is thought that under some circumstances, even though a stimulus has been considered to be too small to be registered, a person may nonetheless be influenced by unconscious mental processing of the information. Evidence for this is conflicting.

Synaesthesia: an apparently rare but interesting phenomenon first described by Francis Galton (1822–1911). Certain individuals seem to get an overlap between two or more senses, which gives them a very different perception of the world from the majority. Many people occasionally experience some overlap or may make meaningful connections between different sensations, such as describing colours as warm or cool, or numbers as coloured. The term synaesthesia is reserved for where the overlap is very marked and stimulation of one sense organ gives rise to sensations associated with a different sense, dominating the individual's way of perceiving the world. It was originally believed that the nervous system was operating in an unusual way. However, Cytovic (1994) argues that, at a basic level of neural processing, a similar kind of comparison and evaluation of all sensory associations takes place in all people, and that a greater understanding of marked synaesthesia will assist in an understanding of normal mental processes.

The effect can be pronounced in some drug-induced states. This is presumed to result from the reduction in normal inhibitory mechanisms that isolate the central processing of the senses (Gregory, 1987).

Taste (gustation): this is a 'chemotactile' sense in which a large number of chemoreceptors are present in humans in a special region of the mouth and tongue (Messenger, 1979). It used to be thought, from early psychological experimentation, that only four types of receptor were present on the tongue, responding to saltiness, sweetness, sourness and bitterness. These areas can be clearly mapped out on the tongue in simple taste tests. It was believed that all other aspects of what we consider taste when responding to the flavours of foods arose from the sense of smell. A person who loses the sense of smell, either through damage or through applying a clip or clothes-peg to the nose, cannot readily distinguish between the taste of pieces of apple and onion. However, it is now acknowledged that taste may be more complex than formerly realised. Ageing, illness, mood, experience and hormonal changes, such as in pregnancy, can all affect the sense of taste, and individuals may find they can no longer tolerate previously liked foods. This can cause frustration, especially if carers are not aware of the perceptual changes that can take place and put the new dislike down to faddiness or fussiness.

Touch: touch is one of the most important senses in health care as it can be used positively in the communication of empathy and sympathy. Sense receptors in the skin respond to pressure, warmth and cold and can also detect chemical or electrical stimulation. These receptors activate specific nerve fibres, which may be activated singly or in parallel. Neural processing takes place within the spinal cord, in the brain stem and in the thalamus on the way to the somatosensory area of the cerebral cortex. This can be related to the gate control theory of pain, which looks at changes in the neural processing within the spinal cord. Perceptual processing is assumed to take place in adjacent areas of the cortex (Gregory, 1987). Perceptions may range from mild to strong feelings of pleasantness or unpleasantness, or from generalised smooth touch to distinct pinpoints or tingling and can distinguish between steady pressure, vibration and light touch.

A distinction can be made between 'haptic' touch and passive touch. Haptic touch is active exploration, especially with the fingers. Gregory (1987) says that it is rarely used except in the dark or by blind people. However, it is extensively used in professional health care for detecting bodily changes such as the extent of a pregnancy or the existence of lumps or obstructions. Haptic touch makes use of single neural channels. Passive touch refers to all other kinds of touch when external objects press on the skin on any part of the body. This makes use of *parallel processing* of neural channels.

When using touch as communication, carers need to take into account any loss or change in sensory ability and perception. Different parts of the body are more sensitive than others. For example, fingers can detect minute spacing between stimuli, which is utilised in learning Braille, whereas in the centre of the back, pinpricks several inches apart may be interpreted as being in the same place. Ageing may result in a loss of sensory acuity. Disease, depression, schizophrenia or autism may result in oversensitivity, making touch unpleasant. See also Chapter 9.

Vestibular sense: the sense of balance in the inner ear, which provides information about movement in relation to the horizontal and the vertical. Fluid in the semicircular canals moves in response to movements of the head so that the amount and speed of movement can be 'calculated' mentally. This can be explained as the effects of gravity and inertia.

Vision: this can variously be described as an *exteroceptor, telereceptor* or *photoreceptor* sense (see senses). The eyes enable us to pick up information from a distance by the action of light on receptors in the retina. There are two kinds of receptors: rods and cones. Rods contain a pigment (rhodopsin, or visual purple) that responds to low levels of illumination. Cones contain a range of pigments that respond to different colours or frequencies of light (see colour vision). Changes in the chemical nature of the pigments create *action potentials* that travel via the optic nerve to the visual cortex at the back of the brain. Information from one side of the visual field travels to the opposite hemisphere (see Chapter 5). Gregory (1971) argues that the eye and brain developed simultaneously during evolution to allow the processing of information. It is not well understood how visual images are interpreted.

Vision is normally the dominant sense, and most imagery is described in visual terms, which socially disadvantages those with limited or no vision in addition to any other problems they may experience.

15 PERCEPTION OF SELF AND OTHERS

Studies of our perception of ourselves and other people are usually separated into chapters on interpersonal (person) perception, self-concept and personality. However, since our perception of ourselves is directly dependent on how we view other people and these perceptions generally include notions such as personality, this chapter will put together some of the related concepts. Those aspects of personality which are specially relevant to lifestyle and health-related behaviours are given in Chapter 7.

Definitions	
Peck and Whitlow (1975)	some psychologists have defined personality very widely so that it covers virtually everything a person does, from how he solves problems and how he deals with incompatible thoughts, to changes in physiological functioning in response to emotion-rousing situations.
Ryckman (1989)	Despite the plethora of definitions, there is basic agreement among investigators that personality is a psychological construct: that is, a complex abstraction that includes the person's unique learning history and genetic background... and the ways in which these organized and integrated complexes of events influence his or her responses to certain stimuli in the environment. Thus, many investigators see the study of personality as the scientific study of individual differences that help to account for people's unique ways of responding to various situations.
Eysenck (1947)	Character denotes a person's more or less stable and enduring system of conative behaviour (will); temperament, his more or less

Definitions (cont'd)	
	stable and enduring system of affective behaviour (emotion); intellect, his more or less stable and enduring system of cognitive behaviour (intelligence); physique, his more or less stable and enduring system of bodily configuration and neuroendocrine endowment.
Millon and Everly (1985)	personality... refers to the pattern of deeply embedded and broadly exhibited cognitive, affective, and overt behavioural traits that emerge from a complex biological-environmental formative matrix. This pattern persists over extended periods of time and is relatively resistant to extinction. Temperament, on the other hand, may be viewed as a biologically determined subset of personality... [and] character may be thought of as the person's adherence to the values and customs of the society in which he/she lives.
Price (1990)	We should like to believe that our self-image is congruous with, and is an expression of, our personality. Yet we also guess that our self-image is strongly affected by what other people think of us. Self-image then, is our own assessment of our social worth. It is composed of ideas of whether we are 'true unto ourselves' and whether others think we are worthwhile people. Self-image is important for our confidence, our motivation and our sense of achievement.
Rogers (1961)	Self-concept includes self-image, ideal self and self-esteem.

Approaches, Arguments and Applications

Studies of personality, self-concept and interpersonal perception generally include the consideration of how we see ourselves, how others see us, how we think others see us and how we see others. Approaches are derived from social psychology, cognitive psychology and humanistic and psychodynamic therapies. Although the definitions above point towards personality as consisting of stable and enduring characteristics, most people are aware of their own fluctuations and variations with mood, the situation and other people who are present. Attribution theory illustrates how important the context is in determining what we notice about a person and how we interpret our own and other people's behaviour. Studies of groups show how adherence to group norms and expectations influences behaviour irrespective of individual differences. The effectiveness of psychological interventions and therapies is dependent on certain characteristics being amenable to change, and it is open to debate whether the constructs of personality that have developed during the twentieth century are really the most useful ways of describing individuals.

Most approaches to the study of self-concept and interpersonal perception involve descriptions of personality traits such as friendly, warm, withdrawn or shy, but there is considerable controversy over whether such traits can be measured systematically, and whether they occur in clusters that can be identified as 'personality types' or are essentially individual. As with other aspects of self-concept, we may gain an awareness of our personality through feedback from others and by comparing ourselves with others. In addition, we may choose to fill in questionnaires purporting to assess personality, either from a professional psychometric agency or in a popular magazine, or even accept descriptions given by astrology. When we look at other people, we use all our social and personal understanding of how people think, feel and act in order to make sense of their personalities.

It can be argued that the better we know a person, the less we want to say in description. There is always so much that could be said that describing personality in terms of a type or a collection of traits somehow misses what the person is really like. Trait descriptions, profiles or 'thumb-nail' sketches of types, however well grounded in research, do not seem to do justice to the complexity of personality, although they might help with a quick listing of those factors (especially the ones Allport, 1962, calls central traits) which are thought to be important. Different traits might be emphasised in different circumstances.

Nevertheless, in practice, in many situations, particularly when meeting a person for the first time, most people sum up the characteristics of the other person and tend to retain this initial judgement on subsequent occasions. It is this tendency to simplify and pigeonhole observations that forms the core of interpersonal perception.

Key Terms and Concepts

Adolescence: a period of great change in self-concept, in relation to both changing appearance and bodily functions, and to personality, social roles and expectations, the development of new interests, friendships, educational levels and possibly new spiritual and aesthetic values. According to Gross (1996), children prior to puberty are relatively unconcerned with the appearance of their bodies, and it is only in adolescence that such awareness emerges. It could be argued that this notion no longer holds true, as fashion clothing is now directed at young children. Incidences of anorexia nervosa are found in children as young as 8 years old. However, it could still be true that, for many, there is an increase in bodily awareness during and after puberty.

Altered body image: a change in the perception of one's appearance, bodily functions or state of health with the potential for a change in self-esteem. This may be triggered by an actual physical change such as injury, surgery, illness, the effects of drugs, a loss or gain in weight, an increase or decrease in exercise, maturation and ageing. In some cases, however, an altered perception can arise with no actual change of appearance or state but from a situation or event that simply leads the person to view his or her body differently. Most interventions focus on negatively altered body image and lowering of self-esteem, and look for ways in which to help a person cope with changes that have given rise to perceived unattractive appearance or a loss of function. Interventions may include non-directive listening to fears and worries, cognitive restructuring to help correct any distortions of perception or unrealistic ideals, and practical advice about confronting the change. They may inform about camouflage or prostheses and help to shift attention away from the undesirable change towards other aspects of the person's self-concept. Interventions may address personality, social roles and interests that give rise to positive self-appraisal.

It is helpful to remember that an alteration in body image is not always negative. A change in fitness, weight or state of health may be for the better. This may still require some adjustment as it takes time for the new body image to replace the old. For example, it can take time for a person who has lost a lot of weight through careful dieting and exercise to get used to having a more attractive body, discover a rise in self-esteem and self-efficacy, and replace old habits with new ones. This can be particularly true if the person had placed an unrealistic expectation on the effects of losing weight and did not realise that other aspects of lifestyle, such as interpersonal relationships, might have to be dealt with separately. Corrective heart surgery for a child may result in a sudden ability to take part in normal games and activities. This may require an enormous social adjustment as peers who formerly used to provide sympathy and attention may lose interest and drift away. The child may need support and guidance in making new friendships.

Ambisexual: a term used either to refer to a person who is erotically attracted to people of both sexes (Masters and Johnson, 1966), more usually called bisexual, or to refer to the overlap between the sexes of sexual characteristics such as erogenous zones (for example, Ruse, 1990).

Animism: treating inanimate objects as if they are alive and have intentions towards the person. It appears that we see all behaviour as intentional, and we like to look for intentions. Cartoonists make use of this, and the effect has been studied systematically (Heider and Simmel, 1944). Children are particularly noted for imbuing toys with personality and judging them to be blameworthy or praiseworthy for their actions. This tendency is utilised in such experiments as Bandura's work on aggression towards an inflatable bobo doll (Bandura, 1965), and McGarrigle and Donaldson's (1974) use of the Naughty Teddy in exploring cognitive development. However, it is not just children who indulge in animism. Many adults like to refer to cars by personal names and praise or blame them for their performance; others get angry with objects that get in their way and blame the traffic lights for changing to red just as they approach, as if they had done it deliberately. Other examples include blaming the rain for re-wetting the dried washing on the line or blaming a cup for falling and breaking.

Attribution: attribution theory, from Heider (1958), includes a basic assumption that people tend to see the social environment as predictable and controllable according to what is perceived as the cause of events or behaviour – what we attribute behaviour to. A number of effects can be identified: fundamental attribution error (which varies with the seriousness of consequences), animism, actor–observer effect, self-serving bias, false consensus, false consistency, primacy/recency effects, halo/horns effects, self-fulfilling prophecy and stereotyping. Some of these effects can be viewed as *errors in person perception* that can be corrected through increased awareness and the development of *perceptual skills*.

Authoritarian personality: a term derived from work by Adorno *et al.* (1950) to refer to people who favour an authoritarian and hierarchical social structure and are particularly prone to stereotyping and prejudice against minority groups. The term 'authoritarian personality' does not necessarily mean 'in authority' but can apply to a person anywhere in a hierarchy, in either a low or a high position. Within nursing and other caring professions, people who submissively accept a low position within a hierarchical organisation, follow conventions and obey instructions without question and who prefer a highly structured, rule-bound environment to a flexible, innovative one might be said to have an authoritarian personality. As with all labels, classifying someone in this way is open to misunderstanding, and alternative explanations for the behaviour are possible. See also Chapter 3.

Bisexual: a term used either to refer to a person having both male and female physical characteristics (also called hermaphrodite) or to a person who feels erotically attracted to people of both sexes (in this case also sometimes called ambisexual). In the latter case, the term 'bisexual identity' may be more useful when referring to a person who takes part in sexual activity with people of both sexes and who openly lives a bisexual lifestyle. People with a bisexual identity are often not accepted in groups with either a strong heterosexual or homosexual identification.

Body boundaries: we seem to have quite distinct boundaries between self and non-self. Much of early child development is concerned with learning these boundaries and identifying what things in the world belong to self and what are 'other'. There are recognisable developmental changes in knowing and understanding limits of bodily self.

As adults, we are not usually aware of these boundaries until something happens to upset them. Allport (1955), cited by Gross (1996), points out that bodily fluids that we accept comfortably while in the body cause different reactions after elimination; he describes the difference between swallowing saliva while it is still in the mouth and when it has been spat out into a cup. The change in acceptance of blood, urine and faeces from inside to outside the body is considerably greater. This has important implications for people with stomas. Less obvious are the body boundaries associated with monitoring and support equipment. When a person is attached to a machine, the machine may seem part of the person's self, although this may not be consciously recognised. If an attached machine is moved, or someone happens to balance a cup of coffee on it, the patient may feel distinctly uncomfortable. Visitors often find that there are significant changes in communication when new attachments are added or when accustomed machines are removed. It may help if these changes are openly discussed and recognised.

Body image: perceptions of self that relate specifically to the body. These can include anything to do with appearance and also the physical state or state of health or bodily functions. Thus body image might include a description of facial features, or the current position in the menstrual cycle or pregnancy, the extent of a suntan, fitness, or whether one is constipated or has any other condition. Strictly speaking, following Carl Rogers' (1961) usage of the terms 'image' and 'concept', body image could refer only to pure description without any comparative or evaluative aspects. However, in most usage, the term 'body image' covers both description and evaluation, together with the associated self-esteem, that is, how people feel about how they look or what they can do.

Price (1986) lists the following factors that contribute to body image formation:

- genetics
- socialisation
- fashion
- mass media
- peer group pressure
- culture/race
- health education.

Camouflage: anything that helps to reduce the visibility of something against its background. This may include the use of skin-coloured lotions and creams to mask or disguise visible blemishes, burns or scars.

Character: a term that is difficult to define in a way that distinguishes it from personality. Often, no such distinction is made or attempted. It can be argued that the term 'character' refers to those aspects of personality which are most relevant to health-related behaviours. Millon and Everly (1985) define character as the person's adherence to the values and customs of the society in which he or she lives. Eysenck (1947) sees character more as a matter of will or volition (*conative* behaviour). In common language, it is often associated with moral qualities, and we can talk of having a 'good' or 'bad' character and of activities being 'character-building'. Such aspects of willpower, strength of character and cultural values may be seen as contributing to notions of self-efficacy and the kinds of lifestyle that are valued. In a more general sense, it may be useful to think of character as being that part of personality which is learned, in contrast to temperament, which may be seen as inborn. However, as with the whole nature–nurture debate, it is the interrelationship of genetic inheritance and experience, rather than any notion of something being due solely to one or the other, that is important. Nevertheless, as with any learned behaviour, there is a possibility for unlearning or relearning, so that if aspects of personality which are detrimental to health can be identified as learned, a programme of relearning or learning more beneficial behaviour can be designed.

Cross-dressing: any activity which involves wearing clothes that are considered by the culture to be more appropriate to a member of the opposite sex. This may be for entertainment, as in pantomimes and other comedy, or simply be a personal preference. Cross-dressing can range from wearing a few garments while retaining same-sex identity to wishing to appear as the opposite sex. When there is an intention to achieve erotic arousal, the label 'transvestism' is usually used (Ruse, 1990).

Depersonalisation: the sense of a loss of personal identity often felt by people who are subjected to labelling as a member of a readily recognised subgroup of society. This is particularly noticeable for people who use wheelchairs or those with a disfigurement, who may be viewed as non-persons and find that others do not know how to approach them or may regard them as unable to communicate. As with any visible form of discrimination, an affected person may be advised to try to take the first step in establishing communication with others who appear hesitant (Rumsey, 1991).

Errors in interpersonal perception: interferences with subsequent social interaction that result from an over-hasty or restricted judgement of a person's characteristics. Burton and Dimbleby (1995) list the following errors:

- attribution bias
- false consensus
- false consistency
- primacy and recency effects
- *halo and horns* effects
- self-fulfilling prophecy
- stereotyping.

Extroversion (alternatively spelt extraversion): a term used by a number of theorists, particularly Jung and Eysenck (cited in Ryckman, 1989; Gross, 1996; and others), to describe people with an outgoing and relatively confident approach to life. In these theories, extroversion tends to be linked with an acceptance of conventions, a willingness to yield to peer pressure, shallowness of feeling with a change in emotions from one situation to another, pleasure-seeking and impatience. Jung identifies four extroverted types: extroverted feeling type, extroverted intuitive type, extroverted sensing type and extroverted thinking type. Eysenck identifies two extroverted types: stable extroverted (sanguine), and neurotic extroverted (choleric). Eysenck (1965), cited by Ryckman (1989), argues that extroverts have strong inhibitory processes in the nervous system and a large capacity to tolerate stimulation so that they seek out a greater variety of experiences. He found that when electric shocks are administered to participants, the pain tolerance of extroverts is greater than that of introverts. A contrary finding in practice is that sometimes people with extrovert tendencies make more display of emotions and pain behaviour.

False consensus: this term has two important uses: first, that we have a tendency to see our own behaviour, feelings, beliefs and opinions as typical, that is, similar to those of others; and second, that we assume that everyone shares the same view when only a few have actually stated a view. This is related to the common finding that we expect much more consistency than actually occurs. It can lead to generalised assumptions such as 'Everyone else would have done the same', 'Everyone acts like this' and 'We all think the same', and to statements such as 'I know just how you feel'.

False consistency: a tendency to see people's behaviour as more consistent than it really is and to expect them to behave in much the same way on different occasions irrespective of the context. Nisbett and Ross (1980) suggest that this helps to make it easier to deal with people and predict what they will do. In practice, it may lead to carers and patients being ill-prepared to cope with changes in behaviour due to medication or to changes in state of health, which can in turn lead to impatience and frustration. On the other hand, it can contribute to the *self-fulfilling prophecy* effect so that expectation of consistency may bring about such consistency.

Fundamental attribution error: this expression was first used by Ross (1977) to refer to the tendency to attribute cause and blame to people rather than circumstances. Although almost all behaviour is the product of the person and the situation, it seems that there is a tendency to be biased towards attributing negative intentions and fault to the person. For example, if someone carrying drinks in a pub trips and spills some, many people tend to make the immediate assumption that the person is clumsy or drunk rather than look for an outstretched foot or stray bag. This bias gets worse with greater damage and when the onlooker making the judgement is involved. The difference in perception of an event from the point of view of the one involved and an onlooker has been called the actor–observer effect. See Jones and Nisbett (1971) and Nisbett *et al.* (1973).

It is an important concept in health care as how the patient's actions are perceived may make a difference to the quality of care. For example, even a comatose patient might be perceived as deliberately being awkward and falling out of bed 'on purpose'. It makes a great difference whether an alert patient is seen as responsible for his or her state of health, 'difficult' behaviour or failure to comply with advice. This sort of bias is particularly noticeable in professional care where repeated episodes of self-harm or Munchausen's syndrome are involved. Many carers feel frustrated and annoyed when they feel that their time is being taken up by people who are 'to blame' for their condition. The bias can be reduced by increased knowledge and understanding of the condition and the circumstances so that there is increased awareness of all the contributing factors. Zebrowitz (1990), cited by Gross (1996), shows that when participants are encouraged to empathise with the person displaying negative behaviours, attribution bias is less pronounced.

Gender: this term is commonly used interchangeably with 'sex' to refer to biological characteristics, but in the social sciences is now used to describe the extent to which a person identifies with cultural constructions of femininity and masculinity, that is, has a sense of gender identity.

Gender identity: the extent to which individuals conform to the cultural and social norms and ideals corresponding to either biological sex and think of themselves as masculine or feminine.

Throughout history, cultures have described what it means to be a typical or ideal man or woman. These descriptions can be seen either as archetypes (for example, Jung, 1964), the pure idealised form, or as stereotypes, which are oversimplified generalisations based on a few extreme examples. See also Chapter 17.

Talcot Parsons in the 1950s described how, traditionally in Western society, masculinity and femininity are defined in terms of a dichotomy: instrumental versus expressive. Men are seen as instrumental, aggressive, dominant, powerful, competitive, independent and self-assertive. Women are viewed as expressive, dependent, conformist, subjective, intuitive, sensitive, co-operative, tender and nurturing. Until relatively recently, theories of personality and self-concept tended to categorise people as either masculine or feminine 'types' or as somewhere along a masculine–feminine continuum (for example, Eysenck and Wilson, 1976). In contrast, Sandra Bem (1981) describes more recent thinking as rejecting the masculine–feminine continuum and describing individuals as having a measure of masculinity and a measure of femininity that are independent of each other, that is, a position on each of two separate scales. Yet others reject the whole notion of attributing gender labels to any of the above-listed characteristics and would like traits such as being expressive, nurturing, assertive and independent to be regarded as unrelated to sex or gender, being equally applicable to men or women and in any kind of mix.

There is ample evidence to suggest that gender-linked characteristics are encouraged from birth and are generally only rewarded when they are the 'right way round'. It is not at all clear whether this social conditioning *causes* the observable differences between males and females who would otherwise behave indistinguishably, or whether it merely fosters natural differences, in which case it creates problems for only a few non-conformists. However, the cultural notion of what is desirable and natural is constantly changing, and this can be seen as supporting the view that conditioning causes the differences. Images of men have undergone several transformations from male chauvinist to new man to reconstructed man and back to macho man. The image of women has moved from predominantly compliant, child-rearing and home-based to assertive and independent. It could be argued that these changes can be interpreted as either altering what is meant by masculine and feminine or as supporting the notion that men and women are now expressing their opposite-gender characteristics more openly.

Hairstyle: a feature of body image that is readily changeable and can be used in a deliberate way to express personality or conformity to a group identity. Lack of attention to hair care can act as a signal to carers that a person is not coping well with the current situation. Helping a person with restricted mobility to achieve an attractive hairstyle can contribute greatly to a positive body image and feeling of well-being. Loss of hair due to chemotherapy can have a dramatic effect on body image and self-esteem. Interventions may include providing emotional support, practical solutions and a refocusing on other positive aspects of appearance and self-concept.

Halo and horns effects: a positive or negative evaluation in one particular area leads to similar generalisations being made. That is, a halo effect arises when knowledge of one good characteristic leads to a perception that the person is also good in other areas about which nothing is yet known, and a horns effect when being poor in one area generates beliefs that the person is also poor in other areas. This has repercussions for care. For example, Nordholm (1980) found that patients who are seen as physically attractive are often judged to have a better 'prognosis' and to be more intelligent and better motivated than their less attractive counterparts.

Heterosexuality: the prefix 'hetero' means 'other', the usual meaning of heterosexuality being a sexual preference for, or sexual activity with, someone of the opposite sex. It is only since the nineteenth century and the introduction of legal references to homosexuality that the term has come into common usage. The term need not imply exclusively heterosexual behaviour and it is not uncommon for those who regard themselves as heterosexual to have engaged in some homosexual activity.

Homosexual identity: a term that has been recently coined to refer to people who adopt a homosexual lifestyle and share characteristics with others who do the same. This identity is undergoing continuous change as society's attitudes towards homosexuality are altering. Discussion in popular magazines reflects these changes and indicates how different people identify with different images of what it means to be homosexual.

Homosexuality: the prefix 'homo' in this word means 'the same'. Ruse (1990) uses a general definition that a homosexual is a person, male or female, who is erotically attracted to members of his or her own sex and that such erotic attraction can range from fantasy about sexual encounters to actual sexual activity. He distinguishes between people who have homosexual inclinations and those who take part in homosexual acts. This distinction accepts that some people with homosexual inclinations or a homosexual orientation may not engage in any homosexual activity and that some may engage in heterosexual activity. Similarly, a person with heterosexual orientation may engage in homosexual activity. The terms 'bisexual' or 'ambisexual' can be used for a person who is erotically attracted to both sexes. The distinctions are not at all clear. It is not always easy to distinguish between sexual activity that is accompanied by erotic attraction and that which is not. Other writers may use the terms differently.

Foucault (1978) has argued that, throughout history, men have engaged in sexual acts with other men or boys and that such acts, referred to as sodomy, are regarded in many communities as forbidden. These can be a form of rape or bullying. It is only since the nineteenth century that such activity has been regarded as an 'orientation' and certain people identified as homosexual. The situation has been rather different for women, particularly as Queen Victoria did not acknowledge the existence of sexual activity between women. The term 'homosexual identity' can be more useful.

Ideal-self (ego-ideal or idealised self-image): this is one of the three components of self-concept identified by Rogers (1961) and included by Price (1990) in his approach to altered body image. In general, this would refer to the sort of person one would like to be. Specific features can also be identified, referring to particular desired attributes, such as length of hair, body shape, fitness, personality, lifestyle and occupation.

Image: in the context of person perception, this term is often used for a symbolised representation of appearance or patterns of behaviour associated with a particular group in society. For example, prevailing and contradictory images of women include 'woman as child-rearer', 'woman as housewife' and 'woman as temptress'. Images of men include the macho footballer, skinhead, yuppie, city gent, gentle giant and so on. People who choose to identify themselves with a particular image take this on as part of their self-image. The concept is closely allied to stereotype but usually emphasises one particular aspect that has a characteristic visual appearance that is readily copied and recognised. At the time of writing, the description 'anorak' is being used as a derogatory image for someone who prefers the pursuit of knowledge to following clothes fashions.

Implicit personality theory: most introductory psychology texts describe how nearly all people have an individual way of categorising and pigeon-holing characteristics in themselves and others. This idea has been extensively developed in personal construct theory.

Interpersonal perception: in many situations, particularly when meeting a person for the first time, most people sum up the characteristics of the other person and tend to retain this initial judgement on subsequent occasions. It is this tendency to simplify and pigeonhole which is meant by the term 'interpersonal perception'. Burton and Dimbleby (1995) give the following reasons for this process:

- to remember information
- to make sense of the other person's behaviour
- to predict others' behaviour
- to organise social understanding
- to plan communication
- to maintain sense of self and reality
- to reduce anxiety
- to satisfy needs of inclusion, control, affection and so on.

This process, although useful, can lead to significant errors and interfere with more open awareness of what other people are like in different circumstances. See errors in interpersonal perception and perceptual skills.

Introversion: a term complementary to extroversion in some theories of personality, particularly those attributable to Jung and Eysenck (cited in Ryckman, 1989; Gross, 1996; and others), to describe people with an inward-looking and seemingly quiet approach to life. In these theories, introversion tends to be linked with a strong conscience, reliance on personal values and a tendency to guilt and anxiety. Jung identifies four introverted types: introverted feeling, introverted intuitive, introverted sensing and introverted thinking. Eysenck identifies two introverted types: stable introverted (phlegmatic) and neurotic introverted (melancholic). Eysenck (1965), cited by Ryckman (1989), argues that introverts have weak inhibitory processes in the nervous system with a small capacity to tolerate stimulation. They avoid variety of experience. He found that when electric shocks are administered to participants, the pain tolerance of introverts is less than that of extroverts. Some people with introvert tendencies may, however, hide their feelings and display less pain behaviour.

Make-up: like hairstyle, make-up is a feature of body image that is readily changeable and can be used in a deliberate way to express personality or conformity to a group identity. Lack of attention to make-up in a person who previously used make-up regularly can act as a signal to carers that the person is not coping well with the current situation. Helping a person with restricted mobility to achieve an attractive make-up can contribute greatly to a positive body image and feeling of well-being.

Menarche: (pronounced as three syllables, men-ar-key): the onset of menstruation. This signals a significant change in a girl's process of growing up and may bring about problems with adjusting to the altered body image. Professional care interventions may include providing information about the changes that are taking place, emotional support, exploration of perceptions of key members of the family or significant others, peer relations and whether the individual is ahead of or behind those with whom she associates.

Mid-life and menopause: mid-life is commonly defined as occurring between the ages of 40 and 60 years (Platzer, 1988) and has been increasingly recognised as a stressful time of life for men. Women in this age group normally reach the menopause (the cessation of menstruation or menses), which is recognised as sometimes being associated with unpleasant symptoms. The term 'perimenopause' may be used for the transition stage before menstruation finally ceases. Current debate is concerned with whether symptoms are due to biological or social factors. Farabaugh (1988) concludes that only three symptoms of menopause can be directly attributed to biological causes: cessation of menses, hot flushes and vaginal dryness. She argues that other symptoms in women, such as insomnia, mood swings, irritability and feelings of hopelessness and worthlessness, are more likely to be due to changes in lifestyle as children leave home and to worries about growing older. Parallel patterns are found in men who may negatively assess their achievements in life.

Ontological insecurity: a term borrowed from philosophical *paradigms* to refer to feeling unsure of what is real about one's self or one's being.

Perceptual skills: Burton and Dimbleby (1995) suggest the following ways of improving skills and avoiding common errors in person perception:

- attention to detail as well as overall view, avoiding mere impressions
- withholding judgement, keeping an open mind
- seeking further information
- looking for alternative causes
- modifying assessments in the light of new evidence
- checking evidence
- comparing information from different sources and in different ways
- empathising.

Personal construct theory: a theory originating from Kelly (1955) and further developed by Bannister over a number of years. They believe that all people build their ideas of the world in a complex hierarchical network of *bipolar* constructs, similar in some ways to scientific classification systems. Constructs related to perceptions of people form a person's *implicit personality theory*. Constructs such as good–bad, polite–rude and happy–sad can be used in a predictive way to judge how people will behave. Constructs are essentially individual; different opposites, or different shades of meaning, may be used. For example, one person may construe others as being either friendly or withdrawn, another might judge in terms of friendly versus aggressive. Unlike scientific systems, this is not normally done in a conscious way. Kelly and Bannister (see Fransella, 1990) developed a repertory grid technique for revealing constructs. The simplest technique is to ask the participant to list about 20 familiar people. Three of these are selected, the participant then naming one way in which two of the three are similar but the third different. A bipolar label is then chosen for this similarity–difference construct and applied to all other people in the list. Three different names are then selected and the process repeated. This continues until a grid of constructs has emerged.

Personality: a term widely used in attempts to explain individual differences but with little agreement about what is meant by the word. Some definitions are given at the start of this chapter. The concept seems to encompass descriptions variously called 'temperament' and 'character', and may overlap with other such concepts as attitudes, intelligence, motivation, interests, skills (particularly social and communication skills) and lifestyle. Like attitudes, personality may be seen as having cognitive, affective and behavioural components, although the emphasis is often on the behaviour alone. Focus on behaviour is usually considered within a social or interpersonal context, but some approaches also include solitary behaviour. Explanations range from the purely biological to the purely social; most are a mixture.

Despite these differences, definitions of personality are consistent in referring to enduring characteristics or patterns of behaviour rather than fleeting moods or fluctuations in behaviour (although the frequency of mood changes might in itself be regarded as contributing to a personality trait).

It can be useful sometimes to distinguish between normal and abnormal personality patterns. Millon and Everly (1985: 32–3) assess normal personality patterns through personal appearance, interpersonal conduct, cognitive style, affective expression and self-perception. They derive eight basic normal personality patterns: forceful, confident, sociable, co-operative, sensitive, respectful, inhibited and introverted. They believe that these patterns can then be used as the basis for looking at abnormalities in terms of 'syndromal continuity' or position on a continuum rather than as qualitatively distinct mental processes. They suggest that a person possesses a normal and healthy personality when:

- the person displays an ability to cope with the environment in a flexible and adaptive manner
- his or her characteristic perceptions of self and the environment are fundamentally constructive
- the individual's consistent overt behaviour patterns can be considered health promoting

and that a person may be said to have an abnormal and unhealthful personality pattern when:

- the person attempts to cope with average responsibilities and everyday relationships with inflexibility and maladaptive behaviour
- his or her characteristic perceptions of self and environment are fundamentally self-defeating
- the individual's overt behaviour patterns can be shown to be health eroding.

In relation to health issues, although the term 'personality' is used, the behavioural characteristics that are felt to be of significance usually fall into quite limited categories. It is more usual to label these as behaviour patterns rather than personality types. See Chapter 7.

Primacy effects: the tendency to judge others in terms of first impressions.

Q technique: a technique developed by Stephenson (1953) for studying *attitudes* by means of *questionnaires*, cited and adapted for the study of *self* by Butler and Haigh (1954).

Recency effects: the tendency to judge others in terms of their latest words or actions.

Self-concept: in general, our self-concept is what we think, feel and want about all aspects of ourselves. The following six areas, derived from several existing models, for example James (1890) and Kuhn and McPartland (1954), help to sort some of the different aspects of what might be included in perception of self. The same categories can also be applied to perception of others:

- body image: physical appearance and state of fitness and health
- sexuality: sex and gender (attributes and expression)
- roles: social, occupational and family positions
- interpersonal behaviour: personality, emotional traits, temperament and character
- spiritual: educational, intellectual, aesthetic and moral attributes and values
- lifestyle: activities, skills, interests and possessions.

Price (1990: 11) focuses on body image and identifies three aspects:

- body reality – the way in which our body is constructed, namely the way it really is. This is affected by both nature and nurture factors
- body ideal – how we think we should look. We hold a personal body ideal that may also affect how we think other people 'should' look. At a professional level, the carer's body ideal may be informed by health standards. Body ideal is constantly changing and susceptible to a variety of influences
- body presentation – how we present our body appearance (dress, pose and action) to the social world. We are able to control body presentation within certain limits and to reflect actively on how body presentation was received by others.

One limitation of this approach is the reliance on the notion that there is an absolute 'reality'. All perceptions are coloured by previous experience, knowledge and beliefs, and it can be hard to be absolutely objective about what a person is 'really' like.

In everyday interactions, particularly in the professional context, it is helpful to know something of other people's self-concept as this makes their behaviour more understandable and predictable. Gross (1992) suggests that we cannot fully understand a person's behaviour unless we also understand what it means for the person. He also states that part of what we mean when we say we know people well is that we know how they feel about themselves. This can lead to a better understanding of what it feels like to be in their position. To achieve this kind of empathy, it can help to examine one's own self-concept.

Carl Rogers (1961) sorts out three separate components of self-concept – the descriptive (self-image), comparative (ideal self) and evaluative (*self-esteem*) – and emphasises that it is not just how we describe ourselves that matters but the assessment we make, how we feel about ourselves and whether or not we like what we are. Rogers suggests that how we feel depends on whether we believe we measure up to our personal and cultural expectations and ideals. His work suggests that, when there is a gap between self-image and ideal self, the size of this gap contributes to self-esteem (Figure 15.1). The greater the gap, the lower the self-esteem. Interventions can work in two ways: either focusing on the self-image to see if there are distortions in perception, or focusing on the ideal self to see whether this is realistic and attainable. Counselling would aim to reduce the gap by facilitating the adjustment of both self-image and ideal self until they are closer.

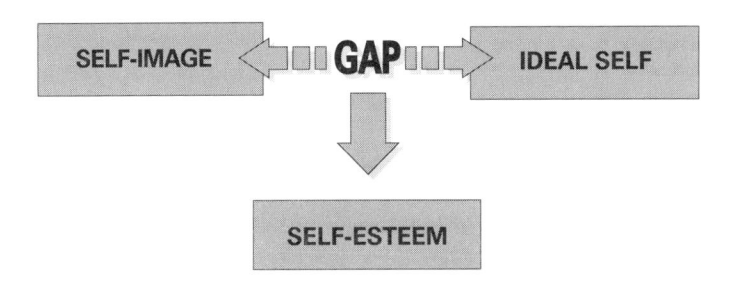

Figure 15.1 Self-concept *(derived from Rogers, 1961)*

Self-fulfilling prophecy: Burton and Dimbleby (1995) summarise this as 'What you want is what you get.' It is observed that behaving in a particular way indicating that a particular outcome is expected is likely to bring about that outcome. This can refer to our expectations about others or about ourselves. For example, if a parent, teacher or carer repeatedly praises a child for being brave, careful or thoughtful, the child is likely to develop those attributes more strongly. Conversely, if a child is constantly in trouble for lack of ability, laziness or clumsiness, these traits are likely to become more noticeable.

Sexuality: in popular usage and the mass media, the term 'sexuality' is generally restricted to mean either sexual activity or sexual orientation/

preference. In the social sciences and professional usage, sexuality has a much wider meaning and includes all aspects of experience and expression that have anything to do with sex, gender, sensuality and attractiveness. Thelan *et al.* (1994: 111) define sexuality as:

> a unique, highly individual expression and experience of the self as a sexual, erotic being. It is an holistic experience in that it encompasses both the mind and the body and a part of the character of a person also termed the personality.

Burt (1995) cites Watson and Royle (1987) and lists four components of sexuality:

- biological sex (hormones, chromosomes and genitalia)
- core gender identity (an inner sense of being male or female)
- sex role imagery (learned behaviour from an early age)
- sexual behaviour (the expression and action of sexual feelings and beliefs).

There is some confusion of the terms 'sex' and 'gender' in their list. It can be rephrased and extended as follows:

- biological sex (defined by genetic coding, sex chromosomes, hormones, visible sexual characteristics and functioning sexual organs)
- core sex identity (an inner sense of being male or female)
- gender identity (conformity to the cultural and social norms and ideals corresponding to masculinity and femininity)
- sexual identity (adopting the lifestyle and sharing characteristics of a particular group, such as heterosexual, homosexual, bisexual or transvestite)
- sexual behaviour (the communication, expression and action of sexual feelings and beliefs)
- sexual thoughts (desires, fantasies, frustrations and anxieties)
- attractiveness (the self-perception of how one looks to other people; this can apply in all social interaction but has particular relevance in finding and relating to partners and the perceived ability to meet their needs)
- personal boundaries (the limits of what is found to be acceptable sexual behaviour, including attitudes to abuse, harassment and rape).

Other sources (for example, Webb, 1985, 1994) give lists that can usefully be compared. The subject of sexuality is a recent addition to the literature for professional health care. Many professionals are reluctant to initiate conversations about sexual activity or other aspects of sexuality, are uncomfortable about witnessing certain kinds of sexual activity and do not feel competent to advise clients on issues to do with sexuality. The 'sexuality box' on patient assessment forms causes a great deal of difficulty and embarrassment for nurses: many avoid the issue by writing something banal and meaningless or leaving it blank. Sexual problems among patients with cancer are often ignored because sex is seen by medical staff as a minor issue for those with such a serious physical disease (Baldwin, 1990; Lamb, 1995). Single people and adolescents are often excluded from body image or sexuality counselling (Auchincloss, 1989, cited in Barraclough, 1994).

A greater awareness of the wider issues, such as those listed above, and increased openness in discussing all related issues may lead to more appropriate and helpful care. Where nurses take the initiative, ask questions tactfully and confidently and come to the point quickly, patients may feel more trusting (Burt, 1995). Some educational programmes are now including opportunity for discussion and the sharing of information.

Poems by Grace Nichols (1984) illustrate a strong positive sense of sensual and sexual identity. An example is included here (Figure 15.2), partly to 'allow' thoughts and conversation about sensuality, sexuality and body image. Readers may find the images disturbing and embarrassing or powerful and uplifting, and may be prompted to ask why.

Social roles: positions one occupies within groups or society as a whole, either by choice or by circumstances. Roles can be roughly classified as follows:

- family/partner relationships and positions
- neighbourhood relationships
- educational/professional/occupational positions
- clubs and group memberships and positions of responsibility
- age, gender, sexual orientation and ethnic identity.

How one acts within each role depends to a large extent on expectations about what it means to be a member of that group. What does it mean to be a mother, neighbour, manager or counsellor? Moreover, what does it mean to be a good mother, good neighbour, good manager or good counsellor? Rogers' (1961) model of self-concept helps to identify any gap between a person's perception of himself or herself in a particular role and what he or she thinks is required of the role in order to be seen as 'good'.

Temperament: a term used for aspects of personality that are regarded as fundamental characteristics, usually viewed as innate rather than acquired, and related to levels of energy and physiological responsiveness to the environment. Early personality theories such as those of Kretschmer and Sheldon (cited by Pitts, 1991) classified people into types that were seen as biologically determined, such as active/passive and relaxed/assertive/restrained, and related to inherited body type (see introductory psychology texts). It is argued today that body type and other aspects of physiological responsiveness can be strongly influenced by lifestyle, and there is no consistent evidence of a correlation between body shape and personality. Buss and Plomin (1975) give four dimensions of temperament:

- activity
- emotionality
- sociability
- impulsivity.

Invitation

1

If my fat
was too much for me
I would have told you
I would have lost a stone
or two

I would have gone jogging
even when it was fogging
I would have weighed in
sitting the bathroom scale
with my tail tucked in

I would have dieted
more care than a diabetic

But as it is
I'm feeling fine
feel no need
to change my lines
when I move I'm target light
Come up and see me sometime

2

Come up and see me sometime
Come up and see me sometime

My breasts are huge exciting
amnions of watermelon
    your hands can't cup
my thighs are twin seals
        fat slick pups
there's a purple cherry
below the blues
        of my black seabelly
there's a mole that gets a ride
each time I shift the heritage
of my behind

Come up and see me sometime

Grace Nichols
The Fat Black Woman's Poems

Figure 15.2 Sexuality – a poem for discussion

Thomas and Chess (1977) expand this list to nine temperament dimensions for describing a child's behaviour:

- activity level
- rhythmicity
- approach/withdrawal
- adaptability
- threshold of responsiveness
- intensity of reaction
- quality of mood
- distractability
- attention span
- persistence.

Traits: Cattell (1965) cites Allport and Odbert as having found over 3000 trait words for describing personality but suggests that, of these, there are a limited number of traits that can be identified by factor analysis as natural, unitary structures in personality. Cattell distinguishes source or underlying traits from surface traits and developed the Sixteen Personality Factor (16PF) Questionnaire. Allport (1962) refers to cardinal, central and secondary traits and warns against 'pseudo-traits'. William Stern (1912), and mentioned by Holt (1962), emphasised that particular traits, however precisely described, are meaningful only in the context of the whole person.

According to Allport (1962), there are personality traits of major significance and traits of minor significance. A person's central traits are those few which stand out and can be readily distinguished. Allport suggests that these are what are normally included in letters of reference, in some rating scales or in brief descriptions of a person. Less conspicuous traits are said to be secondary.

Transsexual: a person whose sex and gender are not the same (Ruse, 1990: 3). This can happen by accident, when a baby whose sexual characteristics are not well defined is wrongly 'sexed' at birth and brought up a child of the sex opposite to what later becomes apparent. Such a person may have to make a choice of whether to continue with the accustomed gender identity or to develop a new one.

Some people feel that they are simply the wrong sex; they have an inner sense of being male or female that does not correspond with their visible characteristics. This may be rather different from what we normally mean by gender identity. It is quite common for people to feel that they do not have the personality or social characteristics that society associates with being male or female, that is, they have an imbalance of masculine and feminine characteristics in the 'wrong' direction, as defined by society. Some people in this position simply reject the social stereotypes and are content to be labelled as masculine women or feminine men. Others, who feel a greater need to conform, may hide or attempt to change their social characteristics to fit in with others' expectations. When individuals feel deeply, however, that they are the wrong biological sex, living as the wrong sex can become unbearable.

It is possible for such a person to make a deliberate switch to the opposite sex. Sexual characteristics are evenly distributed throughout a person's genetic coding rather than just determined by the X and Y sex chromosomes, so the potential for characteristics of either sex are potentially present in everyone. Visible secondary sexual characteristics, such as facial hair, musculature, breasts and the distribution of body fat on the hips and thighs, are influenced by hormones. Hence, modern surgical techniques and hormone supplements make it possible for someone of either sex to acquire the physical appearance, and some functional ability, although not the reproductive functioning, of the opposite sex. Social, moral and ethical considerations have led to this surgery being made available through the British National Health Service only after a person has lived for some time as the opposite sex, is totally convinced that the biological sex is not how he or she 'feels' and has received specialist counselling.

Such deliberate choices may be regarded as unnatural and viewed with suspicion, fear, disgust and other negative emotions by many people in society, and it can be difficult for a transsexual person to find acceptance in social groups if the change is openly declared or suspected. In professional care, it can be helpful for carers to share their experiences and explore feelings so that hidden emotions do not inadvertently get in the way of providing the best possible care.

Transvestite: someone who dresses in the clothing their culture considers proper to a member of the opposite sex in order to achieve some kind of erotic arousal – if no erotic arousal is intended, the person is better known as a cross-dresser (Ruse, 1990). Sexual orientation is not related to being a transvestite, except perhaps that most transvestites consider themselves heterosexual whether engaging in sexual activity with someone of the opposite sex or with another transvestite of the same biological sex (Kinsey *et al.* 1953; Pomeroy, 1975; Stoller, 1975; all cited by Ruse, 1990).

Types: a way of classifying people into a small number of distinct groups. This is a popular way of pigeonholing people and is common in management training, in selection for careers options and in magazines and horoscopes. Its usefulness as an approach depends on the thoroughness with which trait analysis has been carried out. This should determine the clusters of traits involved in each type. It also depends on whether a typology attempts to provide a general theory of personality or a 'narrow-band' picture concerned with a more specific and restricted content area. Types thought to be related to health outcomes are discussed in Chapters 7 and 20.

16 Planning, Playing and Problem-Solving

Planning care is a complex process that involves all kinds of thinking, playing with ideas, trying them out and learning from experience. Thinking is a distinctive characteristic of mankind and is considered to distinguish humans from other animals. How do children learn to think? What are we referring to when we say we are thinking? What are the links between inherited characteristics and environmental influences? How do language, cognitive development and problem-solving skills interrelate? Is intelligence fixed at birth, or does it change through life? Can a person learn to think? Is creativity a type of problem-solving, and can it be learned? How is playing related to thinking and planning? In what ways can play contribute to development and therapy? Would adults benefit from more play or different kinds of play? How can education be improved? This chapter gives information on some of the approaches which attempt to address these questions.

Definitions	
Thomson (1959)	We all think from time to time... We know very well how some of our thinking sticks to the point and moves steadily to its conclusion while other thinking runs round in circles or drifts off into blind alleys or gets bogged down. Some answers to problems come in a flash, while at other times we are confused and befuddled in spite of hard efforts. ...thinking can be regarded as a disposition – a complex coordination and integration of specific activities... There are typical operations and systems or groups of operations examples of which can

Definitions (cont'd)	
	be recognised in any thought process... The psychologist is interested in describing what people actually do when they are thinking and what conditions determine the precise pattern of their performance.
Barron (1965)	A man may think a thought which for him is a new thought, yet it may be one of the most common thoughts in the world when all thinkers are taken into account. His act is a creative act, but the 'something new' that is produced is something new in the population of thoughts he can claim as his own, not something new for mankind as a whole.
Runco and Albert (1990)	There is a growing awareness of the complexities of the field of creativity, both conceptually and methodologically... It would be helpful to teach all persons that failure is intrinsic to creative behaviour, and that continuous effort tailored to the lessons of failure, rather than the emotions of it... would help remove, or at least reduce, a sense of helplessness and a passive belief and reliance on inspiration, chance, or blind luck as necessary elements of creativity.
Bransford and Stein (1993)	an ideal problem solver is someone who continually attempts to improve by paying attention to his or her processes and by learning from any mistakes that are made.

Approaches, Arguments and Applications

Reasoning and problem-solving include all those diverse kinds of thinking that involve dealing with some kind of information or data and making something of it, for example planning a schedule of visits, organising a meeting, planning care for a patient, working out how to dispose of sharps safely, implementing a scheme for avoiding cross-infection on the ward, sorting out the family budget to allow for a holiday, organising that holiday, thinking over an argument or debate, studying, writing an essay, novel or sermon, translating languages, composing music, using mathematical analysis and designing a new building or department.

A number of different ways of thinking can be identified: inner speech, mental images, thoughts without recognisable speech or images, logical processes, lateral connections, insight, intuition, acting out or doing, visual representation in writing, pictures and models, and talking through. Some of these processes can be clearly linked to activity in different parts of the brain, and there is evidence that the left and right hemispheres of the cortex process information in different ways (for example, Springer and Deutsch, 1993).

Each individual may use many or all of these methods, according to mood, interests and the type of task. Problem-solving abilities may depend on specialised knowledge in a particular discipline. The same individual may be both good and poor at problem-solving, depending on the sort of problem.

Some people may notice they have a preferred method of working, with a tendency to neglect other methods. It is suggested by various authors, for example de Bono (1971), Buzan (1988) and Bransford and Stein (1993), that all types of thinking and problem-solving can be regarded as skills that can be practised and improved, and that awareness of one's own processes (metacognition) greatly assists development.

It is the category of rational thought that is usually referred to in psychology textbooks on thinking and problem-solving, and this is usually classified under cognitive psychology. Other related activities and experiences will be found under headings such as dreaming, perception, memory, learning, playing, attitudes and so on, and will involve contributions from all perspectives.

Biopsychological and ethological approaches: largely the study of activities of animals that lead to them satisfying basic needs, such as for food, shelter and exploration and the satisfaction of curiosity. Play can be seen as striving towards goals and may be: the practice of skills; using up surplus energy and filling a vacuum because there is nothing else to do; a displacement activity when other more desirable activities are not available; a persistence of activity through habit (for example, toying with food even when sated); or incomplete activity that does not reach a recognisable goal.

Psychodynamic approaches: much thinking and problem-solving is related to resolving anxieties; play can be seen as the symbolic enactment of unresolved conflicts and can include free association and fantasy. This may occur in particular association with sexuality. Play may explore notions of right and wrong associated with praise and shame and guilt. Some play may represent regression to earlier psychosexual or psychosocial stages.

Behavioural and social learning approaches: thinking and problem-solving can be seen to develop to some extent through conditioning, habit and copying what other people do. Play may be regarded by some behaviourists as totally vague, inane or empty, not worthy of specialised study since it may only be a response to rewarded behaviour. For example, a child may respond to praise by repeating actions and saying, 'Look what I can do!' Much of children's play involves watching and copying others. The play of adults can be seen to involve social contact, competition and co-operation, physical exercise, the development of skills, and emotional and intellectual expression.

Cognitive and social approaches: the study of thinking and problem-solving has been traditionally considered to be largely the province of cognitive psychology. Other psychological perspectives had little formal relevance, but it is now recognised that all perspectives can be seen to be important in terms of social interaction, communication and emotional content and, as with most psychology, the trend is towards integrating ideas. There are a number of particularly prominent theorists associated with this field.

Jean Piaget (1896–1980): Piaget observed that children give answers to problems that are different from those given by adults. They do not seem to think logically. They get things wrong! Piaget reasoned that children think differently from adults (for example, 1926, 1929, see 1989, 1990). He believed that children are *unable* to reason logically or abstractly but that they pass through a series of stages, involving sensorimotor and concrete operations, after which logical thinking emerges if the right information has been correctly absorbed.

Piaget recommends that education should not introduce reasoning at an early age. The main educational method at early stages should be unguided discovery learning, which provides experience of handling objects, observing events and allowing the development of language. In a hospital setting, this might mean providing plenty of toys related to procedures, such as bandages or syringes, and allowing a young child to play freely with them under supervision but without giving explanations.

Vocabulary associated with Piaget includes: schema, assimilation, accommodation, equilibration, sensorimotor, concrete operations, formal operations, egocentricity and conservation.

Problems with Piaget's approach include that his set tasks are obscure and remote from reality, that children cannot pay attention or remember for long enough, particularly when they are confused about expectations, that it is not clear how children move from one stage to the next, and that children are found to use logic in many contexts; even intelligent adults do not stick precisely to formal logic on most occasions.

Jerome Bruner (1915–): Bruner became interested in the processes by which a child progresses. He suggests that there are no distinct stages but instead a gradual development of competence in mental representation and integration. Bruner (1964) identifies three ways of mentally representing recurrent regularities of the environment: enactive, iconic and symbolic. At first, the child thinks only through actions but gradually develops the ability to hold mental images in the form of pictures of objects and activities, and then use substitute objects and language to stand symbolically for the objects and activities. Bruner suggests that all activity is intentional and that the child learns to make links between an intention to do something, the activity itself and the feedback he or she receives about the success of the activity. This happens more readily if surprising and conflicting events are observed. Bruner believes that concepts can only develop if attention is paid to language. That is, language comes before thinking. He recommends a spiral curriculum in which students revisit topic areas according to a carefully planned timetable so that the same content is repeatedly covered at new levels of understanding and language. He argues that early development will be assisted if education does not try to introduce logical reasoning at an early age but centres on discovery learning in which the teacher makes full use of language and introduces opportunities for observing similar and contrasting situations. In a hospital setting, this might mean introducing a child to some of the language associated with treatment without attempting rational explanations.

Vocabulary associated with Bruner includes skilled activity (intention, activities, feedback), representation (enactive, iconic, symbolic), integration (comparing and contrasting, sorting) and spiral curriculum.

George Herbert Mead (1836–1931): Mead was interested in the social context in which children learn rather than in the precise nature of logical thought. He discussed how children develop a sense of self and others through interactions with others (Mead, 1934). His work indicates how children can see things from another's point of view and are not purely egocentric in the way in which Piaget describes. Mead's approach has influenced other psychologists, who have analysed why children fail in a task such as the 'three mountains' (Piaget and Inhelder, 1956) but cope well with similar tasks that are more obviously related to normal social experience.

Margaret Donaldson (1926–): greatly respects Piaget's work but rejects certain features. She has investigated why some children find school work difficult or boring and strongly believes that education based on Piaget's theory of stages severely underestimates children's capacity for rational thought. She has shown that if children are in a meaningful setting and are able to use language that makes sense to them in ordinary human terms, they are very often able to perform tasks and explain what they are doing in ways which Piaget would have thought impossible. Donaldson (1978) recommends that teachers should take account of children's conceptions by listening carefully to each child's explanation and then building on what the child already knows. For example, when trying to explain a procedure, the teacher must listen carefully to how a child describes what happens. What the teacher then says or does will depend on each individual child's preconceptions. Explanation should encourage reasoning and problem-solving skills carefully linked to concrete examples using appropriate language. Tasks can be devised that assist attention and concentration, memory and imagination. Donaldson also stresses the importance of reading in the development of language and thinking. The teacher should be clear about the intentions of a task so the child understands what is expected. It is also important for the teacher to give 'real' explanations, based on a thorough understanding of the concepts, rather than something superficial, learned by rote, muddled up with faulty preconceptions or using 'baby' language that obscures meaning. In a health-care setting, this would mean listening carefully to each individual child to discover what preconceptions he or she has and what kind of language the child uses. Play preparation might involve interacting closely with the child, building on previous knowledge and understanding, encouraging the child to work out explanations, introducing useful language and guiding towards appropriate concepts.

Peter Bryant (1937–): like Donaldson, Bryant is indebted to Piaget for setting the scene, since the controversies arising from the early theory have led to much exciting and productive exploration of children's and adults' minds (Bryant, 1982). Bryant rejects Piaget's conclusions about why children fail in certain set tasks and argues that children can think logically providing they know what is being asked and can concentrate and remember for long enough. He has demonstrated that children use different strategies at different times and, like Donaldson, suggests that education needs to take account of individual differences. His ideas can be compared with those of Wason (Wason and Johnson-Laird, 1968), who has demonstrated that adults also use different strategies in different situations and for different tasks. Wason argues that adults pay more attention to the overall meaning of a situation than to the rules of pure logic. When given a task that is removed from social reality, adults make the same logic errors as children and give an answer that is personally meaningful rather than strictly logical. The differences between children and adults, both Wason and Bryant would agree, result from experience, attention span and memory rather than being a fundamental difference in choice of strategy or ability to think logically.

Key Terms and Concepts

Abilities: problem-solving abilities often depend on specialised knowledge in a discipline. Bransford and Stein (1993: 4) point out that the same individual may be both good and poor at problem-solving, depending on the nature of the problem: a brain surgeon may be brilliant in the operating theatre but unable to solve a plumbing problem. Most problem-solving depends on general thinking and problem-solving skills in conjunction with specialised knowledge and skills. Bransford and Stein stress that when assessing people's problem-solving abilities (including one's own), it is important to ask whether the problem is relatively routine or non-routine for the problem-solver. See also expertise.

Abstract thinking: being able to think about things that are not actually present or that do not exist in material or concrete form. This sort of thinking may be in visual images (iconic) or in words or other notation, such as mathematical (symbolic). Adult problem-solving demands that children learn to make the transition from concrete, common-sense reality to coping with abstractions. This process of moving beyond the bounds of common sense does not appear spontaneously but is made possible through education based on the product of long ages of culture. At the present time, only a small minority of people ever develop intellectually to a high level of competence. The question for educationalists is whether this should be accepted as inevitable or whether teaching methods should be changed.

Accommodation: a term used by Piaget and others to describe the process by which a child or adult adapts existing schemas or conceptions when new information is assimilated that contradicts previous notions. Bruner extended the ideas behind this concept and suggested that children learn most effectively when they are confronted with contrasting evidence and have to develop new mental representations in order to make sense of the contradictory data. In the absence of contradictions, new learning may only take place at a superficial level.

Analysis: the breaking down (resolution) of anything complex into its simple elements, the opposite of synthesis. Much health-care research involves the careful observation of complex care processes and interactions, which can then be analysed to reveal the basic elements.

Assimilation: a term adopted by Piaget to refer to the process of taking in new information. If new evidence contradicts what has been previously learned and understood according to the person's individual schemas or preconceptions, the person may do one of three things: reject the new information and soon forget it, assimilate the new data at a superficial level alongside the previous schemas with no shift in understanding, or accommodate the new data by developing new more effective schemas. Assimilation of contradictory ideas, without accommodation, can lead to *cognitve dissonance* and in turn to distortion or later rejection of one of the ideas, forgetting or *denial*.

Cognitive development (cognitive growth or intellectual growth): the ongoing process of learning to think, organise thoughts and generally make sense of the world. Until the late 1960s it was strongly believed that cognitive development only really took place during childhood and that a person reached the peak of ability in late adolescence or early adulthood, thereafter starting to decline. This formed the basis of early models of ageing (for example, Bromley, 1966), which are now known as 'decrement models'. It is now acknowledged that cognitive development continues throughout life, which has given rise to a 'personal growth model' (Rapaport and Rapaport, 1980). Even when some short-term memory and attentional processes deteriorate in old age, this does not prevent a continued improvement in wisdom and overall cognitive appraisal of the world.

Cognitive styles: an expression used in relation to Bruner's approach to thinking. Bruner (1964) suggests that we use different cognitive styles, or ways of representing the environment, for solving different tasks. During early development, a child uses only an enactive style and then gradually adds the iconic and symbolic styles as memory and language develops. As adults, all three styles may be used, starting, perhaps, with enactive, then adding iconic and then symbolic representations, repeating and refining these as appropriate. See also problem-solving.

Concept: an abstract idea, mental image or word picture (Talbot, 1995: 652) usually derived by looking at a set of examples and working out what it is that they have in common. For example, a carrot, a parsnip and a cabbage have something in common, that gives rise to the concept of vegetable. Apple, orange and peach contribute to the concept of fruit. Concepts often give rise to classification systems and precise definitions. Items may be differently classified for different purposes, depending on what concepts come to mind or are useful. A tomato may be classed as a fruit or a vegetable, according to the context.

Many concepts, such as justice, pain, stress, personality, caring and nursing, are difficult to grasp or define precisely. One way to understand a new concept is to look at lots of different examples and learn by trial and error to recognise when a particular example belongs to a given class. The accurate identification of similarities and differences forms the basis of much scientific work. In many contexts, it is not always necessary to be able to give a precise definition of what examples have in common or what makes them different from items that do not belong. By sharing experiences and comparing examples over a long period of time, a culture invents words to stand for concepts and gradually builds a more and more useful language.

Concrete operations: the second main stage of intellectual growth described by Piaget, lasting from about 18 months to 11 years. According to Piaget, thinking during this stage is restricted to concrete or real objects and examples, without any facility for abstraction or formal operations. Piaget believed that a child in this stage was unable to think logically or cope with abstract ideas. The stage can be subdivided into preconceptual, intuitive and operational. As the child moves through these substages, thinking becomes clearer and more systematic, concepts such as conservation become established and the child can describe and manipulate observations.

Conservation: a term used by Piaget to describe whether children have reached a stage in their development at which they can correctly answer questions relating to changes in the appearance, but not the quantity, of objects. Using tasks related to length, area, volume, number and mass, Piaget identified the order in which children develop concepts of conservation. According to Piaget, children in the preconceptual stage respond to all tasks incorrectly and therefore cannot conserve any quantities. During the intuitive stage, children begin to conserve length and area. For example, they can tell that a piece of string stays the same length whether it is curled up or straightened out. However, these children cannot tell if liquid poured into a different shape container still comprises the same amount. They appear distracted by either the height or the width of the container and do not seem to be able to pay attention to both dimensions at the same time. Conservation of volume and weight or mass develops during the operational stage. Alternative explanations of the faulty answers are given by Bruner (1964), Donaldson (1978) and Bryant (1982), who suggest that the questions are misleading, that children do not understand what they are being asked, that they cannot remember what has taken place or that they do not understand words like 'more' and 'less'.

Convergent thinking: a style of problem-solving that is intended to reach one particular solution, all efforts being directed towards that.

Creativity: a difficult concept to define precisely, as ideas about creativity range from regarding a creative act as one in which an individual produces something new only to the individual, to something which is new to the culture or the world as a whole. Moreover, being different does not necessarily mean being seen as creative; the merely eccentric is not necessarily creative even if it is statistically uncommon. Evans and Deehan (1988: 11) argue that common conceptions of creativity derive from beliefs in a divine Creator and a conviction that creative people are 'gifted' or 'touched with genius', leading most people to think that they cannot be creative.

The study of creativity is concerned both with attempting to measure personal attributes and with examining the processes by which people are able to produce novel solutions to problems, whether on an individual or a global basis. Early models, for example Wallas (1926), which seek to outline the stages in the creative process, can be compared directly with those of Thomson (1959) and Bransford and Stein (1993) for problem-solving. No differences are found between creativity in art and science, and it is now widely held that, although the end products are different, the processes involved in achieving them are the same. Like all thinking and problem-solving, the creative process may involve a combination of conscious rational processes and flashes of inspiration derived from unconscious connections.

Other approaches have reviewed biographies and autobiographies in a attempt to isolate the features of a specially creative personality. In both of these approaches, researchers now look for the skills involved and how these can be developed. This change has shifted the emphasis away from considering creativity as an inborn special ability, available only to a select few, towards a belief that creativity can be taught.

Deduction or deductive reasoning: the reverse of induction, so that thinking progresses from general principles to individual examples. That is, if a person knows how things work and is asked to predict what will happen in a particular situation, that person can use the knowledge to deduce the answer.

In professional care, it is very important to distinguish between truth and logic. Even using sound logical processes, a practitioner can arrive at a faulty conclusion about a patient or client if insufficiently informed. For example, if a practitioner believes that all type A behaviour pattern (TABP) people have heart attacks, a new patient with TABP will be expected to be vulnerable. This premise is not true. Some research suggests that the likelihood is greater, but this does not mean that all TABP people have heart attacks.

Alternatively, the premises may be true, but the logic faulty. It might be stated that research has shown that some people with TABP have heart attacks, so, since Mr Y has had a heart attack, he must have a type A behaviour pattern. It is helpful if such thoughts are written as *syllogisms* (see below).

Dichotomous reasoning: presenting both sides of an argument or dividing an argument into two parts. See also Chapter 6.

Discovery learning: a *learner-centred*, self-directed approach to learning that is associated with Piaget (1926, 1929, see 1989, 1990) and Bruner (1960, 1964). This approach requires learners to take an active role in the teaching and learning process, drawing upon their own experiences and researching information. Discovery methods favour experimentation by the learner. They allow for learners with different kinds of knowledge to work at different speeds and may be achieved by presenting learners with problems and challenges.

Questions that contain an element of controversy or contradiction may prompt the learner to reflect on the subject matter. A question phrased:

Mrs X has agreed to accept treatment on the ward. Have we the right to insist that she gets out of bed to attend the ward meeting when she wants to lie in?

rather than:

Do you think we should insist that Mrs X gets up for the ward meeting?

will encourage the learner to consider the personal rights of Mrs X as a patient, in association with her need to receive treatment.

The same is true of simulation exercises, which the teacher can use to present the learner with imaginary problems designed to mimic those they have faced in reality. This can promote debate and understanding and may encourage the learner to adopt a problem-solving approach.

Divergent thinking: a style of problem-solving that is intended to find as many alternative solutions as possible. Divergent thinking may be the most important ingredient of the initial processes of problem-solving. The alternative solutions can be compared and then convergent thinking employed to select the most suitable solution for a particular case. See also lateral thinking.

Egocentricity: according to Piaget, a newborn baby is totally egocentric, unable to make any distinction between itself and the outside world. The baby does not know that anything else exists or even that he or she exists. In the course of the sensorimotor period, the child slowly manages to reduce this unawareness and begin to distinguish between self and the rest of the world (decentring). Egocentric play and an egocentric view may continue for several years until after a child has started school, so the process of decentring can take some time. Piaget's timescale for development can be called into question, particularly as new evidence is accruing on what the perceptual world of the fetus is like. It is unlikely that a newborn baby is as lacking in experience as Piaget assumed. Moreover, observation of children indicates that although children may play alone, they are watching and copying each other.

Enactive representation: the first of Bruner's ways of describing mental representation of the environment in order to think or solve problems. This involves actions. For example, if asked how many pieces you would get if you cut an apple across the middle, one way of finding the answer would be to get an apple and cut it. Bruner describes young children as using this as the main way of discovering how the world works. In developing health-care skills, a great deal of attention is paid to carrying out and practising procedures as part of the learning process. Without a firm foundation in enactive processes, theoretical explanations make little sense. It would seem that Bruner's notion that enactive thinking is one possible mode for people of all ages is more useful than Piaget's assertion that the sensorimotor stage of thinking is only the first stage and will be replaced in later years by reasoning.

Equilibration: a term from Piaget's work to describe the process by which a child tries to stay in balance, accommodating new information by changing schemas to suit new experiences or rejecting new information that will not fit.

Expertise: in general, experts have a greater store of memorised solutions to problems within their domain than novices. They tend to work 'forwards' towards a solution by making inferences about what is needed rather than backwards from the goal or by means–end analysis. Experts sometimes spend time on constructing a concrete representation of the abstract problem before attempting to solve it but also relate the items mentioned in the problem to underlying concepts (Bhaskar and Simon, 1977, cited by Kahney, 1993).

Fantasy play: Lucariello (1987) gives four dimensions of fantasy play (action, roles, objects and organisation), based on Piaget's stages of cognitive development. The list below is modified slightly to help avoid the notion of stages as a fixed sequence and to integrate ideas from other theories.

Action: play becomes more complex as a child becomes able to integrate a sequence of actions. Activities that are at first restricted to simple sensorimotor or enactive movements, babbling, manipulating objects and scribbling, later extend to include a more elaborate use of artefacts, making and playing with three-dimensional action models, talking, drawing pictures and, later, writing.

Roles: as children develop, the focus shifts from self to fantasies involving others and later to the creation of multiple roles. This kind of play becomes more elaborate as children are exposed to an ever-increasing variety of real-life situations and events and have greater opportunity for interaction with others. Solitary play may extend and enrich role-play with toys, telling stories to oneself and later writing stories.

Objects: children use objects at first in a way that is closely linked to the normal daily function. Later, substitute objects may be used symbolically to represent something else. For example, a cardboard tube may serve for a telescope. It can be argued that this simple symbolic representation, and the realisation that one thing can stand for another even when it does not bear much resemblance, is essential to the development of language, which, by its nature, is symbolic. Accurate miniature replicas (such as a realistic looking telescope) are, in some ways, less effective in helping this development than is pure fantasy based on unrealistic substitutes. This may help to explain why small children are often more interested in playing with the cardboard box than the toy that came in it!

Organisation: as children develop, the planning and organisation of play becomes more complex and depend on elaborate sets of rules. Dynamics within a group become more complex; leaders may emerge.

Formal operations: the last of the stages of intellectual growth identified by Piaget. He believes that this starts in adolescence and becomes the chief style of thinking of the intelligent adult. According to Piaget, thinking at this stage is characterised by systematic experimentation, isolation of variables, looking for relationships and explanations, recognising contradictions, making logical deductions, reasoning with abstracts and distinguishing between truth and logic. This is strongly criticised by other theorists who argue that children can use these operations at any age given the appropriate conditions and, moreover, that even intelligent adults do not think like this much of the time.

Group of displacements and reversibility: the development of the object concept is closely tied up with the progressive organising of movements in space: the movements of the child and the movements of the objects. At first the baby drops toys out of the pram and waits for an adult to pick them up. This is non-reversible action. Gradually, the child learns to make a group of displacements, moving himself or herself or the objects in a sequence of actions, taking objects from one place to another and retrieving them, or moving to another part of the room and returning. Piaget suggests that this develops during the sensorimotor stage of development.

Heuristic strategies: heuristics are (imperfect) rules of thumb that guide a search for a solution to a problem (Kahney, 1993: 49). Heuristic strategies are those which a person can work out without instruction.

Iconic representation: the second of Bruner's ways of describing mental representation of the environment in order to think or solve problems. Iconic representation involves forming mental images of objects and the activities that the child (or adult) wishes to carry out. The term is usually used to refer only to visual images but could be extended to cover all sensory modes (see Chapter 14). It depends on having sufficient memory for the objects and activities to be held in the mind long enough for the activity to be thought through. This approach can be readily compared with Baddeley's ideas on working memory, which he describes as using a visual 'sketchpad' or 'scratchpad' as part of the short-term memory processes designed to handle information that has been temporarily recalled from long-term storage (Baddeley, 1990).

If you imagine a cube and think of cutting it in half and then half again, you might be able to say how many freshly cut faces each of the pieces has. How easy you find this task will depend on how clear your iconic imagery is and how readily you can carry out this kind of activity in your mind. You might like to consider what your cube was made of and what colour it was, what you cut it with and so on. Many people do not make a particularly clear picture. Others imagine a specific material such as cheese or one with a distinct colour, which is different inside from outside, and may even evoke a smell and a taste. Others may imagine sawing a wooden cube with a power saw, complete with sound effects, the smell of the sawdust and the pull on the arm muscles. Notice how much easier this task becomes if you think of cutting an apple into quarters. Your experience and memories of cutting apples is significantly greater than for cubes. See also Chapters 11 and 14.

Differences in the ways in which people make use of iconic imagery can result in difficulties in communication, as two people may find they are just 'not on the same wavelength'. It is important in professional care to try to match descriptions and explanations of procedures to the kind of language and imagery the client uses.

Induction or inductive reasoning: reasoning from particular observations to a general belief or, in more formal terms, from empirical data to a model. This involves noticing what things have in common and arriving at a general principle or concept (see Chapter 18). In most areas of life, despite sound reasoning, people are likely to arrive at only partial truths and faulty conceptions owing to incomplete knowledge. It is helpful to realise that wrong answers are not usually the result of an inability to think logically but merely of insufficient data. See also Chapter 15.

Insight: in the context of problem-solving, this term is used for a sudden solution to a problem where the steps involved in reaching the solution are not known. This may also be referred to as an 'aha' experience, in which a person has been struggling unsuccessfully to solve a problem and then abruptly sees what is needed.

Intelligence: an abstract concept with no agreed definition. Alice Heim (1954) discussed over 40 definitions of intelligence. Some early definitions stressed rational, convergent thinking. For example, Guilford (1967) defines intelligence as ability in dealing with problems that require one, clearly defined and correct answer. Others recognise the need to include imaginative divergent thinking. Use of the term 'intelligence' now usually refers to a person's ability to learn from experience. This will include adapting to the situation, both in dealing with familiar situations and in solving new problems. This view of intelligence appears to be related to the rate at which a person can assimilate information and the ease or effectiveness with which this can be related to previous knowledge, skills or experience.

It was once commonly believed (for example, Eysenck, 1962; MENSA) that intelligence was determined by inheritance. However, much of what used to be thought of as intelligence can now be identified as problem-solving skills that can be learned at any age. It is sometimes useful to distinguish between crystallised and fluid intelligence. Crystallised intelligence is associated with well-established patterns of thinking, habits, knowledge and skills. Evidence suggests that this continues to develop throughout the lifespan and that most people continue to get better and better at their chosen occupations and hobbies and to provide accurate answers to familiar problems. Fluid intelligence is concerned with responding to new situations and making use of previously learned knowledge and skills in new, creative and adaptive ways. There is some evidence that this adaptability declines with age, as most people settle into habitual ways of dealing with situations and find it difficult to come to terms with new events and experiences. Fluid and crystallised intelligence are sometimes abbreviated to 'wit and wisdom'. The concept of intelligence has largely been replaced by a focus on intellectual modes (for example, Donaldson, 1992) and problem-solving styles.

Lateral thinking: thinking that does not follow logical constraints but introduces novel solutions. This may involve shifting to another 'frame of reference' such that the answer belongs to a different set of expectations from what seems to be indicated by the task. Many jokes are based on a lateral thinking approach in which the story seems to be leading in a certain direction but the punchline is a surprise. Edward de Bono (1971) argues that lateral thinking produces a much richer set of possible solutions than pure logic and can be use productively to find the best solution. Lateral thinking represents the extreme in divergent approaches. In some problem-solving procedures, brainstorming of a lateral kind can throw up many interesting and creative, often deliberately odd, ideas, which may in turn give rise to a usable solution.

Means–end analysis: means–end analysis involves determining the differences between the current state of a problem and the goal state (the differences between what the situation is now and what is required) and depends on problem-solvers having an awareness of the means (operators) at their disposal for achieving the desired ends (Kahney, 1993).

Examples can sound unappealingly pedantic and long-winded, but means–end analysis is a powerful tool for breaking down a problem into goals and subgoals until specific activities can be identified which can be used to solve the problem. Such task analysis underlies much of behaviour modification therapy, in which the individual steps need to be clearly identified. See also Chapter 4.

Metacognition: an awareness of one's own thinking processes. The prefix 'meta' suggests a higher logical plane, a change of position or something beyond the regular condition.

Object concept: children develop a sense of a world of objects that is independent of themselves and their actions. For example, a young baby learns the difference between being able to control the movements of his hands into his field of view and not being able to control toys hanging on the cot. The baby gradually comes to know that things can go on existing when he cannot see them or sense them in any way.

Piaget tested this stage of development by hiding a toy behind a pillow. Up to 6 months of age, the young baby loses interest as soon as the toy disappears. At a slightly later stage, the baby waits for it to reappear. However, personal experience has shown that babies, apparently at the earlier stage, show surprise if the object reappears from the 'wrong' place. This indicates a more sophisticated object concept than Piaget assumed.

Play: play has traditionally been generally considered to be any activity engaged in by children or adults that does not appear to serve a 'useful' purpose or satisfy basic physiological needs. However, it is now believed that play can contribute to many facets of cognitive and emotional development at all ages. Fantasy play can be helpful in exploring emotions. The relaxation of logical constraints and 'playing with ideas' can be a significant part of problem-solving. Harvey and Hales-Tooke (1972), the Department of Health (1991), Newman and Newman (1991), Slade (1995) and Bee (1997) identify many types of play and how these can be used in hospital. For example, stages of play can be seen, relating to ideas from Piaget, Bruner and social learning theory:

- sensorimotor play (infancy)
- first pretend play (from 12 months)
- constructive play (approximately 2 years)
- substitute pretend play (2–3 years)
- sociodrama (preschool)
- awareness of the roles (6 years and above)
- games with rules.

At any given age, the child (or adult) may engage in a variety of play activities, drawing on whatever is available in his or her current repertoire and exploring and experimenting with new things. Many therapeutic approaches that use creative arts encourage adults to take part in child-like play in order to give new expression to emotions and bring release from stress.

With children in health-care settings, play can be used constructively to help to reduce anxiety. A variety of approaches is possible, all of which will help in some way. In general, a mixture of unguided play, the introduction of appropriate language, guided play and fantasy will enable the child and carer to play together. This may help to explore beliefs and preconceptions, develop appropriate concepts built on accurate information and explanations, and provide opportunity for emotional expression. See also fantasy play.

Problem: according to Bransford and Stein (1993: 7), a problem exists when there is a discrepancy between an initial state and a goal state, and there is no ready-made solution for the problem-solver.

Problem-solving: Bartlett (1958) suggests two processes:

- closed-system thinking, characterised by the application of a particular solution that is already known to similar problems
- adventurous thinking, characterised by a new formulation of a problem and obtaining a solution by original or creative thinking.

An early behaviourist, Thorndike (1931) suggests that problem-solving is an aspect of trial-and-error learning. His experiments with cats in a 'puzzle-box' generally seemed to support this view. This was strongly challenged by the Gestalt psychologists, especially Kohler (1925), who emphasised that solutions to problems were sometimes reached quickly, rather than gradually by trial and error. This explanation utilised the concept of insight, which refers to a sudden reorganisation of a problem and completion of a solution without trying out all the possible alternatives.

Some of these ideas were put together in early ideas about the process of problem-solving (Thomson, 1959: 32, 49):

- The person first has to decide what the central problem really is
- He or she searches or explores the situation, trying out various things, by trial and error, handling materials and so on
- Then analysis of the problem is needed, constructing a plan and systematically working through (formal operations); if this does not work, it is necessary to restate the problem and search again
- Then attack; this can sometimes lead to immediate or 'insightful' solutions, sometimes to more trial and error, sometimes to following the plan, but usually to a mixture of these.

All these states are affected by prior knowledge and emotional factors such as anxiety, tension, disappointment, anger, boredom, satisfaction and relief, according to success or failure and the previous experience of success or failure.

Bransford and Stein (1993: 20) set out a model of the stages in problem-solving with the acronym IDEAL to assist in remembering the stages:

- **i**dentify problems and opportunities
- **d**efine goals
- **e**xplore possible strategies
- **a**nticipate outcomes and **a**ct
- **l**ook back and **l**earn.

Bruner suggests that a sequence of enactive, iconic and symbolic representations is needed when faced with a new problem. That is, three-dimensional action models can be made, which can be handled and experimented with. Then the problem can be represented as drawings and diagrams. Finally, the problem and possible solutions can be talked and written about, possibly with mathematical or other symbolic representations.

Reflective practice: the process of reviewing events in the light of theoretical knowledge in order to gain insight into what was done and learn from successful outcomes and mistakes. This can be linked to Bransford and Stein's (1993) definition of the ideal problem-solver and metacognition.

Schema (plural schemas or schemata): Piaget's term for an internalised representation or conceptualisation of experience. The process of developing schemas starts in the sensorimotor stage, in which each schema is simply a mental representation of a sequence of actions. Through the processes of assimilation and accommodation, a child adapts to the environment and develops more complex schemas.

Sensorimotor: the first stage of intellectual growth or cognitive development identified by Piaget. Lasting roughly from birth to 18 months of age, it includes the reduction of egocentricity, the development of object concept, group of displacements, reversibility and the beginnings of language. The period can be summarised by the expression 'Thought is internalised action.'

During this period, the baby is gaining experience through all the senses and absorbing it in patterns of behaviour. By using a combination of assimilation and accommodation, the baby adapts to the environment in such a way as to achieve success.

Seriation: putting things in order or a series according to some rule. An activity for children in the intuitive or preschool stage would include putting building blocks or saucepan lids in order of size.

Set (fixity) in problem-solving: once a person has found a suitable procedure for solving a problem, there is a tendency to keep to this procedure for all similar problems. This can be a successful technique and may save time and effort. However, a simpler solution may sometimes be missed. Moreover, as a habit, it will not lead to novel or creative solutions.

Skilled activity: Bruner (1964) lists three basic components of skilled activity:

- intention: where the end state to be achieved is specified
- activities: which are identified and serially ordered
- feedback: by which the effectiveness of each activity is judged.

When a child's interest is aroused, he or she can try out various activities. Successful activity will be repeated the next time an intention is felt. Skill-learning is linked with problem-solving and can later be refined into the higher mental processes. After a great deal of experience in learning new skills, a child begins to think.

Syllogism: a simple three-part representation of a sequence of logical deduction. A syllogism consists of two premises and a conclusion. The syllogism can be examined in a number of ways to see whether the conclusion is true, whether it follows logically from the premises and whether both premises are true. Representing a logical argument in the form of a syllogism can help to distinguish between truth and logic and help in identifying what has led to faulty conclusions. The following two syllogisms can be compared. The first has correct logic but is based on a false premise. The second is based on true premises but uses faulty logic.

- All people with TABP (type A behaviour pattern) have heart attacks
- Mr X displays TABP
- Mr X will have a heart attack.

- People displaying TABP are more prone to coronary heart disease than are non-TABP people
- Mr Y has coronary heart disease
- Mr Y must be type A.

Symbolic representation: the third of Bruner's (1964) ways of describing mental representation of the environment in order to think or solve problems. Symbolism means using one thing to stand for another even when it does not look like it. This can include using a cardboard tube as a telescope, putting symbols on a map to show the positions of churches and using words to stand for objects, activities and concepts. Where the object or mark looks like the thing it stands for, as in a model telescope or a drawing of a church, it is referred to as an icon rather than a symbol. Symbols belong to a system that has been agreed by people who wish to use them for communication, and the meanings have to be learned. The use of language depends on a fundamental understanding that something can stand for something else, and it is felt that symbolic imaginative play with children accelerates language development.

Synthesis: the putting together of parts or elements in order to make up a complex whole. The converse of analysis. In thinking processes, it normally refers to putting ideas together in a new arrangement or relationship that produces a new 'whole'. Models in nursing and health psychology often involve putting together elements of theory or practice into a meaningful list or diagram that shows the whole picture and the relationships between the elements.

Transfer effects: positive transfer refers to improved performance as a result of solving a number of similar problems. Negative transfer occurs when previous experience interferes with the solution of a current problem. Kahney (1993) gives the example that motorists would soon learn new traffic light signals if the green were changed to blue since these are similar but would have frequent accidents if the red and green were reversed. See also Chapter 11.

17 PSYCHODYNAMIC PSYCHOLOGY AND PSYCHOTHERAPIES

This approach is based on the belief that it is possible to interpret what is going on in the unconscious mind, using theories of the structure and dynamics of emotional development.

Some writers regard all in-depth therapeutic approaches, including client-centred and cognitive strategies, as psychodynamic. In this book, the term 'psychodynamic' is reserved for those therapies which are based on a coherent theory of unconscious processes and are inclined towards a medical or therapist-centred model of the therapeutic relationship.

This chapter attempts to give information about some of the named theories that may be used by psychodynamically trained members of a multidisciplinary team. Terms and concepts that are useful to those within the caring professions will be defined.

A word of caution is needed. As with all specialist terms, there is a danger of misuse by professionals who risk increasing a client's fears and distress by introducing concepts that may be heavily laden with cultural and personal connotations. This is particularly true of psychodynamic terms, which evoke powerful associations but are little understood.

Definitions

Robbie (1988)	The conscious is 'whatever is in the consciousness right now' and as demonstrated by Miller (1956), it has limited 'channel capacity' and can only process seven (plus or minus two) 'chunks' of information at any given time. The unconscious is not so easy to define. One

Definitions (cont'd)	
	version is 'everything which is not in consciousness right now'....
Freud (1924)	'Consciousness' is what we are aware of at any given time, and the 'preconscious' refers to mental experience just beyond consciousness, which can be readily brought into awareness. The 'unconscious' is deeply repressed experience, the emotional content of which continues to exert an influence and which can only be brought into consciousness with difficulty.

Approaches, Arguments and Applications

Psychodynamic theories attempt to explain all experiences but in particular why people sometimes behave irrationally or in ways that are (or appear to be) dangerous or unpleasant for themselves and others. Conscious awareness is viewed as only the tip of the iceberg of the mind. The whole of the rest of the mind is not conscious and is perpetually processing thoughts, emotions and behaviour without conscious awareness or control.

This is a view that is shared to some extent by all psychologists, but psychodynamic theories go further than the mainstream perspectives in attempting to create a comprehensive interpretative structure based on the dynamics of emotional development. Psychodynamic theories are not normally considered to belong within mainstream scientific or experimental psychology as they are based on speculation derived from qualitative data and individual case histories, and are not seen to be supported by objective, statistically quantifiable research.

The most prominent theory is that of Sigmund Freud who, over a period of many years, proposed and continuously refined an elegant psychoanalytical theory of the mind that was intended to explain all the vagaries of human experience. Freud's books are fascinating to read but can be difficult to understand. Much of what he says seems odd, or even stupid or irrelevant to current lifestyles. Many secondary sources paint lurid pictures of Freud's psychosexual models while missing the point of what he was suggesting.

A key assumption is that who we are at any stage in our lives, and how we feel, depends entirely on all our previous experiences and that the first few years of life are crucial in determining what follows. Each new experience builds on the ones before as our expectations shape our new perceptions. What we take notice of, and how we interpret it, depends on what we have met before and what happened in a similar situation last time. Put like this, psychodynamics does not sound very different from behaviourism, which suggests that all behaviour is determined, or conditioned, by the outcome of previous experiences. Both perspectives are deterministic. What makes the difference between the two approaches is that behaviourism ignores the workings of the mind (the black box), concentrating solely on visible actions, whereas psychodynamics examines the inner mind and focuses particularly on emotional experiences. In psychodynamics, emotions, particularly anxiety, are what matters, more so than overt cognitions or behaviour.

Psychodynamic approaches also support a belief that detailed and thorough analysis can trace the ways in which previous experiences have shaped the current state of the person. Analysis of an individual's experiences will lead to that person having a better understanding of himself or herself and hence a greater ability to cope with problems. However, even Freud admits that his style of psychoanalysis does not necessarily make a person feel happier: it just helps with understanding the causes of unhappiness.

There are now many different psychodynamic theories or styles. Most can be seen to have been influenced by Freud in one way or another, but each theory is based on different sets of beliefs or interpretations of behaviour, each adding something new to our overall understanding. Important names include Alfred Adler, Wilfred R. Bion, John Bowlby, Erik Erikson, Eric Fromm, Karen Horney, Melanie Klein, Jacques Lacan and Donald Winnicott.

Alfred Adler (1870–1937): Adler developed a psychodynamic approach to personality, based on detailed case histories, which he named 'individual psychology'. He used early recollections, dream analysis and knowledge of birth order to analyse childhood experiences. A key principle is that faulty response patterns have developed to safeguard the person from the burden of excessive feelings of inferiority. In particular, the theory focuses on the idea that personality is influenced by birth order, particular characteristics being linked to this. Adler (1927) proposes four major personality types: the ruling type, the getting type, the avoiding type and the socially useful type. Ryckman (1989) suggests that Adler offered this typology reluctantly, as he strongly believed that each individual is unique, but found it useful in explaining the nature of healthy and unhealthy personalities.

Wilfred R. Bion (1897–1979): Bion was trained by Melanie Klein and has developed ideas relating to the carer as a 'container for emotions'. He considers that 'No mother is bad at everything', an idea related to Winnicott's description of the 'good enough mother'. Other ideas associated with Bion include the need to know when to stop digging, the recognition that it can sometimes be helpful to give back feelings, and the separation of person and behaviour, which helps people to clarify attributions. These ideas are developed in humanistic approaches. Bion is best known for his studies of groups, during which he took the role of passive observer and waited to see what would happen. This upset many participants, who did not know how to respond positively to a non-directive approach. Their complaints and other behaviour led him to identify three types of group behaviour: fight–flight, dependent and pairing (Bion, 1961).

John Bowlby (1907–1990): Bowlby, a paediatrician, has replaced earlier Freudian notions of instinct by studying mother–child relationships and considering the effects on the child's behaviour when bonds are prematurely broken, unduly strained or not properly formed. He combines ethological concepts from the study of animals with psychoanalytical theory. He is associated with explanations of juvenile and adult delinquency in terms of the problem of the 'unwanted child'. His work (for example, 1951, 1953, 1988) has had a powerful influence on the hospital practice of allowing parents to stay with their children.

Erik Erikson (1902–1994): Erikson has developed a psychodynamic theory of psychosocial development, identifying eight stages. This can be compared with Freud's psychosexual stages, but Erikson puts emphasis on social influences rather than sexual causes of conflict, and extends the stages beyond adolescence to the whole of the lifespan. The eight stages can be summarised (Erikson, 1979, 1982) as:

- basic trust versus mistrust
- autonomy versus shame and doubt
- initiative versus guilt
- industry versus inferiority
- identity versus role confusion
- intimacy versus isolation
- generativity versus stagnation
- integrity versus despair.

Therapy using this model is not limited to psychodynamic analysis but involves social and cognitive elements aimed at helping clients to understand their emotional development and cope with problem areas.

Sigmund Freud (1856–1939): Freud developed a method of psychoanalysis based on a predominantly biological approach to mental functions. He believed that psychology would eventually be explained in purely biological terms. However, he used a mental model to explain clinical observations for which biology could not account. He used it for treating patients whose symptoms could not, at that time, be explained in terms of organic disorders. Freud labelled three distinct aspects of mental activity. He used the term 'id' for biological instincts related to psychosexual gratification. The 'ego' is what is normally thought of as the conscious mind. The 'superego' or basis of conscience is partly conscious and partly unconscious.

Freud believed that anxiety can be traced to unconscious conflict between the id and the superego. When anxiety becomes very great, the superego may operate through defence mechanisms to repress memories, fantasies or thoughts because they are too painful to dwell on. However, the distressing emotions remain and may be expressed through dreams and other disguised or symbolic representations.

Through the examination and interpretation of dreams and defence mechanisms, the client may become aware of the repressed material and, as an adult, find a way of resolving the conflict and dispelling the anxiety.

Vocabulary associated with Freud (for example, 1924, 1938) includes id, ego, superego, libido, death-wish (thanatos), pleasure principle (Eros), psychosexual stages, Oedipus complex, penis envy and defence mechanisms.

Eric Fromm (1900–1980): Fromm believes that the strongest motivating force for all people is a need to find a reason for existence. He argues than humans have lost a sense of oneness with nature and lists a number of needs that help us not to feel isolated:

- transcendence
- rootedness
- identity
- frame of reference and devotion
- excitement and stimulation.

Fromm (1947) lists a number of different personality types related to whether people find satisfaction from stimuli within themselves or in the external environment. He suggests (1941, 1956) that problems arise from faulty social relationships and a fear of true freedom.

Karen Horney (1885–1952): Karen Horney developed a psychodynamic approach based on Freudian ideas but stressed that cultural and social conditions, rather than sexual instincts, contribute to neurosis and sexual disturbances. Horney suggests that basic anxiety is common to all people and that extreme or neurotic anxiety comes about as a result of disturbed relationships between parents and children, and that all children are anxious owing to the difficult nature of childhood. She saw anxiety (Horney, 1945: 41) as originating in:

> the feelings a child has of being isolated and helpless in a potentially hostile world. A wide range of adverse factors in the environment can produce this insecurity in a child: direct or indirect domination, indifference, erratic behaviour, lack of respect for the child's individual 'needs, lack of real guidance, disparaging attitudes, too much admiration or the absence of it, lack of reliable warmth, having to take sides in parental disagreements, too much or too little responsibility, overprotection, isolation from other children, injustice, discrimination, unkept promises...

She proposes that there are a number of neurotic strategies that people use to cope with feelings of basic anxiety. In particular, she lists ten neurotic needs (Horney, 1942: 54–60). These are for:

- affection and approval
- a partner to take over one's life
- the restriction of one's life within narrow borders
- power
- exploitation of others
- social recognition and purpose
- personal admiration
- personal achievement
- self-sufficiency and independence
- perfection and unassailability.

These ten needs can be classified into three basic types: compliant (moving towards others), aggressive (moving against others) and detached (moving away from others). Most people can identify elements of these needs in normal personality patterns. It is only when they become overly rigid, distressing or destructive that they are classed as neurotic. As an adult, a client can be helped to understand these anxieties and work through them. This list can be compared with those used in cognitive and rational-emotive therapy (see Chapter 6).

Carl Gustav Jung (1875–1961): Jung uses much of the same language as Freud but defines the terms rather differently. For example, he takes libido to mean life energy in the broadest sense rather than just sexual energy. His principal concern is with people who have been separated from their parents. He considers that people are striving towards psychic wholeness or integration, an idea also developed by Maslow (1962) from a phenomenological perspective. One of the key elements in Jungian therapy can be the recognition and integration of opposite attributes of the self (for example, masculine and feminine) that have previously been repressed. Jung called his method analytical psychology, to distinguish it from Freudian psychoanalysis.

Vocabulary associated with Jung (for example 1964, 1983) includes psyche, principle of opposites, libido, archetype, persona, shadow, alter-ego, anima and animus, individuation, mandala and collective unconscious.

Melanie Klein (1882–1960): Klein worked predominantly with children. She believed that strong emotions are present in children from an early age but that these are not always adequately expressed. She developed her theory in terms of the positions a child must move through in order to accept its mother as a whole separate person and struggle to move from dependence to independence. This can involve ambivalence and unresolved feelings of love, hate, fear and concern. She suggested that it is possible to detect and interpret these by observing play, and she undertook to analyse children's problems at a much earlier age than anyone had thought possible or necessary. Her most significant contribution is her insistence that children adopt 'positions' rather than go through 'stages'. She disagreed with Freud that children pass through a sequence of psychosexual stages and found, rather, that childhood represents a time of development of a particular way of approaching the world. She identified two main kinds of problematic positions: paranoid-schizoid and depressive. The paranoid-schizoid position involves splitting the external world into extreme opposites, a form of *dichotomous reasoning*, so that some things are seen as very good, others as very bad, with little in between. The depressive position represents a turning-in on oneself and internal conflict. Another key principle of Kleinian therapy is that a carer can act as *container* for the child's distressing emotions.

Jaques Lacan (1901–1981): according to Bowie (1991: 7), Lacan, in France, believed that 'Freud was right but not right enough, or not right in quite the right way.' Lacan's theoretical approach is derived directly from Freudian analysis but is developed according to linguistic models, for example those of Levi-Strauss, Saussure and Jakobson. Lacan asserts that the unconscious mind is structured like a language. Bowie (1991) suggests that, for Lacan, psychoanalysis is concerned primarily with understanding human speech, an idea that reappears in neurolinguistic programming. Lacan's ideas can be difficult to understand, and Lacan (1977) says he deliberately makes his writings obscure so that the reader must bring his or her own ideas into making sense of them and must not expect any simple or ready-made answers. He used the term 'jouissance' in various senses, including orgasm or a kind of gaiety, roguishness or 'bloody-mindedness' of the unconscious mind, or with some other meaning according to context.

One of the ideas that Lacan developed is that we are constantly striving towards the things we desire, but as soon as we achieve them, we want something else. This concept is associated with St Augustine (354–430), who said:

> our heart is restless till it finds its rest in thee. (Confessions, Book 1, Chapter 1)

This theme has also been developed by Baudelaire in his poem 'The Voyage' (1859) cited by Jouve (1980). Baudelaire's poem is a metaphor for the journey through life. He describes an insatiable desire to travel and gain new experiences, mixed with ideas of a voyage towards death. Baudelaire uses imagination of a wonderful world seen with a childlike naivety interwoven with disillusionment, jaded experience and an obscure catalogue of horrors and says:

> desire, that great elm, fertilised by lust...
> why are you always growing taller?

Lacan is associated with feminist writings, and his views are widely used in the interpretation of creative arts.

Donald Winnicott (1896–1971): like Bowlby and Klein, Winnicott worked with children. He analysed how children develop attachment bonds with their mother and how these bonds loosen as the child grows. The mother can assist in this process by allowing the child to choose continuously between feeling independent and acknowledging dependence. Winnicott (for example, 1960) suggests that an 'ordinary devoted mother' who offers 'good enough mothering' will allow the child rights over precious feelings of dependence and unity with the mother and will not interfere with the sense of security this brings.

Key Terms and Concepts

Alter-ego: see principle of opposites.

Altruism: unselfish attention to the needs of others, sometimes at some disadvantage to oneself. One explanation for this behaviour is that it can operate as a defence mechanism directing attention away from one's own pain and anxiety. Examples might include that of a grandparent coping with the death of a grandchild by becoming a volunteer at a children's hospital. Vaillant (1977) identified altruism as a healthy defence mechanism.

Anima and animus: the feminine and masculine *archetypes* respectively. Jung was one of the main theorists to argue that individuals have both masculine and feminine characteristics and refers to 'transpersonal' traits. Jung suggests that all people have both anima and animus, but that the anima is predominant in women, the animus in men. In Western history, the archetypal or ideal male is seen as the warrior, bold and strong, the female as soft, pliant and nurturing. These extremes are exemplified by the gods of ancient Greece and Rome. They are also seen in the medieval symbols for iron ♂ (a hard, strong metal) and copper ♀ (a soft, pliable and decorative metal), which have been adopted as the symbols for male and female. Jung suggested that the anima and animus have positive and negative characteristics that can be developed by an individual. An ability to reason and use logic to solve problems is labelled as a positive masculine characteristic, uncritical and dogmatic adherence to certain ideas as negative. Warmth and intuitive understanding are labelled as positive feminine characteristics, moodiness and irritability as negative ones. See also *gender identity* in Chapter 15.

Anticathexis: restraining of energy.

Anticipation: a healthy type of defence mechanism identified by Vaillant (1977). It involves anticipating problems and finding solutions for them before they happen. An example of a healthy anticipation is arranging regular respite care for an elderly or difficult relative before problems arise. Anticipation can become unproductive if the person worries so much that plans are so incomplete or inadequate that the benefits are outweighed by the additional worry.

Archetype: a term used by Jung, among others, for a symbol that represents a universal theme or ideal.

The term 'archetype' may be confused with 'stereotype' in common usage, and it sometimes difficult to distinguish the two concepts even in Jung's own writings. Someone may describe a friend as the archetypal male when seeking to suggest that the friend has characteristics that represent the universal idea of maleness when, in modern terms, the friend simply matches the prevailing stereotype of masculinity and has a strong gender identity. Jung's notions of archetypal masculinity and femininity, anima and animus, are quite likely to be described today as culturally determined stereotypes that are by no means universally accepted.

Art therapy (art psychotherapy): there are various different ways in which art can be used therapeutically (see also Chapter 8). A qualification in art therapy in the UK implies a particular style of training in a recognised institute. The traditional style of training builds on a background in art or art history and is psychoanalytically based, using Freudian-style models of interpretation. The focus of training is on the theory of art and analysis rather than on the development of interpersonal skills of counselling. The art therapist interprets the client's paintings according to the theoretical model in order to analyse emotional experiences and problem areas, and guide the client towards greater insight. Alternative training courses may be based on Jungian or other psychodynamic models. Art therapists generally acknowledge their particular school of thought or bias, although the trend in some institutes is towards becoming eclectic or integrated. Person-centred art therapy rejects this theoretical approach (see Chapter 8).

Asceticism: denying oneself pleasures. Anna Freud suggested that adolescents sometimes deny themselves self-indulgent behaviour by, for example, refraining from eating certain foods because of their uncertainties in growing up. This is one explanation given for the early stages of anorexia nervosa. It used to be offered as an explanation for food fads, including vegetarianism in the days before this became widespread. It is possible that it forms part of many disorders in which an individual feels guilty about overindulging. The term is mainly used in connection with religious sects who observe strict lifestyles.

Blocking: a lay term for being unable to think of or do something because of some not-understood emotional significance. This may include forgetting someone's name when that name is the same as someone else for whom there is an emotional significance. Common usage includes writer's or artist's block, in which the individual is unable to produce new work.

Catharsis: a sudden powerful release of pent-up emotion with a subsequent feeling of calm and well-being.

Cathexis: investment of energy in a particular object.

Collective unconscious: Jung gives various ambiguous descriptions of the collective unconscious. He suggested that because people throughout the world have so much in common in dreams and art, there must be an underlying factor common to all humans. He called this commonality the collective unconscious. He regarded it as to some extent genetically inherited. However, he also seems to have held the belief that the archetypes expressed through creative arts indicate that mankind is in some state of communion with a divine or world mind.

Compensation: finding an alternative pleasure to compensate for missing emotional love, comfort and security.

Complex: a word coined by Jung, but also used extensively by Freud, to refer to the association of an idea with the strong emotions it arouses.

Container for emotions: a concept associated with Melanie Klein and W.R. Bion. They illustrate how a parent or other carer can provide a safe environment for a child who is experiencing ambivalent feelings of love, hate, fear and concern during the difficult period of growing from a position of total dependence to independence. Parents can help in this development by allowing a child to express emotions safely in a warm and secure environment and fluctuate between being independent one moment and dependent the next. This is a useful concept in professional care, in which patients are forced into a position of dependence. They may experience feelings of hopelessness and powerlessness coupled with rage. The carer can help to provide a safe 'container' for the expression of these emotions.

Countertransference: see transference.

Death-wish (thanatos – 'death' in Greek): Freud, and many analysts following him, point to the existence in people of dark and destructive qualities. This is sometimes viewed as a deeply unconscious wish to seek nirvana, the extinction of individual existence.

Defence mechanisms: conscious or unconscious mental strategies adopted by an individual when faced with emotional experiences that are too painful or difficult to be faced directly. They include:

- altruism
- anticipation
- asceticism
- avoidance
- compensation
- countertransference
- denial
- displacement

- fantasy
- identification
- intellectualisation
- projection
- rationalisation
- reaction formation
- regression
- repression
- sublimation
- suppression
- transference.

Of these, anticipation, avoidance and suppression are conscious defence mechanisms. Denial, reaction formation, repression and transference are regarded only as unconscious mechanisms. The others are generally considered to be mainly unconscious mechanisms but ones which can sometimes involve some conscious awareness. Where the mechanism is completely unconscious, the person involved cannot see what is happening, although it may appear obvious to others.

In health-care situations, defence mechanisms often form part of a healthy, beneficial process for protecting from anxiety and give the individual time to adjust to a new painful or frightening experience. It may be important to distinguish between defences that arise in response to new changes and those which may be lingering from early-established and deep-seated anxieties. Simple uncritical acceptance and respect may be all that is necessary to provide support and allow time for healing, but if defence mechanisms persist or interfere with daily living, specialist counselling or psychotherapy may be recommended.

Denial: the inability to believe that something distressing is true even when faced with evidence that everyone else accepts; continuing to act as if something is not true even when others try to convince one that it is. Examples include the belief that a person who has been declared brain dead will eventually recover, searching for a baby who has died and continuing to expect to recover the use of the limbs even after tests have confirmed permanent damage to the spinal cord.

Within the caring professions, denial is the most commonly mentioned defence mechanism. Examples are frequently observed, and there is ongoing debate over how best to be supportive, that is, whether or not to confront the patients with their denial and try to coax them into acceptance. Most short-term forms of denial are part of a healthy, beneficial process for protecting from anxiety, and give the individual time to adjust to a new painful or frightening experience. The assumption that the observed behaviour results from denial may sometimes be misplaced. For example, alternative explanations for searching behaviour after death can be given from an ethological perspective, so the assumption of denial in this context should be used with caution. In cases of severe injury, apparent denial may actually be vigorous resistance to dependence and may lead to an improved lifestyle and even a measure of recovery. When denial appears to persist, it is important to distinguish between a genuine inability to come to terms with reality which is hindering normal living, rituals that are comforting, and healthy avoidance strategies.

Displacement: finding a socially acceptable activity for the expression of psychosexual energy. When the activity is highly regarded by society, as in artistic expression, the term *sublimation* may be used. The term 'displacement' is also used to refer to emotions that are redirected from the real target to another person or object, such as expressing anger towards nurses, other carers or relatives because of anxiety.

Dreams: see Chapter 12.

Ego: a term taken from the Latin for 'I' and used by Freud to refer to the self. The ego is what we normally think of as the conscious mind, or anything available to consciousness, and is active in learning and adapting to the environment. The ego is concerned principally with cognitive processes such as perception and memory, and with the control of speech and intentions or volitions. Freud saw this as the 'executive' of the personality, balancing id and superego, weighing up the pros and cons of all activities and experiences.

Electra complex: sometimes used as the female equivalent of the Oedipus complex, although the Greek stories do not exactly correspond.

Formative years: many psychodynamic, and other, theories stress that the first years of life, particularly the first five, are the most important ones because they determine what will follow. Some interpretations of these theories seem to suggest that early experiences are essentially important because a young child is more vulnerable or impressionable, and that any damage done to the personality in early life is irrevocable, it being always too late to do anything about it. An alternative view is that the first few years of life are crucial, not because the experiences themselves are more important than later ones, but because they shape the ways in which later experiences will be perceived. In this view, self-awareness as an adult can help a person to develop a greater range of alternative perceptions and choices.

Free association: a technique pioneered by Jung and used within some psychodynamic therapies. The client is asked to say the first words that come into consciousness in response to a stimulus word. By looking at the pattern of responses, the therapist may find ways of directing the client along a fruitful line of enquiry.

Freudian slip: errors in speech or 'slips of the tongue' that seem to reveal some hidden thought that has contaminated what the person intended to say. This contamination is sometimes merely mechanical owing to similar sounds between what is intended and what is actually said; sometimes there is a contraction of several sounds into one. Such slips have been recognised throughout history and date back to ancient Greek civilisation. They have been used widely in literature before Freud's time as a somewhat subtle way of revealing a character's inner thoughts.

Wording can be an excellent witticism, a play on words or *double entendre*, or a blunder, depending on whether the utterances are made with conscious or unconscious intention. Freud made use of slips that occurred during psychoanalysis to point towards associations that might reveal hidden emotional conflicts.

Id: Freud used the word 'id', from the Latin for 'it', to stand for all biological aspects of the unconscious mind dealing with psychosexual needs. Freud viewed the id as natural, instinctive and demanding instant gratification. He described it as having no logic or external reality and governed chiefly by the *pleasure principle*, while at the same time incorporating certain destructive elements.

Identification: sharing or taking on the characteristics of another person to the extent that one's own identity is altered. The concept of identification exists within a helping relationship if the health-care professional fails to maintain an awareness of his or her own reality while sharing a client's experiences. It is closely related to empathy (see Chapter 8) but differs in that the carer loses sight of the 'as if' quality that characterises empathy (Rogers, 1961).

Individuation: Jung used this term to refer to the process, which he saw in certain gifted people in the second half of life, of working towards the achievement of psychic wholeness or integration. This is a idea that Maslow (1962) has adapted in his concept of self-actualisation. It is also used in a more general sense to refer to a sense of personal identity. See also 'deindividuated' under *crowds* in Chapter 19 and depersonalisation in Chapter 15.

Instinct: traditionally defined as an inherited and inborn predisposition to behave in a particular way in response to environmental cues. Very few aspects of human or animal behaviour are now regarded as instinctive, and early psychoanalytical ideas based on instincts have been superseded. All evidence now suggests that opportunities for complicated learning processes may start to operate shortly after conception. This means that a new distinction has to be made between things that are present at birth (innate or inborn) or appear alongside maturational development and those which are genetically determined. A few human reflexes, such as rooting and sucking, and a walking response, are present at birth, but it is not yet clear how much subsequent behaviour can be attributed to inherited elements.

Intellectualisation: thinking and reading about life events and giving theoretical explanations in preference to actually experiencing such events or acknowledging the relevance of individual experience. As with asceticism, Anna Freud added this term to her father's list of defence mechanisms in relation to adolescents who may adopt escapist behaviour because they are not coping well with the uncertainties of growing up.

Libido: Freud used this term for the unconscious source of energy associated with psychosexual needs. Jung extended the meaning of the word to cover the whole of life-energy.

Mandala: a symbolic circular figure used as a religious symbol of the universe. Mandalas are associated particularly with Tantric yoga, in which they are used as instruments of contemplation. Jung refers to the spontaneous appearance of mandalas in dreams, which he related to a search for completeness and self-unity.

Oedipus complex: Freud believed that, in the process of growing up, a young child develops a strong attachment to the opposite-sex parent and feelings of rivalry for the same-sex parent. Although this is not expressed overtly as a sexual feeling, and generally passes relatively unnoticed, the deep-seated anxiety that can arise if the situation is not properly resolved can be linked to unconscious associations with incestuous relationships. Revulsion towards incest is felt in most societies (see *taboos* in Chapter 19). The name for the complex is derived from the ancient Greek story of Oedipus, who did not know he had been adopted from birth and inadvertently killed his real father and married his mother. When he discovered what he had done, he was in great anguish and blinded himself as a penance.

Penis envy: a term coined by Freud to describe female feelings of inferiority in terms of a wish to possess male sexual characteristics. In contrast, Karen Horney suggests that women are indoctrinated by social values and norms to see themselves as inferior to men. They may therefore 'unconsciously strive to emulate masculine goals and values and to obtain the advantages and privileges that accrue to members of the male sex' (Horney, 1967, cited by Ryckman, 1989: 147). She regarded the male organ as symbolic of aggressive force (see Figure 17.1).

Persona: a term used by Jung to refer to the part of the personality that people make accessible to other people, the outward mask, allowing them to express their innermost feelings in ways they believe will be acceptable to others.

Pleasure principle (Eros): Freud believed that the id operates only in terms of pleasure obtained through immediate gratification of psychosexual needs. 'Eros' comes from the name of the ancient Greek god of love. When basic needs cannot be met, energy and tension build up, which have to be released in some other way, such as compensation or sublimation.

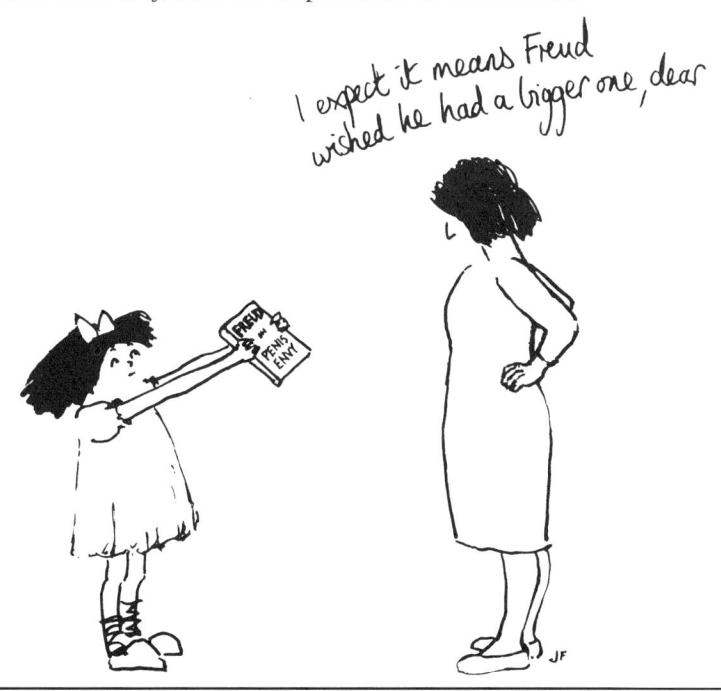

Figure 17.1 Penis envy (© *Jacky Fleming, 1991*)

Preconscious: that part of the unconscious mind that holds and processes information that can be readily brought into consciousness.

Primal integration therapy: this is designed to bring clients to an extreme height of emotion and then release it in order to achieve *catharsis*. It can be described as a regressive technique that brings an adult in touch with feelings that have not been expressed fully since childhood (Rowan, 1988).

Principle of opposites: a key concept in Jungian analysis, based on the idea that personality arises from the relative expression of opposite qualities such as masculinity and femininity. Jung suggested that one half of a pair is expressed strongly through the ego or persona, while the other half is repressed as the alter-ego or shadow. To achieve a sense of personal integration or wholeness, Jung argues that the repressed parts need to be recognised and expressed.

Projection: an unconscious process of attributing to people qualities that you yourself have or that are possessed by other people you have known. This might include liking someone because they unconsciously remind you of someone else. It also applies to disliking someone because of something you perceive in them, a quality or behaviour that is something you do of which you are not aware but which you unconsciously dislike about yourself. In a general sense, it refers to bringing or projecting personal interests and concerns into perceptions of any stimuli.

Projective techniques: standardised procedures for exploring a person's cognitive and emotional world. Stimuli are deliberately vague and can allow a wide variety of interpretations. Normative data are available for some tests. Examples include the *Rorscharch Psychodiagnostic Test* and the *Thematic Apperception Test (TAT)*.

Psyche: (pronounced as two syllables, sigh-key): this term is Latin for soul, mind or spirit, from a similar Greek word. It can be used in a general way to refer to the mind but is particularly associated with the writings of Jung (for example, 1964, 1983).

Psychoanalysis: the particular style of analysis developed by Freud and used by psychoanalysts who adhere closely to his interpretative model. The more general term 'psychodynamic' is used for approaches that are not strictly Freudian.

Psychodrama: a technique involving role-play enactment, role reversal and alter-ego support. It was first developed by Moreno (for example, 1946), who believed that working through problematic relationships and events would lead to insight and catharsis. This is a particular form of drama that involves Freudian and Jungian analytical interpretations. It should not be confused with other uses of drama and role-play in which concepts such as ego and alter-ego are not given any value.

Psychosexual stages: Freud tends to be best known for his description of the psychosexual stages of child development, which he named oral, anal, phallic, latent and genital. He suggested that tensions arising from conflict between the id and the superego during these stages and that are not properly resolved result in lasting emotional disturbance. This has given rise to the notion of people becoming 'fixated' at a particular stage. This model, based on Freud's theory of instincts, has been replaced in many modern psychodynamic approaches by a focus on interpersonal relationships.

Reaction formation: behaviour patterns that express an emotion opposite to the one which is unconsciously felt. Freud described how some of his patients who unconsciously feared their fathers expressed strong feelings of love and devotion. In a more general sense, the term can be used for unconscious or partly conscious devices that may or may not be transparent to another person. This could include insisting that visitors stay longer when you really wish they would go or protesting that you intensely dislike someone whom you secretly or unconsciously fancy. This type of behaviour was used by Shakespeare in *Much Ado About Nothing*, with humorous effect.

Regression: a term used by Freud to refer to people who exhibit behaviour associated with the childhood stages of psychosexual development. In more general terms, it is now used to describe any behaviour that is childish or considered more appropriate to a younger age group. It may be used in a health-care context when an anxious patient becomes angry and shouts in a way associated with childish temper tantrums, or when adults in pain rock themselves to sleep or seek comfort in cuddly toys.

Repression: an unconscious mechanism that keeps anxiety-provoking thoughts and memories hidden in the subconscious mind. The anxiety and other distressing emotions remain and can severely impede normal development.

Rorscharch Psychodiagnostic Test: this is perhaps the best known of the projective techniques. It consists of a set of apparently random designs or 'inkblots'. The final set was selected from a large number used in pilot investigations as these designs proved to be particularly useful. The patient or client is invited to look for recognisable patterns, pictures or objects, in the same way that many people like to look for meaningful shapes in clouds. The test may be used in a client-centred way as a convenient device for helping the client to talk freely. Alternatively, a therapist may use the client's responses in a structured way and develop interpretations according to the theoretical model being used for the therapy, directing the client towards fruitful lines of enquiry. The test may also be used by clinical psychologists or psychiatrists to examine cognitive patterns and help towards diagnosis of cognitive impairment. Standardised data are available.

Subconscious: a popular term for the unconscious mind but one not used in Freudian or other psychodynamic theories.

Superego: the term used by Freud to describe the aspect of the mind that is constantly in conflict with the id, attributing praise to good behaviour and guilt and blame to bad behaviour. The 'superego' is partly conscious and partly unconscious, and is learned through social constraints. It forms the core of conscience and adult morality.

Suppression: a conscious effort to avoid thinking about stressful or anxiety-provoking things. This defence can be a healthy one if nothing can be done to solve the problem. For example, when waiting for medical tests, it can be healthy to avoid thinking about the tests since nothing can be done until after the results are known. However, it would be unproductive to use suppression and ignore the results if action is required.

Thematic Apperception Test (TAT): this is another of the more well-known projective tests and consists of a set of pictures that can be used to determine a person's patterns of thought and emotional concerns. The pictures, mostly of people, are deliberately vague and ambiguous, and the client is invited to talk about the picture or tell a story.

Transference: in therapy, clients may unconsciously treat the therapist in the same way in which they have responded to a significant figure from their past, typically a parent or sibling. This may lead to resistance to therapy or to overdependence or exaggerated feelings of attachment. The therapist can make use of this by helping clients to look at patterns of behaviour and relate this to past experiences.

Countertransference can occur when the therapist loses sight of professional objectivity and begins to respond to the relationship in a personal way because of unresolved emotional difficulties. Training normally includes intensive analysis to enable the trainee to recognise signs of personal interests, feelings of attraction or anxieties that might interfere with therapy.

18 Research, Statistics and Psychometrics

Research can be scientific or non-scientific, quantitative or qualitative. Traditionally, only quantitative research has been regarded as scientific, being seen as systematic, objective, based on clearly defined hypotheses, examining cause and effect, seeking general laws, using statistical analysis when necessary and seeking to be reliable and valid. The chief experimental design related to health professions is the randomised controlled trial (RCT). Qualitative research tends to be exploratory, based on research questions rather than hypotheses, does not involve experiments and is less rigid.

Definitions	
Allport (1947)	[science provides] understanding, prediction and control above the levels achieved by unaided common sense.
Wright *et al.* (1970)	The term 'experimental psychology' has been used for several decades to refer to scientific psychology, which uses mainly experimental methods, as opposed to kinds of psychology based mainly on philosophic or therapeutic considerations… Psychology bridges the gap between the biological and the social sciences.
Searle (1989)	all sorts of disciplines that are quite unlike physics and chemistry are eager to call themselves 'sciences'. A good rule of thumb to keep in mind is that anything that calls itself 'science' probably isn't – for example, Christian science, or military science, and possibly even cognitive science or social science… There is only knowledge and understanding… some disciplines are more systematic than others, and we might want to reserve the word 'science' for them.

Definitions (cont'd)	
Hannigan (1982)	Statistics is concerned with scientific methods for collecting, organising, summarising, presenting and analysing data, as well as drawing valid conclusions and making reasonable decisions on the basis of this analysis.

Approaches, Arguments and Applications

To qualify as scientific, studies are expected to follow scientific methods and satisfy accepted criteria for good theory and research practice. These criteria include:

- falsifiability or refutability
- validity or truth value
- clarity
- the ability to predict
- internal consistency or coherence
- simplicity or economy of ideas
- fertility or generating of ideas
- aesthetic or intuitive appeal
- practical guidance
- the impact on our self-concept.

When compared with the physical and biological sciences, there is a great deal of argument over whether psychology can be truly considered as a science, particularly in relation to health care, since so much social science research is exploratory and qualitative, and sometimes cannot establish laws for which conditions can be exactly defined. Mainstream psychological perspectives, such as behaviourism, biopsychology and cognitive and social psychology, are generally considered to be more scientific, and therefore more reliable, than psychodynamic and humanistic approaches. Psychodynamic and humanistic psychology are usually considered non-mainstream as they are more concerned with individual case histories and a qualitative approach, and are not conducive to experimental research.

A division can be made between 'process' and 'holistic' approaches. Biopsychology, behaviourism and cognitive psychology are concerned with separate processes that do not need to take into account the whole person. Social psychology and humanistic psychology are more inclined to view the person as a whole, although much research in social psychology concentrates on one particular aspect at a time. Psychodynamic psychology can be seen as viewing people holistically, but it is sometimes accused of making interpretations of hidden dynamics in a way that seems detached from real life.

In pure research, some current approaches are recognisable as following a particular school but most have many influences. It is usual for an individual to study the contributions of different schools and then take an eclectic approach to the research issue, drawing on both quantitative and qualitative methods.

Psychiatry, psychoanalysis, psychotherapy and various branches of applied psychology, such as health psychology, medical psychology and clinical psychology, are usually regarded as separate and distinct disciplines, each with its own theory, methods and practices.

In addition to orthodox perspectives, there is a growing awareness of the ways in which complementary approaches can contribute to psychological well-being and reduce pain and stress. There is little research evidence to provide explanations of how and why these work, but it is hoped that increasing research into coping strategies and the concept of self-efficacy will bring new understanding.

Key Terms and Concepts

Analysis of variance (ANOVA): this is a statistical method for comparing samples to see whether there is any significant difference between them that can be attributed to the different experimental conditions. It is used for tackling problems for which the simple t-test is insufficient and can reveal whether sampling errors are confusing the results. Like the t-test, ANOVA is only useful for data that are selected from approximately normal (Gaussian) distributions. Special tables are used to compare values with normative data.

Baseline observations: initial measurements of physical and psychological factors, taken before intervention and against which the effectiveness of the intervention can be evaluated.

Bimodal (bi-modal) distribution: a set of numbers that has two modes. The prefix 'bi' means 'two', as in bicycle and bilingual. When shown as a diagram or graph, a bimodal distribution has two humps.

Central tendency: the formal mathematical term for an average or typical value in a set. There are three main types – mean, median, mode – each of which is an attempt to summarise the whole set of figures in one representative figure. The mean is the arithmetical average. The median is a central value with as many observations that are greater as smaller. The mode is the most commonly occurring value. Although these are all called a measure of central tendency, they may not actually occur at the midpoint of a distribution graph. The choice of which to use depends on the nature of the figures and the purpose of the study.

The mean is most useful where the numbers cluster closely around a central value but is misleading where there is a large spread or uneven distribution. The median is useful for small samples and is likely to be more stable than the mean, particularly where the values at each end (outliers) change dramatically. That is, if the mean and median are calculated for a set of figures and one or two more values that are at the extreme ends of the scale are then added to the sample, the mean will change noticeably but the median will stay roughly the same. The median can be time-consuming to calculate or a nuisance to use with large samples or where the middle values move. The mode is rarely used in statistical analysis but can be useful in everyday situations if decisions are to be based on the most commonly occurring values.

Chi-square (X^2) measure of association: a group of tests based on the calculation of X^2 that provides numbers to show relationships between variables in groups of observations. It is useful where data can be arranged in a *contingency table*, in which each cell represents a variable. For example, the simple chi-square test could be used to indicate whether there is a relationship between body weight and susceptibility to heart attack. In this case, there might be four cells arranged in a 2x2 table, that is overweight/underweight x have/have not had a heart attack (Clegg, 1982: 94). By referring to special tables, the observations in each cell can be compared. The chi-square test cannot say whether relationships are certain but can put a number on their degree of certainty.

Like tests of correlation, the chi-square measure does not indicate whether one thing precedes or causes another but only that the data show an association.

Contingency table: this is a way of presenting data so that the frequencies of two variables can be 'cross-tabulated'. Polit and Hungler (1995: 387) give an example of participants' gender and their responses to a question asking whether they are non-smokers, light smokers or heavy smokers. The raw data are presented as a table that lists participants and shows whether each one is male or female and non-smoker, light smoker or heavy smoker. This can then be arranged as cells in a 3x2 contingency table. Totals may also be given.

	female	*male*
non-smoker		
light smoker		
heavy smoker		

Data may be presented as frequencies or percentage frequencies. When presented in this way, data in each of the subgroups or cells can be compared to see whether there are significant relationships. A common statistical calculation for determining significance is the chi-square measure.

Control group: a group that is used for comparison in an experimental investigation. The control group does not receive any intervention or treatment.

Correlation: a measure of the relationship between two variables. A measured correlation only shows that two variables are related; it does not indicate that one causes the other.

Correlation coefficient: the number between 0 and 1 that represents the degree of relationship between two variables. A high correlation coefficient, for example, 0.8 or 0.9, indicates a high level of relatedness. A low one indicates that the variables are not noticeably related. A negative correlation indicates an inverse relationship; that is, when one value increases, the other decreases.

Cross-sectional study: an investigation for comparing performance at different ages, which is carried out at a single point in time, based on groups of different age or development. For example, investigations of how memory changes with age might compare groups of 20-year-old, 40-year-old, 60-year-old and 80-year-old people. Difficulties with this approach include problems with isolating or compensating for differences in education, familiarity with measuring equipment such as computers and the use of language, all of which will affect individuals' responses and may yield misleading data.

Data (singular datum): data are things which are known or assumed to be known as a basis for inference. Statistics is concerned with the systematic collection of numerical data or facts and their interpretation.

Degrees of freedom (df): a concept used in tests of statistical significance, referring to the number of sample values that cannot be calculated by knowing the other values or a calculated value, such as the mean. Degrees of freedom represent the number of factors that have to be taken into account when calculating correlations and that affect the way in which findings are interpreted. Usually, the number of degrees of freedom is $N - 1$, that is, one less than the number of values in a sample. Where there is more than one sample, the smallest sample is used. Degrees of freedom can be calculated in different ways in different tests.

Dependent variable: whatever is being observed to see whether the independent variable has any effect on it, that is, whether it is dependent on the conditions. For example, in a simple experiment to test the effect of alcohol on performance, the dependent variable is the performance of the participant, the independent variable (manipulated by the experimenter) the consumption of alcohol by the participant.

Descriptive statistics: 'statistical methods which summarize, organize, and describe data, providing an organized visual representation of the data collected' (Talbot, 1995: 653). These include frequency distributions, measures of central tendency (mean, median and mode) and measures of dispersion (range and standard deviation).

Deviation score: the difference between an individual value and the mean. Where each value is symbolised by X and the mean is $\overline{X}$ (called X bar), each deviation score is $(\overline{X} - X)$.

Dispersion (variability or spread): the degree to which values in a set of scores are widely different. Measures of dispersion include the range, mean deviation, standard deviation and variance. See standard deviation.

Double-blind design: in order to avoid bias and experimenter effect as much as possible, a double-blind method may be used. In this method, in which an experimental condition is compared with a control condition, neither the experimenter nor the participant knows who is in which group. For example, in testing the effects of a new drug, one group is given the drug, the other group a *placebo* (see Chapter 7). Neither the experimenter nor the participants know who has been given the drug. In this way, the experimenter has less chance of affecting observations by anticipating or expecting certain effects, and the participant has less chance of inadvertently behaving differently because of beliefs or expectations about the drug. Only when all the observations have been made and correlated is it revealed who was in each group.

Experiment: in a 'true' experiment, the relationship between two variables is investigated under conditions in which all variables are controlled, except the one being investigated (the dependent variable). There are three defining characteristics of the true experiment: randomisation, control and manipulation. Five basic experimental designs can be identified: single-subject, independent subject, matched subject, repeated measure and complex. When the subjects are people, they are best referred to as participants. In a 'quasi' experiment, one or two of the three defining characteristics are not present.

By deliberately producing a change in one variable (the independent variable) at a time, it can be determined whether a change in an independent variable brings about a change in the dependent variable. By manipulating only one independent variable at a time and by eliminating the possible effects of other variables, it may be possible to conclude that one change is the cause of the other, rather than merely being observed as a correlation. In the social sciences, it is difficult to identify and control all extraneous variables, so that even where experiments are possible and are considered ethically appropriate, conclusions must be cautiously drawn.

Experimental conditions: in simple experiments, two conditions are normally compared. One condition is usually a 'control'. The other 'test' condition introduces the independent variable that is to be tested. For example, in order to test the effects of alcohol on performance in a task, the performance in the 'test' condition is measured once with and once without alcohol, and in the 'control' condition twice without alcohol. This makes sure that other variables such as practice do not confuse the results.

Experimenter effect: there are at least two main kinds of effect an experimenter has on an experiment, the first to do with the way in which the experimenter sees the experiment, the second concerning the way in which the participant sees the experimenter. As Medawar (1963), cited by Wright *et al.* (1970: 29), asserts, 'There is no such thing as unprejudiced observation.' Every experimenter chooses what to look for on the basis of his or her own interests and experiences, and will interpret all observations in the light of those interests and experiences. It is difficult to be truly objective. Moreover, the mere presence of an experimenter may affect the behaviour of participants and it is impossible to know what the behaviour would have been like had it not been observed. To try to avoid some of these effects, a *double-blind* method, if possible, is used. See Hawthorne effect.

Factor analysis: a technique for examining a large number of variables and looking for interrelationships. Items that can be seen to be closely correlated can be gathered into a smaller number of variables. These can then be compared to see whether they can be interpreted according to known concepts or whether they give rise to new concepts or constructs.

Focused (semistructured) interview: an interview in which the researcher or interviewer prepares a list of questions or a topic guide but encourages participants to talk freely about all the questions or aspects of the topic without being closely guided. Interviews are generally recorded so that they can be analysed in depth later.

Focus group interview: a type of group interview that is becoming increasingly used in health research. A small group of people is gathered together and guided by the interviewer in a discussion according to a prepared set of questions. In this way, the interviewer can gather a number of different people's views in a short time. Disadvantages are that not everyone is likely to contribute equally to the discussion, and some people are reluctant to discuss their views in a group.

Frequency distribution: the grouping of data into categories and then counting the number of values or occurrences in each category.

Grounded theory: a qualitative research methodology developed by Glaser and Strauss (1967) based on symbolic interactionism. This can be used when there is at first little known about the subject matter. During initial data analysis, the researcher develops working hypotheses that are tested through the collection of further data. Through further careful analysis of the data, a theory can be developed. Rather than using random sampling, the researcher initially uses purposive sampling. As categories begin to emerge from the data, a move is made to using theoretical sampling (see sample). Glaser and Strauss (1967) used this strategy for looking at types of awareness of impending death (see Chapter 10). Another example might be looking at health-care professionals' perceptions of an aspect of their practice that has not been previously researched from the same perspective.

Hawthorne effect: an important example of an observer or experimenter effect that has been found in industrial research, in which increases in productivity may be found to occur in response to the mere fact that attention is being paid by the investigator, irrespective of what changes in practice are actually implemented. It is named after a study in 1927–29 in the Hawthorne plant of the Western Electric Company in Chicago (Gregory, 1987: 303).

Hypothesis: an idea or hunch that a relationship between variables might exist, expressed as a statement of an expected relationship between the dependent and independent variables, which it is possible to investigate systematically. For example, it has been hypothesised that people chose partners who are similar to themselves in attractiveness (Murstein, 1972). In quantitative research, it is usual to identify one or more hypotheses from previous experimental work and then test these systematically. In qualitative research, hypotheses may emerge as data are being collected and analysed. The word hypothesis is derived from the Greek word 'hupothesis', meaning a foundation for argument (Partridge, 1958). See also null hypothesis.

Hypotheticodeductive: a short-hand term for referring to the highly structured type of research that is based on one or more hypotheses and uses processes of logical deduction for deriving conclusions. It is usually contrasted with more open phenomenological methods.

Idiographic: studies and theories that consider each individual as an individual rather than looking for statistical norms and general laws, hence including all members of a population rather than only those who behave according to the norm. The idiographic approach can be just as systematic, and hence considered as scientific, as nomothetic studies but yields a very different type of description and analysis of behaviour.

Lazarus (1976) argues that both nomothetic and idiographic approaches are needed for a full picture and that they should be considered supplementary rather than contradictory approaches.

Independent variable: the variable that the experimenter controls or manipulates, that is, the factor that is being systematically altered to see whether it has any effect on behaviour. For example, in a simple experiment to test the effect of alcohol on performance, the independent variable (manipulated by the experimenter) is the consumption of alcohol by the participant, the dependent variable the performance of the participant.

Inferential statistics: parametric and non-parametric statistical tests that are used for testing hypotheses.

Law: a statement of a relationship that is always found to exist under certain conditions and that will stand even if a more sophisticated investigation shows that there are limits to its applicability which had not been known about. As long as the conditions are specified under which the relationship can be observed, the law still stands. Laws and general principles are common in the physical sciences. In the social sciences, there are few relationships that can be stated as laws: most social science statements are better referred to as 'confirmed hypotheses'. There are approaches that are described as nomothetic, seeking general laws and principles, but social science is, at best, based on statistical analysis rather than absolute numbers, and the general principles can only be roughly applied to a percentage of the population. Findings cannot be used to predict individual cases but only used to estimate how many examples are likely to be found in any given sample. It would be inappropriate to publish as a *law*, the conclusion that partners are similar in attractiveness. Since this finding is not always replicated for different samples, the conditions under which it does apply cannot be firmly established, and it cannot be applied to individual cases. Murstein (1972) felt that the evidence he collected confirmed his hypothesis that partners are similar in attractiveness more often than would be expected by chance.

Likert scale: a commonly used type of scale for recording responses to a questionnaire. The respondent is usually given an odd number of boxes (usually three, five or seven) from which to choose one response to each statement. The boxes may be numbered in either ascending or descending order of importance, may be labelled from true to false or from strongly agree to strongly disagree, or may use some other relevant wording. The middle choice is usually arranged to be of neutral importance, for example, 'neither agree nor disagree'. A choice of 'not applicable' may be placed in the middle or at one end. A variety of arrangements is in common use. Examples might be given as follows:

strongly agree/agree/neither agree nor disagree/disagree/strongly disagree

[ ]strongly disagree [ ]disagree [ ]agree [ ]strongly agree [ ]not applicable

disagree [ ]　　　　　undecided[ ]　　　　　agree[ ]

least important　1　　2　　3　　4　　5　most important

true　7....6....5....4....3....2....1　false

Problems may be found in collecting data in this way. Since the format can vary, the order of importance may not be immediately apparent, and respondents may misinterpret the boxes. Pilot studies should reveal most of these difficulties so that the instructions can be made clear and unambiguous. It is vital that respondents understand what is needed of them.

Longitudinal study: a study of a group or groups of people that takes place over a number of years, following the individuals. This has some advantages over a cross-sectional study as real changes in individual people can be measured, but it is by nature time-consuming.

Mann-Whitney U test: a test for comparing two sets of values that are not matched or that do not contain the same number of values and cannot be put into pairs.

Model: a device that helps to organise thoughts. A model may be a series of statements, a diagram, a physical construction or a mathematical formula. It represents an ideal, simplified or scale version of the real thing. It can show the relationships and patterns between constituent parts, indicate similarities and differences, and be used to describe, explain, predict and influence events. For example, communication models such as those of Schramm (1982) are helpful in analysing the communication process. In nursing, the term 'model' is often extended to encompass a whole theoretical framework that demonstrates relationships between key elements such as health, nursing, the patient and the environment.

Nominal data: observations that can be named but are not necessarily assigned a numerical or ordinal value. Examples would be qualitative data such as the colour and make of cars, or the signs and symptoms of an illness.

Nomothetic: the term comes from the Greek *nomos* meaning law and refers to research that seeks general laws or principles. This is done by studying samples and applying statistical tests to compare these with the general population, looking for normal distributions and establishing what most people do under certain conditions. These studies are inclined to ignore the percentage of the population that falls outside the norm.

Normal (Gaussian) distribution curve: a bell-shaped curve representing the way in which values in a normal population are distributed. Its main features are that it is symmetrical and that the mean, median and mode all have the same value and lie in the same place at the centre. The areas under the curve correspond to the number of values occurring within a specified number of standard deviations (Figure 18.1). To be 'normal', it must be a true bell shape, which conforms closely to the mathematical formula derived by Gauss. Real-life variations can be narrower or wider than the normal, skewed, bimodal, multimodal or irregular.

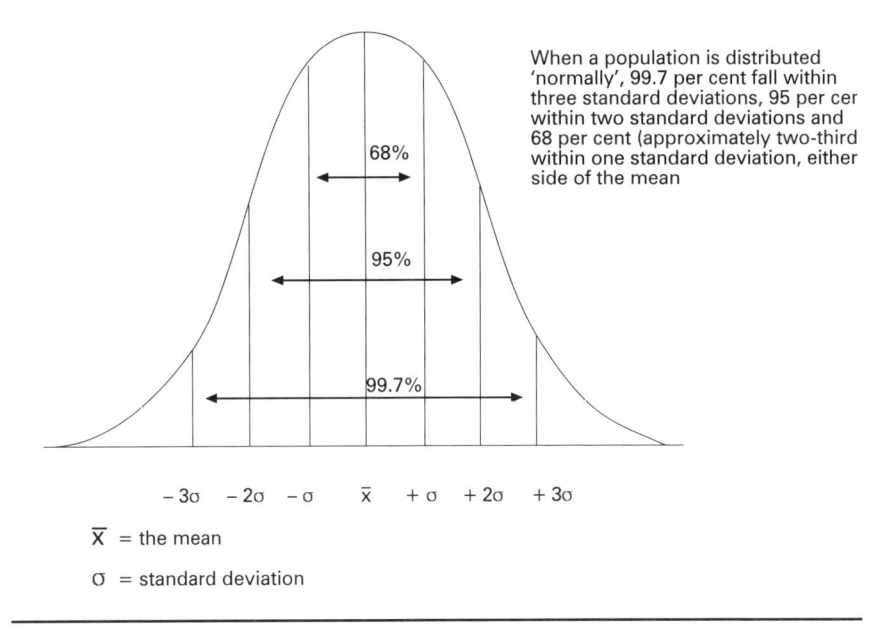

Figure 18.1 Normal (Gaussian) distribution curve

When a population is distributed 'normally', 99.7 per cent fall within three standard deviations, 95 per cer within two standard deviations and 68 per cent (approximately two-third within one standard deviation, either side of the mean

$\overline{X}$ = the mean
σ = standard deviation

Null hypothesis: the statement of no expected relationship between two variables. This can be thought of as the restating of an hypothesis such that no effect is expected more than by chance. In Murstein's (1972) study, the null hypothesis would state that there is no more correlation between the attractiveness of partners than would be expected by chance. Clegg (1982: 60) suggests that the best approach to take to any analysis of statistical data is to assume that 'the experiment has not worked' and that the independent variable has not affected the dependent variable. This can help to avoid bias arising from expectations about the results that are wanted by the experimenter in order to prove a point.

Objective: a viewpoint that sticks as closely as possible to the observable and measurable reality and that is the same for all observers, uncoloured by feelings or opinions.

Operational definitions: before an idea for an experiment can be made into an actual experiment, the independent and dependent variables must be carefully defined. An operational definition is stated in terms of the steps or operations that have to be carried out in observing or measuring whatever it is that is being defined. It is necessary to specify the procedure that is carried out to distinguish between two experimental conditions, the exact nature of the tasks and exactly what is being measured. For example in a simple experiment to determine the effects of alcohol on performance, the type and quantity of alcohol must be defined, as must the task to be performed and how performance is to be measured. This allows different experiments to be compared more meaningfully. For example, the effects of alcohol could be different according to whether beer or spirits are consumed, and care is needed in comparing experiments in which different types of alcohol are imbibed.

Ordinal data: data that can be put in order (rank order) according to the size of the values or some other dimension.

Outliers: values that do not appear to fit with the other values in a set.

Paradigm: a viewpoint or way of looking at natural phenomena that is based on a particular set of philosophical assumptions. For example, one of the main paradigms for enquiry into the relationship between the mental experience and physiological processes is the Cartesian (from Descartes) idea of dualism, which considers that the mind and body are separate entities. There is always considerable debate about the most useful or appropriate paradigm to be used to guide a line of research, or about whether it is preferable to start without making any assumptions.

Parametric and non-parametric tests: parametric statistical tests can be used when the parameters for the population are known, that is, where there are already data available for the population as a whole so that the new experimental data for the sample can be compared with the normal results. Parametric tests usually assume that the scores are normally distributed (see normal distribution). Examples are the two t-tests and analysis of variance. Non-parametric tests are used where the normal parameters are not known and where the data are qualitative rather than quantitative, that is, they require only ordinal, or in some cases only nominal, data. Examples are the Wilcoxon test and Mann-Whitney U test.

Participant: a person taking part in an observation, survey or experiment. This name is now preferred to the previously used word 'subject'.

Participant observation: an observation in which the investigator takes a part in the activity being observed. This is often used in the observation of children where the observers interact with the children, observing the children's responses to their interventions, as well as other behaviour.

Phenomenology: strictly speaking, the study of things and events that can be observed. The term has come to be used for various styles of philosophical enquiry and qualitative research in the social sciences that focus on the wholeness of experience and emphasise the searching for personal meanings and essences of experience rather than quantitative measurement. Humanistic psychology is sometimes called 'phenomenological psychology' because it focuses on behaviour and events as they appear to the client, searching for the client's own meanings and experience. Names associated with phenomenological writings are Kockelmans, Kant, Hegel, Descartes, Heidegger, Weber and Husserl. The differences between their individual approaches are often more significant than is any commonality. The term 'empirical phenomenology' is sometimes used to draw attention to the existence of observable evidence.

Phenomenon (plural phenomena): in the strict sense, this means a thing which can be detected by the senses: an object, an event. Hence the phrase 'visual phenomena' refers to ordinary things that can be seen. However, its usage is broadened to cover things and events that are experienced without obvious sensory input, such as in the expression 'mental phenomena'. In common usage, the term is further extended also to include things that can be imagined or supposed, or are thought to have been seen, and is used for events or happenings that are unusual or remarkable or for which there is no material evidence, as in the phrase 'supernatural phenomena'.

Population: the entire set of people or objects with a common characteristic that is under investigation.

Psychometrics (psychometry): the theory underlying principles of measurement used in psychometric tests or tools.

Psychometric tests: the systematic assessment and measurement of individuals' psychological attributes, such as personality, mental or scholastic ability, family relations, social behaviour, language dysfunction and motor skills, using specific psychological tests or statistically based assessment. Published tests are rigorously researched to ensure that they meet the requirements for reliability and validity. Statistical data provides testers with an idea of what the norms are for particular populations.

Cattell (1965) defines three databases of psychometry: L-data or life-record, derived from first-hand or second-hand knowledge of a person in the form of a rating by someone who knows the person well; Q-data, obtained from questionnaires; and T-data, measured by objective tests. See also Q technique in Chapter 15.

Most published objective tests are controlled and made available only to trained testers; a few are unrestricted. The NFER-NELSON Assessment Library stresses the importance of the thorough reading and understanding of test manuals of unrestricted tests so that the untrained tester is fully aware of the strengths and limitations of the test and can make the best possible interpretation of the scores. Otherwise the test does not provide the proper objectivity but becomes a mere extension of the tester's personal opinions, which in the guise of a test is potentially very dangerous (Beech and Harding, 1990). Many hospital wards or departments devise their own tests for use with patients, for example for the assessment of language difficulties following a stroke.

Qualitative and quantitative variables: Variables are called qualitative when they are described without being given a number value, that is, being types rather than measurements. When a measurement is made so that a numerical value is recorded, the variable is quantitative.

For hospital treatment, descriptions of satisfaction and comfort are qualitative, while waiting list time, cost and length of stay can be quantified. A qualitative variable can sometimes be assigned a numerical value on a rating scale so that quantitative comparisons can be made. For example, satisfaction with care could be assigned a rating on a scale from 1 to 5, going from least satisfied to most satisfied. See also Likert scales, parametric tests and non-parametric tests.

Qualitative research methodology: at least five models of qualitative research can be identified: ethnography, grounded theory research, hermeneutics, empirical phenomenology and heuristics. These approaches focus on the wholeness of experience, searching for individual meanings and essences of experience rather than quantitative measurements and abstract explanations.

Polit and Hungler (1995: 16) suggest that qualitative research generally:

- attempts to understand the entirety of some phenomenon rather than focus on specific concepts
- has few preconceived hunches and stresses the importance of people's interpretation of events and circumstances rather than the researcher's interpretation
- collects information without formal, structured instruments
- does not attempt to control the context of the research but rather attempts to capture it in its entirety
- attempts to capitalise on the subjective as a means for understanding and interpreting human experiences
- analyses narrative information in an organised but intuitive fashion.

Quantitative research: research that involves the measurement of variable quantities and the systematic collection of these numerical data, which can be analysed using statistical methods.

Polit and Hungler (1995: 15) suggest that quantitative research generally:

- focuses on a relatively small number of specific concepts
- begins with preconceived hunches about how the concepts are interrelated
- uses structured procedures and formal instruments to collect information
- collects the information under conditions of control
- emphasises objectivity in the collection and analysis of information
- analyses numerical information through statistical procedures.

Questionnaire: a set of questions or statements, usually presented in written form, that can be used to collect standardised data on a particular research topic. Unlike an objective test, questionnaires do not involve respondents in exercising skill but only in stating a point of view. Most commonly, questionnaires are used to measure attitudes, lifestyles or levels of satisfaction. Responses to statements are usually given according to a Likert-type scale ranging from true to false or strongly agree to strongly disagree. Statements need to be carefully designed to ensure they are not ambiguous or impossible to answer. The following criteria from Edwards (1957) can be useful in constructing statements:

- Avoid statements that refer to the past rather than the present
- Avoid statements that are factual or capable of being interpreted as factual
- Avoid statements that may be interpreted in more than one way
- Avoid statements that are irrelevant to the psychological object under consideration
- Avoid statements that are likely to be endorsed by almost everyone or no-one
- Select statements that are believed to cover the entire range of the affective scale of interest

- Keep the language of the statements simple, clear and direct
- Statements should be short, rarely exceeding 20 words
- Each statement should contain only one complete thought
- Avoid universals such as all, always, none and never
- Words such as only, just and merely should be used with care and moderation when writing statements
- Whenever possible, statements should be in the form of simple rather than compound or complex sentences
- Avoid the use of words that may not be understood
- Avoid the use of double negatives.

Range: the difference between the highest and lowest scores.

Rank order: placing scores (ordinal data) in order according to size or some other dimension.

Rate: the frequency with which something occurs. In the physical sciences, this can be measured in a number of ways according to how many items occur in a certain mass, length, area, volume or time. In statistical analysis, the rate is most commonly given with *time*, that is, how many (or how much) per second, per hour, per year and so on. The rate of deliveries in a maternity unit might be, on average, 40 per week or 2000 per year.

Particularly in social matters, for example the 'birth rate', the standard way of expressing the rate is to give the occurrence per 100,000 in a population for the year in question. Expressing rates or frequencies in this way enables comparisons to be made between groups. Raw data of this kind need to be treated with caution and should never be taken out of context.

Raw data: all the information that has been collected in a research study before any analysis has been undertaken.

Reductionism: when giving explanations for human behaviour, it is possible to give either 'same level' or 'reductionist' types of explanation. Wright *et al.* (1970: 23) say that when we explain a participant's behaviour in terms of the behaviour of other people and the general nature of the experimental situation, we are providing a 'same level' explanation. However, it is also possible, in principle, to explain behaviour by describing the sequence of electrical and chemical events in the brain and nervous system that are correlated with the behaviour. This would be an example of a reductionist explanation, that is, reduced to more fundamental physical laws. An important debate within psychology centres on whether reductionist approaches actually explain the behaviour or merely give a descriptive account of what accompanies the behaviour. The precise relationship between mental experience, behaviour and neural activity is not understood. See also Chapter 12.

Reliability: To be of any use, any measuring device (whether weighing scales or psychometric test) should always measure the same characteristic or produce the same value or score if it is used to measure the same thing on two separate occasions. This assumes, of course, that the thing being measured is stable – that it has not changed between the first and second measurement, or that if it has changed, the test will be able to detect this change. The degree to which a measuring instrument achieves reproducible measurements is called its reliability. Reliability can be statistically defined as a measure of the accuracy with which it measures the 'true' scores. Apart from the self-explanatory test–retest reliability, there are several different ways of assessing reliability, such as delayed equivalence, equivalent form and split-half reliability.

Delayed equivalence: this procedure takes into account changes in the individuals taking the test and changes in the test items introduced in the retest and counts both of these as error. Only lasting general factors are regarded as true variance. It is less frequently used than simple test–retest or equivalence reliability.

Equivalent form reliability: two equivalent forms of the same test are used with the same individuals with very little time delay between the tests. This avoids the administrative problems of retesting at different times and the likelihood that the individuals will themselves have changed between tests.

Split-half reliability: As Wright *et al.* (1970: 460) point out, it is not possible to administer equivalent forms of a test to the same individuals at the same time, and there must always be some delay even in equivalent form assessing, so there may be some change in the individuals taking the tests. To avoid this problem, the items of a test are compared by splitting the test in half and comparing the results of one half with the results of the other. In practice, the items making up the two split halves are usually selected on an odd–even basis. Thus the scores obtained on the odd items are correlated with the scores obtained by the same participants on the even items. Split-half reliability is different from other reliability measures in that it examines the homogeneity, or internal consistency, of a test rather than its reliability from one occasion to another. It is more clearly part of test construction than the other procedures and may be used more often during that process.

A test that is reliable may still not be valid, in the sense that it may give similar scores under different conditions but not actually measure what it is intended to measure. See also validity.

Research process: investigations or projects may involve the following components:

- project justification, decision about area of interest, aims and purposes, ethical aspects and costs
- the choice of research *paradigm*
- the examination of personal assumptions, beliefs and expectations
- information-gathering, a search of relevant publications, consultation and general, pilot or preliminary work
- detailing and categorisation, essential factors, similarities, differences, relationships and hierarchies
- the selection of variables; sorting the dependent and independent variables
- the formulation of hypotheses and the expression of each expectation clearly as an hypothesis or null hypothesis
- the selection of research questions

- project design, choosing or setting up situations for observation, experiments or surveys, and the identification and control of variables
- the systematic and methodical collection of data with regard to safety, resources and ethical considerations
- analysis of the data
- evaluation to ensure objectivity and conclusions
- theories, laws and models, reasons behind the findings and confirmation of the hypotheses
- publication and debate; follow-up work
- consideration of allied fields and the applications of the findings.

Retrospective and prospective studies: Retrospective studies are those which look back to see whether anything in the past can be linked to effects that are currently noticeable. Prospective studies start with the investigation of what is currently happening and then follow through into the future to see whether there is any link with what is observed later.

Sample: It is usually desirable for an investigation to give results that would be applicable to the population as a whole. A sample that is unbiased, in the sense that each member of the population has an equal chance of appearing in the sample, is known as a random sample, and is therefore in theory representative of the whole population. Where a sample is not random, the way in which it was selected must be stated. Convenience sampling uses people who are readily available. Participants in a purposive sample are chosen for their relevance to the information being sought.

Spearman's rho (ρ): a way of calculating a correlation coefficient by placing two sets of values in rank order and comparing whether they appear in the same order in both sets.

Standard deviation (σ, sigma): a measure of the variability or spread of the scores. The standard deviation summarises the average amount of deviation of values from the mean. A large standard deviation indicates a wide spread of scores and the distribution graph is wide. Where the scores are all very close to the mean, the bell shape is narrow and the standard deviation is small.

To find an average deviation quickly, it is possible to use a numerical mean deviation, ignoring whether each deviation is positive or negative and simply summing all the deviations and then dividing by the number of values. However, it is not possible to calculate a true algebraic mean deviation taking into consideration the sign of each deviation, since roughly half the values are above the mean and half below, and this would always come to zero. To allow for this, the deviations are squared to make them all positive. They are then summed, and the mean is calculated. This is known as the variance. The square root of this answer is taken to give the standard deviation. The procedure of squaring the values is derived from the equation defining the 'bell curve' and is related in various ways to the area under the curve. See also normal distribution.

Subjective: an individual personal viewpoint that depends on one's own emotions and capacities or on imaginary elements that are separate from the objective reality.

Subjects: until recently, the people or animals taking part in a psychology experiment were referred to as subjects, the symbol S being used to indicate a subject. The term 'participant' is now preferred. The British Psychological Society (BPS) occasionally print reminders (for example, July 1997) that the term 'subjects' is no longer acceptable in their publications when referring to people.

Symbolic interactionism: a theoretical paradigm based on the idea that people 'act towards things on the basis of the meanings that the things have for them' (Blumer, 1969). The actions of individuals are guided by the way in which they define and interpret what is happening in their environment. Meanings given to events derive from social interaction and are shaped by personal experiences.

In grounded research and other approaches using this paradigm, it is expected that individuals will behave differently, according to their own particular meanings. The research focuses on these individual differences and is not concerned with looking for general laws and principles.

t-test (Student's t-test or Student–Fisher t-distribution): a test devised by W.S. Gossett in 1908, writing under the pen name of Student. There are two types of t-test, the matched t and the independent t. These are parametric tests that are used to compare two sets of data that follow a normal distribution. The matched t corresponds to the non-parametric Wilcoxon test and is used with matched pairs. The independent t-test corresponds to the non-parametric Mann–Whitney U test and is used where sets of scores are not matched. The test gives a number that, in its relation to the numbers of values in the data, allows the probability of correlation to be estimated.

Theory: a coherent system of ideas or statements that can either be an hypothesis that has been confirmed by observation or experiment or an attempt to explain a group of observations or experimental data. A theory can only stand until it is improved or disproved by further study. It was an interesting hypothesis of Murstein (1972) that marriage partners are of similar attractiveness, which he found was confirmed by his data and which he developed into a theory by linking together appropriate explanations for his findings. His work is open to question and would be easily disproved if someone accumulated convincing data to show that there is no more of a relationship between the attractiveness of partners than would be expected by chance. A rival theory could be developed to introduce arguments and explanations for why a person is not likely to marry someone of similar attractiveness. Alternatively, it might be confirmed in repeated observations that partners are of similar attractiveness, but a new theory might be developed, giving different explanations for this.

Thesis: a proposition stated as a theme to be discussed; an understanding of the matter being investigated, to be proved or maintained against attack.

Validity: validity is concerned with what is being measured or investigated and whether the research or psychometric test is true or meaningful. Talbot (1995: 661) defines validity in quantitative research as the extent to which an instrument measures what it purports to measure, and validity in qualitative research as the extent to which the research findings represent reality.

With psychometric tests, it is not possible to guarantee that the final test will actually measure what was intended. Evidence is needed to show what it does test and how well. Validity cannot be defined statistically but 'relates to the appropriateness and justifiability of the things we say about scores on a test and the justification we have for making inferences from such scores to other measures' (Bartram, in Beech and Harding, 1990). There are at least six ways in which the term validity is used: face validity, content validity, construct validity, predictive validity, criterion-related validity and concurrent validity:

Face validity: this refers to the degree to which the test-*taker* sees the test as being reasonable and appropriate for a given situation. In practice, high face validity has no necessary relationship with what a test measures nor with how its scores may be justifiably used. However, it may have indirect results in aiding co-operation between the test-taker and the administrator. People are more likely to take seriously activities that seem reasonable and that they feel they understand.

Content validity: this refers to the degree to which the test is judged to be appropriate by 'professionals', and the extent to which a group of experts agree on, for example, whether the items cover sufficient breadth. Such judgements are best seen as part of the process of test development, as an indication that the testers are on the right track.

Construct validity: many tests are constructed to measure traits that are hypothetical. For example 'intelligence' does not exist in any physical or tangible form, nor do 'extroversion', 'spacial ability' or 'mechanical reasoning ability', yet tests have been created to measure all these qualities. Such physically non-existent qualities are often called constructs, rather than concepts, as they have been deliberately constructed as a means of trying to describe and explain patterns of differences between people's behaviour. There is no one piece of evidence that can prove construct validity. In practice, construct validity is gradually built up as more and more evidence accumulates about its usefulness. Each test should have positive correlations with other tests of the same construct, and it should correlate with real-world measures that are known to involve the construct. It should not correlate with situations known to be independent of the construct. Good test manuals contain a range of detailed information about correlates of a test. Construct validity ultimately relates to how well it is known and understood what a test score means. This knowledge may be gained inductively from individual instances or deductively from general principles. It should allow practical predictions to be made about real-world behaviour if the test is to be any use.

Predictive validity: this involves using scores from psychometric tests to predict future performance. For example, in developing a new test, an ability test may be given to students before they start their college course and the scores later compared with their final academic marks and practice assessments. It can then be calculated how well the test scores correlate with performance in real tasks. A variety of statistical methods can then be used with subsequent cohorts to make predictions from their test scores about the likely scores that new students will achieve at the end of their course. These predictions may be used to assist in deciding which applicants to accept. At the time of writing there are no standardised predictive tests for nursing education: selection is made according to academic qualifications and interview, neither of which have proven predictive validity.

Criterion-related validity (also known as empirical validity): some tests are designed to predict specific aspects of behaviour, for example the degree of success in a diploma of nursing course. In this case, it is not so important what is measured but how well it predicts a criterion. For example, if nursing students are given a whole range of tests before, during and after a diploma course, their scores can be compared with their success rates on the course. A test that correlates well with success could be considered to be criterion-related even if there were no obvious connection between the questions and success. Such a test is not given an overall score for criterion-related validity since it might be good for indicating success on one course (high validity coefficient) but not on another (low validity coefficient). Criterion-related validity is typically measured either predictively or concurrently or both. There is no clear-cut distinction between construct validity and criterion-related validity in many cases since construct validity is related to making predictions on what real-world criteria it should correlate with.

Concurrent validity: when the criterion and the predictor measures are obtained at the same time, the correlation is concurrent. Thus if an ability test is administered to a sample of student nurses at the end of their college course and their scores are compared with final academic marks and practice assessments, the correlation will give a measure of the concurrent validity.

- **Variable:** any characteristic or attribute of an object or person that varies within the population being studied, that is, something that can have different values for each of the observations taken, for example age, height, amount of alcohol consumed, attractiveness or marital status.
- **Variance:** a measure of dispersion or variability. It is calculated as the square of the standard deviation. See standard deviation.
- **Wilcoxon test:** a non-parametric test that can be used to see whether one set of scores is significantly different (for example, higher) than a paired set of scores. The scores are kept in pairs and the differences compared.

19 SOCIAL PSYCHOLOGY, GROUPS AND SOCIAL SKILLS

Social psychology covers all those areas of human behaviour concerned with interaction and communication in everyday social settings and can be considered to be an academic discipline in its own right as well as a subdivision of psychology.

The main topics are language and communication, interpersonal perception and attributions, attitudes and attitude change, group structures and processes, conformity and obedience, organisations, co-operation and competition.

A number of the main topics are covered in Chapters 3, 9 and 15. This chapter introduces some basic concepts and looks at group processes and social interaction.

Definitions	
Tajfel and Fraser (1978)	The aim of social psychology is to analyse and understand human social behaviour... Social behaviour, as we observe it, is the product of [a] balance between the 'universal' and the 'culture-specific'; this is true both of individual behaviour and of certain features of social organization which affect masses of people sharing a common cultural setting of their lives.
Argyle (1983)	In the present state of knowledge it looks as if social behaviour is the product of at least seven different drives... biological needs, dependency, affiliation, dominance, sex, aggression, self-esteem and ego-identity.
Abraham and Shanley (1992)	Social Psychology is about understanding people and what they do. It is the study of how people behave in everyday social settings. It focuses upon what happens between people,

Definitions (cont'd)	
	that is how they interact. It attempts to discover patterns in this interaction and thereby poses questions about the kinds of beings we are; questions about what controls and regulates our everyday activity.
Aronson (1992)	Social Psychology is about social influence.
Stroebe and Stroebe (1995)	Much of health psychology is applied social psychology.
Brown (1988) cites the following definitions of groups:	
Lewin (1948); Campbell (1958)	people experiencing some common fate.
Sherif and Sherif (1969)	members coexisting within some social structure.
Bales (1950); Homans (1950)	people in face-to-face interaction.
Tajfel (1981); Turner (1982); Turner *et al.* **(1987)**	two or more individuals [who] perceive themselves to be members of the same social category.
Brown (1988)	extends Turner's (1982) definition and suggests that a group exists when two or more people define themselves as members of it and when its existence is recognised by at least one other.

Approaches, Arguments and Applications

Most social psychology books are not classified in the library with general psychology (which developed from roots in philosophy) but catalogued alongside other social sciences such as education, sociology and politics. There is considerable overlap with sociology, but whereas sociology provides a wide perspective of groups and organisational structures, patterns and development, social psychology focuses on the individual's day-to-day behaviour within these structures. Moreover, social psychology, unlike the other social sciences, adopts experimental techniques and quantitative research methods wherever relevant.

Of importance for health are the implications of demographic changes (such as the ageing of the population), the impact of stress, health beliefs and attitudes, public health interventions, the ways in which attitudes to health and illness are communicated and how people cope with change and stress through identification with a group.

The study of groups is central to social psychology and of importance to health-care professionals, who are likely to become involved with, or participate in, a variety of groups during their career. Examples of these include families, training groups in which members learn from the group leader and from each other, professional groups that exist to accomplish particular goals and therapeutic groups in which members attempt to help each other in some way.

A group is generally considered to be two or more people who have something in common that links them in some way in a particular context such that they can be seen, either by themselves or by others, to belong to a group. It is usually argued that a group is more than just a collection of individuals and that each individual may behave very differently when in it or outside it. Brown (1988) says it is hard to imagine a group in which its members do not at some stage mentally classify themselves as actually belonging to it. In the health context, this has interesting implications and may be strongly linked to the concept of *labelling*. When a person is diagnosed as having, for example, diabetes, the professional may have a mental classification of 'diabetics' as a group with certain characteristics. An individual may not at first share this conception and not have any sense of belonging to a group. However, continued exposure to the label 'diabetic', media-expressed stereotypes and the awareness of self-help groups may bring about identification as 'a diabetic'. It can be argued that such group identification has some advantages and some disadvantages. Behaviour of group members tends to become uniform, which can lead to stereotyping and expectations concerning the group label. See Chapter 3.

Key Terms and Concepts

Advocacy: promoting the rights of another to be self-determining and autonomous.

Alienation: a feeling of powerlessness and separation from the dominant group, which may be felt by individuals who identify with a minority group.

Altruism: behaviour that one individual engages in which will 'do good' to another, without any apparent benefit to the individual and perhaps even at some cost. Tajfel and Fraser (1978) state that there is evidence that altruism has developed as a result of natural selection since groups that display altruistic behaviour are more likely to survive. This would imply that altruism is today genetically determined rather than being a cultural feature. Other explanations include the argument that although the benefits to the helping individual are not immediately obvious, the altruistic behaviour results in the satisfaction of some of the individual's hidden needs and may contribute to feelings of self-worth and self-esteem. Most evidence points to people wanting to do what they see as fair and expecting others to do likewise. When faced with making a choice between taking a favourable position for oneself or allowing another person that option, the other person's feelings are taken into account (Lerner and Lichtman, 1968, cited by Tajfel and Fraser, 1978). See also Chapter 17.

Autokinetic effect: the illusion of small random movements made by a stationary pinpoint of light when observed in a darkened room. When a point of light is projected onto a wall in a darkened room, it appears to dart about in a random fashion because of activity in the muscles of the eye. This effect has been used by Sherif (1935), cited by Alexander *et al.* (1970), in some classical studies of group norms and social influences. Initially diverse judgements would gradually become more like the others and converge towards a group norm.

Bales interaction process analysis (IPA): a tool developed by Bales (1950) for examining the interaction that takes place when a group is engaged in accomplishing a task. Interaction is classified according to whether it is task-orientated or socio-emotional.

Coding categories are subdivided into problems of (a) communication, (b) evaluation, (c) control, (d) decision, (e) tension reduction and (f) reintegration. These can be seen in terms of four main groups: (A) positive reactions, and (D) negative reactions, which are socio-emotional, and then (B) attempted answers and (C) questions, which are task-orientated.

Bales and Cohen (1979, cited in Brown, 1988) further refined the analysis to include aspects of status and friendliness, and developed SYMLOG – a **sy**stem for the **m**ultiple **l**evel **o**bservation of **g**roups. This separates three dimensions: friendly–unfriendly, dominance–submission and towards–away from goal direction.

A group may be gathered together and set a specific task; then, as people speak, each utterance is classified according to one of the above categories. Analysis can reveal the patterns of communication that take place, individual styles and the triggers that lead to certain behaviours. For example, it can be seen whether anyone tends to take the lead in asking questions or making suggestions, who tends to be more focused on the task in hand, and who engages in social interaction (such as telling jokes or encouraging others to speak). It can be seen whether this helps the group in the task or hinders it, or whether individuals withdraw by silence or unhelpful suggestions.

Brown (1988) points out that SYMLOG is limited in its usefulness by applying only to certain kinds of groups and neglecting intergroup relations. In a classroom situation, a simplified form of the Bales IPA can be used with 'broken information games' in order to give an introduction to the basic ideas and help members to improve *metacommunication*. Used strictly, only the verbal communication is analysed; all body language and *paralanguage* is ignored.

Broken information games: games that have been devised for education and training and that involve the group in solving a task for which each member has only a small piece of information. Only by sharing the information and working together can the group work towards the solution. An example is solving a crime, in which each member has only one or two clues. Analysis, using Bales IPA, SYMLOG or another tool, can reveal some of the processes of interaction. These simulations can be compared with occupational situations such as ward rounds or case conferences.

Cohesion: this refers to the extent to which group members like and are committed to each other. Where cohesiveness is high, the group can exert a powerful influence on the behaviour of members: absenteeism and member turnover will be low. The following factors that promote the development of group cohesion are given by Johnson and Johnson (1994):

- having common rules and norms that are accepted and understood by all members
- the needs of individual members correspond with group goals
- attraction between members
- maintaining a high level of trust among members.

Compliance: a term with many different meanings and connotations. Compliance can refer to the extent to which a patient follows medical advice. In this sense, if the advice is given as a set of instructions, compliance may carry connotations of obedience. If carer and client are in equal partnership and have devised a care plan together, compliance refers to the extent to which the client manages to keep to the plan. See also Chapter 7.

Conflict: disagreement between individuals or groups, which can range from a conflict of interests to use of force. In relation to problems situations, Zander (1982) suggests the following strategies for conflict reduction:

- distancing – separating people so that confrontation is avoided
- removing conditions that cause conflict
- negotiating
- bargaining/compromise
- problem-solving
- mediation
- force.

Conformity: a measure of the willingness of an individual to fit in with or adopt the behaviour of other members of a group despite a difference of opinion or values. A number of classical studies of conformity have been carried out, including those by Sherif (1935) and Asch (1951, 1952), cited in most general psychology texts including Hayes (1994), Cardwell et al. (1996) and Gross (1996) and and in social psychology texts such as Tajfel and Fraser (1978) and Brown (1988).

In controlled studies, it is usually found that participants justify their conformity by saying they did not want to spoil the experimenter's results or that they doubted their own judgement, thinking that there was perhaps a trick of the light or other illusion.

Festinger and others (for example, Festinger, 1957) give three main reasons for conformity: that we rely on others to help us formulate our beliefs and develop an understanding of the world, that achievement of group goals depends on having agreement and uniformity, and that approval is more likely to be achieved by not seeming different.

Consensus: agreement by a group about something. See also social consensus.

Crowds: crowds can be considered either as primitive or as elementary forms of groups. In order to explain how crowd behaviour can lead to riots, it is argued that, within a crowd, either people feel anonymous or become 'deindividuated', losing their sense of personal identity and returning to primitive, barbarous behaviour (Le Bon, 1896; Zimbardo, 1969; both cited by Brown, 1988), or there is a change of identity towards greater cohesion, pride and a sense of defending the territory against outsiders (Reicher, 1982, 1984, cited by Brown, 1988). In the latter case, new group norms may be quickly established, and where two groups are in conflict, these norms may become polarised towards opposite extremes (seen in, for example, rioters in conflict with police).

Most riot scenarios involve more than one group. In some cases, it is possible to identify an 'in-group' and an 'out-group', and point to behaviour by the out-group that may have served to trigger the defensive behaviour of the in-group and later the whole crowd. This may be interpreted as behaviour becoming more regulated and cohesive rather than primitive and chaotic.

Debriefing: following a therapeutic group session, the facilitators may find it helpful to hold a debriefing session. The purpose of such a session would be to enable the facilitators to:

- reflect upon their role in facilitating the session
- consider their position in relation to the development of the group
- identify any prominent issues or agenda that may have emerged within the session and plan ways of focusing upon these and exploring them further, thus helping to provide direction to the group as and when necessary.

Deviates: a label used in social sciences for anyone who is seen not to conform to the normative limits of a group (see norms). On the whole, pressures to conform are most readily observed when study focuses on individuals who are not conforming. It is found that such deviates receive a great deal of attention from other members who try to make them change their mind and that they are also less liked than other members. However, some non-conformists, particularly when they behave consistently, may be tolerated and can influence the majority.

Ground rules: groups may operate according to rules that members identify and agree to abide by. Examples of ground rules are:

- the 'I' rule, each speaker owning what he or she is saying and not assuming that others think, feel or behave in the same way
- speaking to the whole group and directly to others
- one person speaking at a time
- no interruptions.

Group decision-making: Where a task is to be accomplished, it is generally found experimentally that a group outperforms a single individual. However, if the performances of several individuals, working separately on the same task, are added together and compared with a group comprising the same number of people, the group compares less favourably.

This discrepancy can be explained in a number of ways. Steiner's (1972) theory of group productivity indicates that groups fail to optimise their resources, partly because they do not match individual's abilities to appropriate aspects of the task. The social impact theory of Latane (1981) and Latane and Wolf (1981) focuses on the motivation and satisfaction felt by group members and suggests that, in much group work, members feel less motivated than when working individually. In practice, this may be discovered through experience, and members may choose to work individually in the first stages of problem-solving before pooling their ideas and reaching a decision. Alternatively, a group may choose to have a brainstorming session first and then work separately or in small groups before a plenary gathering together of ideas. In some cases, the leader may gather the group's ideas and reach an individual decision, which is then presented to the group for final refinement and approval. As is found in the study of small group networks (see networks below), greater individual involvement leads to greater morale and satisfaction.

Group development: a number of theories have been proposed suggesting that groups evolve and change over time. Most adopt a sequential approach in suggesting that groups pass through a number of developmental stages. Tuckman and Jensen (1977) suggest those of forming, storming, norming, performing and adjourning.

Forming: an initial period of caution in which members meet each other for the first time and try to get to know each other. During this stage, members try to find out about the situation they are in and attempt to discover their role in the group. Some 'testing the water' may take place as members attempt to discover what type of behaviour is and is not acceptable to other members. During the forming stage, group members may experience anxiety, uncertainty and pressure. Trust and self-disclosure tend to be low and limited to safe themes, and achievements are often minimal.

Storming: a period of conflict during which group members explore the relationships between each other, check out roles and try to establish a hierarchy. Friendships and loyalties are tested as members experience tension between individual and group needs. During this stage, authority may be questioned and members may rebel against the nature of the task and the rules of the group. Members may form subgroups or may opt out and leave the group.

Norming: a greater sense of order prevails as members resolve conflict, settle arguments and develop acceptable forms of behaviour. During this stage, members get to know each other better, so a more trusting atmosphere develops and the group becomes cohesive.

Performing: as members accept the individual differences between themselves and support each other, their energies become focused on the task so that they work together and the group becomes productive.

Adjourning: as the task nears completion, members anticipate a change in relationships and prepare to part.

Johnson and Johnson (1994) describe similar stages as follows:

- defining and structuring procedures and becoming orientated: the leader sets the goals, determines the strategies to be used to achieve these and generally organises the group
- conforming to procedures and getting acquainted: members familiarise themselves with the task and with each other but lack a sense of commitment to the group

- recognising mutuality and building trust: trust between members is developed through self-disclosure, and members realise that they are interdependent
- rebelling and differentiating: conflicts and disagreements are evident as members try to establish their independence from each other and the group leader
- committing to and taking ownership of the goals, procedures and others members: group members become committed to each other and to the group goals, and demonstrate this by collaborating with each other
- functioning maturely and productively: the group develops its own identity and becomes productive as members support and co-operate with each other
- terminating: members confront the difficulties of parting.

Two further models provide lists for comparison:

1. Napier and Gershenfeld (1989):
   - the beginning
   - movement towards confrontation
   - compromise and harmony
   - reassessment
   - resolution and recycling.
2. Kiger (1995: 137):
   - meeting: discovering task requirements
   - sorting: beginning work and discovering difficulties
   - accepting: resolving difficulties
   - working: co-operating and progressing towards task completion.

Group dynamics: the scientific study of behaviour in groups. Typically, the focus of study includes the development of the group (see group development), inter- and intragroup communication, the influence of group membership on task performance and decision-making, and relationships between group members.

Group effectiveness: a number of dimensions of an effective group have been identified by Johnson and Johnson (1994: 24):

- Group goals are understood by members and are relevant to their needs
- Communication within the group is clear and accurate
- Participation and leadership is distributed between members
- Procedures for decision-making are flexible enough to respond to the needs of the situation
- Conflicts are encouraged and constructively managed
- Equal power and influence exists between members
- Group cohesion is high
- Problem-solving ability is high
- Members have high interpersonal effectiveness.

Group membership: Johnson and Johnson (1994) differentiate between a collection of people and a group. They suggest that a collection of people do not necessarily constitute a group as they may simply be individuals without any common characteristics who happen to be in the same place at the same time, whereas a collection of people may be defined as a group if they share a number of characteristics. Johnson and Johnson (1994) suggest that members of a group:

- engage in social interaction with each other
- are interdependent in some way
- share common goals
- perceive themselves as belonging to a group (common identity)
- are motivated to be part of the group in order to satisfy personal needs
- are governed by the same rules and norms
- influence each other.

Group polarisation: the decisions made within groups tend to be more extreme than those made by individual group members. Myers and Lamm (1975) suggest that group membership generates a sense of security that enables the members collectively to decide on a course of action that is either riskier (risky shift) or more conservative (caution shift) than that which individual members would have previously chosen.

Group processes: how the group is functioning. Things to look for in groups include:

- participation
- influence
- styles of influence (see client–carer relationships, parenting styles)
- decision-making procedures
- task functions
- maintenance functions
- group atmosphere
- membership
- expression of feelings
- norms.

The following unhelpful processes can be identified:

Pairing: two group members, usually sitting next to each other, talk to each other rather than to the group. This can be a distraction to other group members. Alternatively, two group members form an exclusive relationship and support each other when one of them makes a contribution.

Projection: a group member blames the group for the way he or she is feeling. This may stem from insecurity within the group or from the individual's lack of self-awareness.

Scapegoating: the group looks for someone to blame for the way the group is feeling or behaving, or the circumstances in which members find themselves. The scapegoat may be a quiet or vulnerable member on whom others vent feelings or an outside scapegoat, for example an employing organisation or professional body.

Shutting down: a member may cut off from the rest of the group and become isolated. This often occurs when people cannot face or talk about their feelings.

Rescuing: one person may constantly defend others from attack, thus denying the attacked person the opportunity to learn how to cope with the situation.

Flight: difficult issues or decisions are avoided by strategies such as changing the topic, making jokes, theorising or talking superficially.

Groupthink: a term used by Janis (1982) to describe the process in which members of a group that values harmony and equates disagreement with disloyalty experience pressure to agree with each other.

Individual programme planning: Brechin and Swain (1987) describe how individual programme planning was designed to support people with the label of mental handicap to express their own wishes and make their own decisions about their futures. It was found that planning for each individual in response to particular strengths, needs and circumstances was more satisfactory than were routine provisions. However, as planning developed, so attitudes and circumstances changed and there became greater possibilities within community-based living for independence and self-advocacy. Carers and clients became increasingly involved in planning, and the reciprocal nature of arrangements was recognised, so that individual plans gradually became replaced by *shared action planning.*

Initiation rituals: entry into a group may be marked by some kind of initiation ceremony or ritual, which can range from a warm welcome to embarrassing mocking and teasing or even painful 'rites of passage'. For example 'rookie' recruits into the fire or ambulance service or nursing are often sent on fools errands or ordered to carry out procedures that blatantly contradict rules, regulations or common-sense notions of health and safety. Coping successfully with the teasing marks the recruit as a real member.

Brown (1988) discusses some possible reasons for this. There may be a symbolic function for both the newcomer and the group, and help in the process of identity transition. It can allow the newcomer a reference point to recognise that he or she is no longer quite the same as before. It may introduce the recruit to the standards and norms of the group and perhaps help towards getting the recruit to feel and express some loyalty to the group. Aronson and Mills (1959), cited by Brown (1988), gave an interesting explanation for the painful rites inflicted by some groups, particularly where newcomers are in some doubt as to whether the group is worth joining, suggesting that having to overcome such a trial in order to join the group induces a belief that the group must be worthwhile if it is so difficult to become a member. The experimental findings have been linked to the notion of cognitive dissonance and dissonance reduction. Initiation rituals and teasing can also be seen as bullying that serves to maintain hierarchical power relationships.

Intergroup relations: It has been realised that social identity processes influence intergroup behaviour. Brown (1988) describes how intergroup comparisons contribute to self-esteem: if one's own group can be seen as superior to another, some of that glory can be attributed to oneself. Skevington (1984) found that nurses often display intergroup bias. For example, higher-status registered nurses see themselves as superior in certain task-related skills such as intelligence, confidence and responsibility, whereas enrolled nurses may view themselves as superior in such socio-emotional attributes as being cheerful.

Leadership: the emergence of a leader in a group can be studied in various ways. It may be seen from the point of view of personal leadership attributes, as an outcome of the structure of a group or as an interaction of the two. Leadership may also be regarded as a process of negotiation between leaders and followers. On the whole, leaders are seen as those people occupying high-status positions with a tendency to initiate ideas and activities in the group.

Brown (1988) suggest that leaders are those who influence others in the group more than they are themselves influenced. There are various methods by which a leader comes to be in that position, such as natural emergence, election, appointment, seniority or domination.

It is a common view that people who become leaders have natural qualities of leadership, hence the saying 'Leaders are born, not made.' In particular, political leaders are seen to share certain special traits. Conversely, a politician in a high-status position without these traits may be much criticised for lack of flair.

This can be contrasted with the view that anyone appointed to a leading position can acquire the necessary skills or that anyone aspiring to lead others can learn what is required. Current tendencies in management training are towards identifying skills that can be learned by all members of a group, including the leader, so that groups do not have to be dependent on having a naturally 'good' leader but can work towards developing effective methods. Brown (1988: 88) suggests that the objective of leadership training is to 'improve the fit' between the leader and the situation but that there is controversy over whether to change the leader, the situation or both.

Mediation: a service available through the British social services to couples undergoing separation or divorce. The service does not seek to reconcile the couple, although information about counselling may be given, but to assist in decision-making about the distribution of material goods, care of children and so on. The service mediates between the couple, particularly where communication is difficult, and seeks to assist in arriving at amicable or mutually agreed arrangements with a minimum of conflict.

Networks: a network in telecommunications is a set of channels linked to each other via terminals so that anybody participating in the network can contact others.

In general terms, any group, such as a family, who are constantly in touch with each other can be viewed as forming a network. Brown (1988) points out that it is more helpful to think of the communication channels as 'linkages' rather than in terms of distances.

A number of different patterns of small group networks have been identified and studied by Bavelas and Leavitt, who compared the performances of different networks with five members (for example, Bavelas and Leavit, 1948; Bavelas, 1969; both cited by Brown, 1988 and Gill and Adams, 1992). Five basic networks were investigated: the circle, the chain, the wheel, the 'Y' and open channels. It was found that where many or all channels were open, members expressed high morale and enjoyment but took longer to accomplish tasks. Where a leader emerged from a key position in the network, and communication channels were limited, tasks were completed quickly but were prone to error, and while the leader expressed enjoyment, other members felt less involved and became bored.

In practice, naturally occurring groups do not operate according to a clear single type of network, but elements of each can sometimes be identified and may lead to an understanding of the relative involvement of members in decision-making processes.

Norms: according to Brown (1988: 50), 'all groups evolve systems of norms which define the limits of acceptable and unacceptable behaviours'. As with social consensus, these norms may be subject to change but can be highly stable over a period of time. Norms can provide a way of regulating or controlling the behaviour of members, help each member to make sense of the social environment and predict what is likely to happen. How much each member is expected to conform to the normative limits depends on how important a particular norm is to the group and on the status of the individual within the group.

Obedience: engagement in behaviours determined and demanded by those who are perceived to have power and where the expectation exists that those who possess the power may exercise it by administering punishment for a failure to obey. Milgram's (1963, 1965, 1974) experiments indicated the extent to which subjects would obey commands given by an authority figure and how peer group support enabled subjects to defy an authority figure.

Parenting skills: parents can develop strategies for involving children in activities that are rewarding for parents and children, and help to prevent the development of problem behaviour. Jenner (1993) recommends the following:

- Cut right down on commands: do not give instructions unless they are really necessary
- Decrease the number of times you say 'No': reserve your vetoes for the big issues such as safety and health
- Restrict the amount of factual teaching you do: the most important thing your child can learn from you is that you approve of them
- Drastically reduce the number of questions you ask: only ask a question if you are genuinely going to listen to the answer
- Do not criticise: constructive suggestions can work wonders, whereas criticism often breeds resentment, hostility and angry feelings of rejection
- In play, use the right balance of child-centred attention, especially 'attends' in which you enthusiastically describe what your child is doing from moment to moment and ignore minor naughtiness. This will strongly

encourage them to carry on with whatever activity they are involved in and really works for children who seem to lose interest very quickly
- Let your child choose the game or toys from a selection that you know to be safe, stimulating and fun, preferably for both of you
- Remember to let your child lead the playtime
- Do not compete with your child: playtimes are when we help them to experience interesting activities and are not opportunities for us to show off our own prowess.

Parenting styles: Baumrind (1967, 1980), cited in Pitts and Phillips (1991) and Bee (1997), describes three styles of parenting:
- authoritarian: children are expected to obey unquestioningly
- authoritative: control is exerted, explanations are given, and obedience and conformity are valued, as are independence and self-direction
- permissive: few regulations are imposed and an accepting, non-evaluative role is adopted.

Coopersmith (1967), cited in Gross (1996), found that children of parents who had clear definitions of authority tended to exhibit high self-esteem. Those with parents who seemed unclear about standards and expectations, and whose discipline was unpredictable and inconsistent, or who fluctuated between overstrictness and overpermissiveness, tended to have low self-esteem.

Bee (1997) cites Liebert and Harris (1992), who found little difference between the children of authoritarian and permissive parents. Both of these groups were less motivated to achieve, less independent and more disoriented, distrustful and self-centred. Authoritative parents 'produced' more successful children, who were responsible, self-reliant and friendly. These qualities can be compared with the development of *hardiness* (see Chapter 20).

Peer group: those of the same status as, and associated with, a person; commonly used to refer to those of the same age group.

Peer influence: a tendency to conform to peer group norms is found in all studies of conformity, most notably in the early work of Sherif (1935) and Asch (1951, 1952) cited in most general psychology texts including Hayes (1994), Cardwell *et al.* (1996) and Gross (1996), and in social psychology texts such as Tajfel and Fraser (1978) and Brown (1988). See autokinetic effect and conformity.

Power: 'Social power is the potential influence that one person exerts over another. Influence is defined as a change in the cognition, behaviour or emotion of that second person which can be attributed to the first' (Huczynski and Buchanan, 1991: 192).

Most groups have a power structure, and whenever power is exercised, it can act as a significant motivating force promoting group functioning and goal achievement. Although power is a neutral concept, it is often viewed negatively, probably because of the way in which it can be abused. Power is often thought of in the context of dominance versus submission, and this is highlighted by Marquis and Huston (1996), who suggest that power is used positively when exerted on behalf of, rather than over, someone. This idea is particularly pertinent to health-care professionals who work with vulnerable people as it embodies the theme of advocacy.

Power may also be viewed unfavourably if associated with the notion of power struggles that can disrupt group functioning. A more favourable view of power may be generated if the notion of powerlessness is considered. Few people would welcome an inability to exert influence over aspects of their life as some degree of control is desirable.

The career structure of health-care workers tends to be hierarchical in nature. However, the position of any one person in their professional hierarchy may not reflect the amount of power possessed by that individual.

French and Raven (1959) propose six kinds of power:

Legitimate: one person perceives that another has a legitimate right to order him or her to do something. This includes formal power invested in a role. For example, a manager can order a health-care employee to adhere to the dress code of the employing organisation, or a nurse can ask visitors to leave the ward when visiting time has ended.

Reward: one person perceives that another is able to offer a reward that is valued and that the reward will be given for compliance with instructions. This can include power resulting from control over resources such as wages, respect and co-operation. Supervisors can exercise reward power by allowing a hard-working student study time away from the clinical area.

Coercive: one person fears that another is able and willing to punish. This can include power resulting from control over feared consequences. These punishments or penalties can be physical or psychological in nature. A patient may fear rejection by the health-care professional or the withholding of pain relief if he or she does not comply with therapeutic interventions; a student may fear a poor ward report if voicing complaints about standards of care during a placement; a health-care professional may fear the withdrawal of colleagues' friendship and emotional support if complaining about the behaviour of another worker.

Expert: one person perceives another to have some expert knowledge or skill that is relevant to the task being performed. This is power resulting from special knowledge, skills or expertise. A client may follow the advice given by the health-care professionals, believing them to know what is best for the condition; a student may respond to the remarks of the personal tutor and amend an essay.

Referent: one person identifies with someone else who has power. The greater the attraction, the greater the identification and consequently the referent power. This is power given to others through association with the powerful. A student placed on a clinical area where the staff have an excellent reputation for quality of care may have referent power among his or her peers; a health-care professional may gain referent power through networking with specialists in the field.

Informational: one person believes another to have valuable information. Power results from the ability of an individual to gain and share information that is required by others to accomplish their goal. A shift co-ordinator is often the focal point for information exchange in a ward; the support staff or unqualified health-care workers may have informational power by having the information that a health-care professional requires to perform their work smoothly.

Note that in the second and third items above, the power is inherent in the role itself, but the personality of the role-occupier can play a greater part than is seen in the first point.

Hein and Nicholson (1994) identify charisma as being an additional power base. This type of power results from the possession of particular traits that are seen as attractive to others. The power of leaders who are charismatic may be more important than their nominal or role-related power.

It is possible for one person to use different types of power in different contexts and at different times. The broader the power base an individual has, the greater the power he will exert. However, to a large extent, the power of a leader depends on the beliefs of the followers. Although a leader may have expert knowledge and be able to control rewards and punishments, if the subordinates do not believe that the leader has these attributes, they may not be willing to be led. In contrast, a leader may be able to manipulate subordinates into believing that they possess power that they do not actually have. The types of power are interrelated so that the use of one type may affect the leader's ability to use another. A nurse who uses coercive power may lose referent power.

Problem behaviour: Zarkowska and Clements (1994) have devised the STAR approach for people with learning disabilities who present problem behaviour. This is a planned eclectic mix of biological, social, educational, behavioural, psychodynamic, cognitive and humanistic principles for identifying and managing behavioural problems.

At the centre of the star, the key element is to review progress. Then there are six points to the star:

- assess: the behaviour, skills, motivators and conditions for positive behaviour
- define goals: short-term and long-term change
- alter settings: environmental and personal
- alter triggers: remove triggers, add new ones and alter trigger–action relationship
- alter actions: teach new skills, encourage appropriate alternatives and teach self-management
- alter results: reinforce the absence of behaviour and respond to problematic behaviour.

Rights and obligations: entitlements and duties attached to the various roles that exist within a group. These are interdependent so that the rights associated with the role performed by one group member may be the obligations associated with the role occupied by another. For example, within a therapeutic group, each group member may have the right to speak to the group and the other group members are obliged to listen to what is being said. There may sometimes be conflict between the rights and obligations of a group member. For example, a member of a therapeutic group may have an obligation to participate in the group discussion yet may also have the right to remain silent or to opt out of the group.

Role conflict: this may occur when the demands of two or more roles being occupied by the same person are incompatible or when the expectations held about one role are contradictory. A charge nurse, for example, may fulfil a number of different roles, including those of ward manager, teacher, innovator and change agent.

Roles: Brown (1988: 88) defines roles as 'behavioural regularities or expectations associated with particular members'. He distinguishes between roles associated with the task and socio-emotional aspects, and suggests that role differentiation can help with the division of labour and contribute to people's self-concept. Johnson and Johnson (1994: 18) define a role as 'a set of expectations defining the appropriate behaviour of an occupant of a position toward other related positions'. Formal and informal roles may co-exist in a group. A formal role is one which has been designated and assigned to a particular member. Such roles may be occupied following an election or appointment process and include the role of chairperson, secretary or treasurer. Informal roles tend to evolve as the group develops and members adopt a role on the basis of their interest or expertise. An example may be that of the spokesperson who represents other group members. Other examples can be given:

- leader
- questioner
- scapegoat
- clarifier
- rescuer
- passive follower
- devil's advocate
- jester/clown.

Self-concept and group membership: part of our self-concept involves our view of ourselves as members of different groups or in terms of social roles. Each time we become a member of a new group or review our roles, we are likely to identify ourselves in terms of the group. Our self-esteem may then be affected by our perception of the group and how it fares in comparison with other groups.

Self-help (mutual help) groups: according to Napier and Gershenfeld (1989: 511), these are 'voluntary gatherings of peers who share common needs or problems that are not being addressed by existing organizations, institutions or other types of groups'. A wide variety of self-help groups exists with health-care issues as their focus.

Shared action planning: Brechin and Swain (1987: 132) provide guidelines for the shared action planning process to 'help people with a mental handicap, together with the key people in their lives, to develop and express their wishes and goals, and to control decisions which shape their lives'. They suggest that the process should start with the key relationships and involve joint decisions and the pooling of ideas, always involving the person with a mental handicap.

Social consensus: according to Tajfel and Fraser (1978), social consensus can take different forms, of which the most basic is the wide agreement within a culture about how the information presented to our senses should be interpreted. For example, notions of how the appearance of the sun, moon and other heavenly bodies should be interpreted have each appeared to have had a consensus at certain times but can be seen to have changed throughout history. A noticeable recent example of a change of consensus of opinion in Western society is the interpretation given to body odour. Whereas little attention seems previously to have been paid to this, it is now largely regarded as unacceptable, and a high proportion of media time is given to advertising products that will remove or mask it. An example of a British social consensus that has been lost is the previously widespread acceptance that physical punishment was suitable for the socialisation of children. This notion is now challenged, and many people are seeking alternative methods of influence and control.

These changes in consensus indicate that although we may live our daily lives strongly influenced by the prevailing view, each individual may also create and change his or her immediate social environment, and many different views may exist within one culture. Without such challenge and variety, there would be no change in art, science, technology or value systems. Tajfel and Fraser (1978: 309) suggest that 'when new alternatives are created, the different versions of what is "obvious" begin to clash', and the view adopted by one or another group in the society may then influence the formation of a new consensus.

Social exchange theory: an idea proposed by Homans (1961) that people engage in relationships when each perceives that the relationship will bring more rewards than costs. Tajfel and Fraser (1978) suggest that rewards can include approval and that costs may be expended effort and a loss of personal or cultural identity.

Sociograms: a visual means for recording the patterns of interaction between members of a group. These may range from a simple tally of the number of times each person makes a contribution, to a complete map showing the number and direction of all contributions (Figure 19.1). Sociograms may be used in clinical practice to identify communication problems within a dysfunctional family.

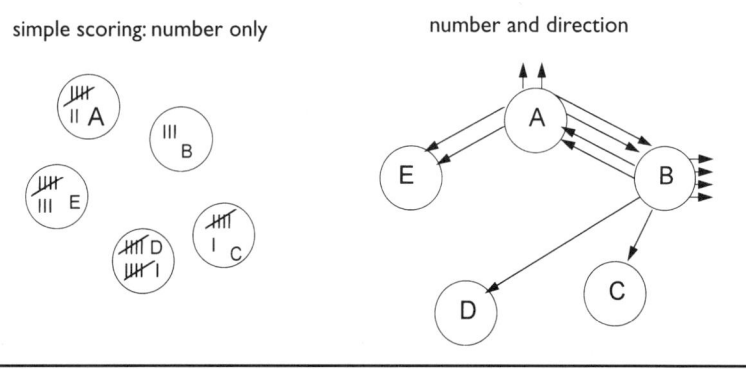

Figure 19.1 Sociograms

- **Status:** both 'role' and 'status' refer to expected patterns of behaviour associated with the position occupied by an individual within a group or organisation, rather than to attributes of the particular individual. Role refers to any position independent of any worth or value attached to it; status suggests that the position is valued in some way relative to other positions. Brown (1988) believes that group members have different levels of power and prestige, giving rise to status hierarchies in most groups. This can be linked to processes of social comparison whereby individuals make appraisals of their abilities. As with other social comparisons that contribute to perceptions of self and others, this can affect actual behaviour and task performance.
- **Subjective norm:** an individual's personal perception of the social norm, the predominant set of values chosen, from a range perceived in the society, by the individual as the norm, or the individual's own particular set of values, which form the normal pattern for that individual.
- **Taboos:** Radcliffe-Brown (1952) defines taboos by noting the word's derivation from the Polynesian term *tapu*, meaning 'forbidden'. The term can be applied to many types of prohibition. However, in another sense, it is related to the word 'sacred' (see Morris, 1987: 130–131). Examples include incest, child abuse and talking about death, particularly suicide.

    Incest is sexual activity between people who are closely related, usually parent–child or brother–sister. There are very strong taboos in most societies against incest, and although it is not clear why this is, several main reasons are usually given. These include using marriage outside the group to give more available mates, being able to keep track of generations for the functioning of society and determining lines of inheritance, seeing incest as a violation of trust and dependence within families, and the increased risk of recessive genetic diseases through inbreeding.

    In practice, as with other activities that are regarded as taboo or as perversions, majority attitudes tend to be coloured by a sense of revulsion that overrides rational considerations of whether the activity is in fact harmful, unlawful or immoral (Ruse, 1990), and incest avoidance is generally regarded as 'natural'.

    Greenberg and Littlewood (1995) report some interesting findings concerning post-adoption parent–child incest, in which relationships have developed after adults who were adopted when young have traced their relatives. In these cases, the usual revulsion is often not felt, which suggests that it is the closeness of upbringing and the formation of early attachments, rather than the actual blood tie, that dictate whether or not sexual activity is acceptable. Greenberg and Littlewood also argue that, perhaps, with so many changes in family structure, we no longer 'need' to avoid some forms of incest.

    Revulsion is more likely to be felt towards parent-child incest than brother–sister incest and will include notions of harm in which one person is seen as younger or less socially mature than the other so that the incest is viewed as abuse. In general, incest survivor groups have developed to provide support for people who, as children, have been sexually abused by a parent or step-parent.

Child sexual abuse is defined as 'the involvement of dependent, developmentally immature children and adolescents in sexual activities they do not truly comprehend, to which they are unable to give informed consent and that violate the social taboos of family roles' (Beezley-Mrazek and Kempe, 1981). A conspiracy of silence is often found to occur when social taboos are broken. The subject itself is taboo, as is the specific behaviour. This is particularly well documented in the case of child sexual abuse, over which it has been difficult to engage in clear open debate.

20 STRESS AND STRESS MANAGEMENT

Stress is used as a general label for a vast, complex, interdisciplinary area of interest and study, much of which is health related. Most often, stress refers to the personal discomfort associated with an overdemanding or distressing situation or lifestyle. It should be recognised that too little activity, demand or challenge is also stressful.

Discomfort may be physical in the form of tension, agitation, aches and pains and serious stress-related illness, or psychological in the form of mood swings or disturbances in social and work-related functioning. Individuals may not be aware of changes until someone else convinces them there is something wrong, or a crisis occurs.

What constitutes stress depends on the individual. What is too demanding for one person may be invigorating for another or even humdrum for a third. The management of stress may involve a change in the stressful circumstances, a change in perception or behaviour, or a modification of physiological arousal responses.

Definitions	
Lazarus (1966)	Stress is the result of an individual's perception that a disturbance has occurred in the person–environment relationship.
	The individual perceives challenge/threat/harm, judges that resources may not be sufficient to manage the disruption, and considers the outcome important to well-being. That is, the person perceives the circumstances as stressful and feels stressed.
Monat and Lazarus (1991)	the stress arena refers to any event in which environmental demands, internal demands, or both, tax or exceed the adaptive resources of an individual, social system, or tissue system.

Approaches, Arguments and Applications

Engineering model: in engineering terms, the word 'stress' is used for the forces acting on a particular object to distort it (the cause). The word 'strain' is then used for the amount by which the object becomes distorted (the effect). Taken together, stress and strain can be used to work out how well the material will withstand the forces on it. It is also possible to measure the elasticity or resilience of a material, which is its ability to spring back into its original shape after bending, stretching or compression. In common usage, the words 'stress' and 'strain' are not thus distinguished, and both are used to refer to either effects or causes.

It is often important to distinguish between cause and effect, so the word 'stressors' is usually used for pressures, forces or demands. The words 'distress', 'stress' and 'strain' can then be used for uncomfortable effects. We can say that a person with greater *hardiness* or *toughness* feels less stress under the same stressors and is likely to show greater resilience.

Hence, it can be seen that there are internal and external factors involved in stress (Figure 20.1): internal factors involve the reactivity of the physiological system (how fast and how strongly it reacts to change) and the personality of the individual; external factors (stressors) include all social and environmental influences and events.

Biopsychological approach: this covers all aspects of physiological change and physiological arousal systems in relation to the psychological experience of stress and the accompany feelings and cognitions. Cannon (1915, 1929) identified the *fight or flight mechanism*, which uses adrenaline. Selye (1956) added the *general adaptation syndrome* (GAS), which involves noradrenaline and adrenocorticotrophic hormone (ACTH) in controlling blood glucose levels.

More recently, the effects of emotional arousal and stress in connection with growth hormone, the insulin system and the immune system have been explored. Dienstbier (1989) describes how some of the physiological systems can be 'toughened' by exposure to heat and cold and through exercise. Other coping strategies might include drug therapy to alter the action of adrenaline, or maladaptive behaviour such as substance misuse.

Ethological approach: this branch of natural history studies animals in their natural wild habitat, their emotional expression and responses to stressful conditions.

Behavioural and social learning approaches: these look at ways in which people are conditioned throughout life to respond to demanding circumstances, through association, copying others and reinforcement. Behaviour related to career demands, hard work and material possessions are highly valued and rewarded by Western society. For example, it may be that type A behaviour pattern (TABP) and the style of the 'workaholic' develop because they are rewarded by social approval and financial gain, and because successful role-models are regularly featured in the media and in advertising. Helpful strategies involve recognising illness- and health-related behaviour, indicating alternative role-models, identifying new rewards, setting new goals and reshaping behaviour in manageable steps. Maladaptive strategies including adopting a persistent sick-role behaviour, particularly when this is reinforced by attention from others, or engaging in ritualistic or compulsive behaviours that disrupt daily living.

INTERNAL FACTORS affected by stressors and affecting resilience	Physiological	Systems: SNS-adrenal-medulla Pituitary-adrenal-cortex Pituitary-gonadal Growth hormone Insulin system Immune system Toughness
	Psychological	Temperament Perception of events Perception of self Locus of control Learned helplessness Vulnerable personality Hardy personality
EXTERNAL FACTORS 'STRESSORS'	Environment/ society	War Earthquake Financial depression Noise Heat Air pollution Wind Crowding Housing conditions The city Discrimination
	Personal circumstances	Bereavement Divorce Marriage Responsibilities Changes at work Pregnancy Arguments Changes in diet Changes in health Daily hassles

Figure 20.1 Factors in stress

Cognitive approaches: these look at perceptions, knowledge, beliefs and values. The ways in which an individual regards circumstances will determine how stressful the demands will be. Lazarus (1966) regards stress as an imbalance between a person's perceived resources and demands. Desirable coping strategies involve a re-examination of beliefs to alter perceptions both of one's own resources and of the demands, and hence redress the balance. Superstitions, myths and cognitive distortions (see Chapter 6) can interfere with this process. Cognitive approaches are often used in conjunction with behavioural programmes for identifying goals and the appropriate steps to take.

Psychodynamic approaches: these see stress-related responses as resulting from unresolved conflicts earlier in life. This may possibly be due to an overdemanding upbringing with conflicting or ambiguous rewards, defective communication and an overemphasis on guilt and shame associated with failure. Unconscious mental processes such as defence mechanisms (see Chapter 17) may develop, which can have short-term benefits but may be detrimental in the long term. Psychoanalysis can help the person to examine past experiences and look at how such patterns have developed. This may enhance the ability to resolve the anxiety-provoking conflicts in the light of adult perceptions. Once the hidden dynamics have been brought to light, positive coping strategies may overlap with cognitive and behavioural approaches in choosing preferred behaviours and trying out new patterns.

Humanistic approaches: these empower the person to take control over events and develop more effective coping and management strategies by using techniques such as non-directive counselling and negotiation.

Complementary therapies: there is a growing awareness that a range of interventions not based on traditional Western medicine can help some people to develop new patterns of behaviour and cope more effectively with the stressors in their lives. Therapies include autogenic relaxation training, massage, aromatherapy, the Alexander technique, acupuncture, shiatsu, yoga, hypnosis and creative arts therapies.

It is not fully understood how these approaches work, but there is a growing interest and body of research literature that helps towards an understanding. Each therapy may contribute something towards the development of a person's ability to relax and may lead to increased awareness of what is influencing stress responses and stress-related illnesses. Different techniques suit different people. In general, it could be argued that anything that interrupts the previously harmful lifestyle, introduces new self-awareness and teaches techniques for relaxation and the efficient use of the body is likely to lead to greater self-efficacy and better stress management. Multimodal stress management centres sometimes include one or more complementary therapies.

Key Terms and Concepts

Adrenaline: a hormone secreted by the medulla of the adrenal gland. Stimulation of the sympathetic nerves activates the medulla and promotes the secretion of adrenaline. The adrenal medulla normally secretes small amounts of adrenaline into the blood. However, the increased activity of the sympathetic nerves that accompanies physical and mental stress causes large quantities to be released. The main effects are to prepare the body for action by stimulation of breathing, increased heart rate and shutting down of the digestive processes. See also *fight or flight mechanism*.

Adrenocorticotrophic hormone (ACTH) (also known as corticotrophin or corticotropin): a hormone secreted by the anterior lobe of the pituitary gland. Its function is to control the production and secretion of certain adrenal cortex hormones, such as cortisol, which control blood glucose levels. Secretion of ACTH increases in response to stress. It is regulated by corticotrophic releasing hormone (CRH), which is influenced by stimuli such as low blood glucose or noradrenaline. See also *general adaptation syndrome*.

Aerobic exercise: vigorous exercise that involves the increased use of oxygen. Sutherland and Cooper (1990) believe that aerobic exercise provides a useful antidote to stress by decreasing the level of physiological arousal, discharging physical excitation and inducing relaxation. See also *toughness*.

Alexander technique: a technique devised by Alexander (1969) that can be used to reduce stress by enhancing awareness of variations in posture, body movements and breathing. David Gorman, director of the Centre for Training in London, describes his approach to teaching the Alexander technique thus in a workshop leaflet:

> We want to be whole, yet we still find ourselves in parts... What we need is a new model of human function which is truly holistic; a model that reveals our design as inherently integrated creatures... a model which shows that when we interfere with this natural integration, we become divided into parts (creating separate mind and body) and inevitably end up with chronic pain, tension, joint damage, strains and other organic problems.

Training involves a blend of practical activities, experiential work, information and discussion, based on knowledge of the major structures and functions of the body.

Anxiety and stress: anxiety is a common counterpart to stress or one of the outcomes of stress. The terms 'anxiety' and 'stress' are often used interchangeably when referring to the emotional distress experienced in a new situation, such as being admitted to hospital. This mixed usage can make it difficult quickly to locate related research studies, and both words need to be used in literature searches. See Chapter 2 and also *hospitalisation*, below.

Assertiveness training: see Chapter 1.

Autogenic relaxation training (autogenic regulation training): a self-instructed relaxation technique originated and formulated by Dr Johannes Schultz in the 1920s in Berlin. This system combines muscle relaxation with meditation in order to support and facilitate the homeostatic self-regulatory mechanisms that exist in the mind and body. Training consists of a series of simple, easily learned exercises. It can be seen as a way of achieving an altered state of consciousness or 'autogenic state', the aim being to replace an internal state of arousal or conflict with one of harmony and peace. It is believed by practitioners to boost the workings of the immune system and promote healing. A medical history is taken to ensure that people at risk or who require special supervision can be identified. It is used mainly as a stress management technique.

Burn-out: Maslach and Jackson (1986) define burn-out as a syndrome of emotional exhaustion, depersonalisation and reduced personal accomplishment that can occur among individuals who do 'people work' of some kind. Burn-out is often thought to be an outcome of chronic occupational stress.

Coping styles: a tendency for a person to deal with a stressful event in a particular way. Miller and Mangan (1983) and Miller (1987, 1989) studied the information-seeking behaviour of patients and identified two coping styles: monitoring and blunting. 'Monitors' use information-seeking strategies to gain a sense of control over the stress-inducing situation and will ask many questions about their health problem, prognosis and treatment options. In contrast, 'blunters' will ask few questions, preferring not to be reminded of the stress-inducing situation.

Miller (1989) found that a person's preferred coping style influences the response to information about the stress-inducing situation. A person who favours a monitoring style tends to experience greater stress if information is withheld, whereas a person who uses a blunting style tends to experience greater stress if provided with information. It is therefore important for health-care professionals to be sensitive to the information-seeking cues given by people.

Roth and Cohen (1986) propose two types of stress coping style – approach and avoidance – which differ according to the amount of attention given to the stressor. People who adopt an avoidance style tend to use strategies such as selective inattention and defence mechanisms to avoid thinking about the stressor. People who favour an approach style tend to use strategies such as seeking information to confront and cope with stressors.

There are advantages and drawbacks associated with both styles. Anxiety levels tend to be lower when avoidance strategies are used, and these can therefore be beneficial if little can be done to remove the stressor. However, if the stressor can be dealt with, avoidance strategies can prove to be harmful. For example, a physical condition may deteriorate if the person fails to acknowledge it and seek medical help promptly.

These models can be usefully compared with such concepts as locus of control, emotion-focused and problem-focused coping, and pain behaviours. See also Chapters 7 and 13.

Daily hassles: relatively minor day-to-day events that cause annoyance, frustration or distress. Examples of hassles include misplacing something, congested traffic conditions, having to meet deadlines and noisy neighbours. Kanner *et al.* (1981) have found some association between a hassle score and health status.

Environmental stressors: environmental or external stressors can be described in terms of duration, quality, quantity and type:

Duration (Elliot and Eisdorfer, 1982):
- acute, time limited, such as an interview, or a visit to the dentist
- sequences or series of events that occur over an extended period of time as the result of an initiating stress trigger, such as divorce, which brings multiple residential, financial, job, parental and social changes
- chronic intermittent stressors, such as periodic arguments with a partner or weekly project meetings
- chronic stressors such as permanent disabilities and long-term marital strife.

Quality (Lazarus and Cohen, 1977):
- major changes, often cataclysmic and affecting large numbers of people (such as war, earthquake or economic depression)
- major changes affecting one or a few persons (bereavement or divorce)
- daily hassles such as running out of coffee and arguing about who was supposed to buy it.

Quantity (Yerkes-Dodson, 1908; Holmes and Rahe, 1967)
- the accumulation of stressors is significant in stress-related disorders
- both desirable and undesirable changes can have stressful effects
- both too much and too little in the way of demands can be stressful (see Figure 20.3 below).

Type: examples of environmental stressors:
- noise
- heat or cold
- wind
- air pollution
- personal space and territoriality
- responsibilities at work
- unemployment
- crowding
- the city, housing conditions
- discrimination and harassment.

Eustress: Selye (1974) differentiates between good stress (eustress) and bad stress (distress):

Eustress:
- a growth-enhancing reaction
- stressors are perceived as opportunities and associated with strength and resistance.

Distress:
- stress overload
- stressors associated with weakness and vulnerability.

This can be compared with the Yerkes-Dodson (1908) inverted U-curve relationship, which shows that when the demands on a person are right for that person, performance will be at an optimum level (see performance). It is only when the demands increase beyond the optimum, or fall too far below, that the person feels distress. Similarly, Lazarus (1966) talks about the balance of demands and resources. When there is an even balance, the perceived demands are healthy, but when they exceed the perceived resources, the person experiences distress.

Fight or flight mechanism: the popular name for the workings of sympathetic nervous system (SNS)-adrenal-medullary (or adreno-SNS) arousal system. According to Cannon (1915, 1929), when stress is sudden, the body reacts with a set of responses that prepare for physical action.

1. Threat is perceived
2. Cortical activity triggers the hypothalamus, which governs the SNS,

which in turn activates the adrenal medulla
3. Adrenaline is secreted from the adrenal medulla so that:
   - the pupils dilate
   - salivary secretions reduce
   - the bronchi dilate
   - respiration deepens
   - arterial pressure rises
   - the heart beats more rapidly
   - blood is shifted away from the stomach and intestines towards the heart, central nervous system and muscles
   - digestive processes in the alimentary canal cease
   - emptying the bladder is inhibited
   - the interest in sexual activity is reduced
   - the spleen contracts and discharges concentrated blood
4. noradrenaline is released from SNS synapses
5. noradrenaline continues to stimulate the SNS.

Adrenaline and noradrenaline (catecholamines) continue to circulate, so that even if the stress is short lived, SNS-adrenal-medullary arousal will continue in a closed-loop, self-perpetuating process, dying away only slowly unless physical activity dispels the catecholamines and the parasympathetic nervous system can restore normal activity. For this reason, a good brisk walk is recommended after driving in frustratingly slow traffic. Regular exercise and exposure to extremes of heat and cold can affect the rate at which the arousal system comes into effect and recovers (see toughness). The amount of adrenaline and noradrenaline in the urine reflects the amount of SNS activity and correlates with how much stress a person reports experiencing. See Figure 20.2.

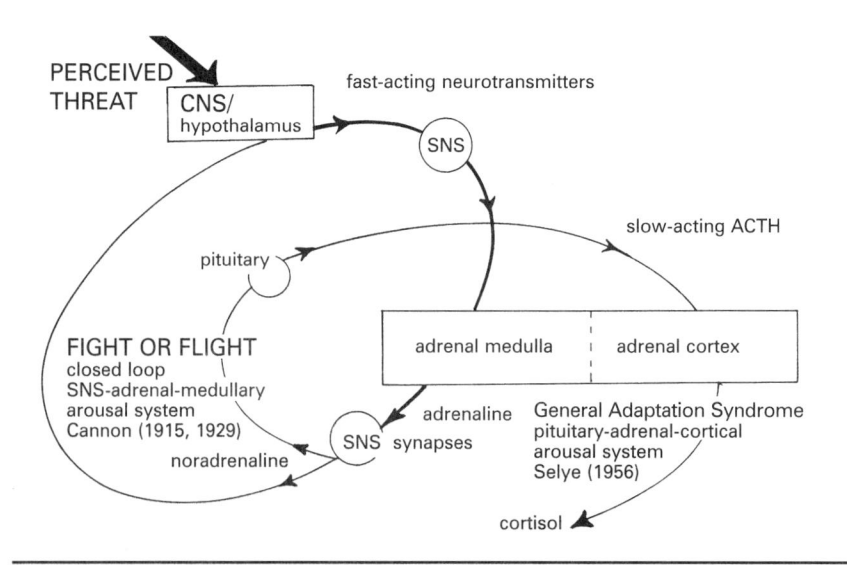

Figure 20.2 Physiological arousal systems

General adaptation syndrome (GAS) or adaptation level theory: Selye (1956) identified a second arousal system, after Cannon's fight or flight mechanism, and developed the concept of the general adaptation syndrome (GAS), which involves the pituitary-adrenal-cortical arousal system (Figure 20.2). This has three stages:

Alarm reaction: the noradrenaline triggers the pituitary gland, which produces ACTH (adrenocorticotrophic hormone or adrenocorticotrophin), this then stimulating the outer part of the adrenal gland – the adrenal cortex. The cortex in turn produces hormones, such as cortisol (a glucocorticoid), which control and conserve the amount of glucose in the blood. Sugar is freed from the reserves in the liver.

Recovery or resistance: if the stressor is not removed, the body begins to recover from the initial alarm reaction and cope with the situation. Increased activity of the pituitary-adrenal-cortical arousal system gradually brings blood sugar levels back to normal under continued moderate stress. Few outward signs of stress are visible although the ability to resist new stressors is impaired and vulnerability to health problems increases.

Exhaustion: under prolonged or extreme stress, the body's resources become depleted and the adrenal cortex no longer functions properly. Severe psychophysiological disorders may develop. The liver may deteriorate. Blood sugar levels drop, and in extreme cases hypoglycaemia may result in death.

Hardiness: Maddi and Kobasa (1991) believe that they have identified conditions in early life that will lead to hardiness or a hardy personality. These include a family atmosphere of variety with many moderately difficult tasks, warm parental encouragement of attempts to succeed, and the expression of individuality. They identify three main elements of psychological hardiness:

- a sense of commitment rather than alienation
- control rather than powerlessness
- challenge rather than threat.

They argue that children brought up in a supportive family atmosphere will deal with demands in a non-stressful way. They add that these qualities of commitment, control and challenge are important throughout the lifespan, at school, college and in the workplace, and that it is possible for adults to develop them even if early experiences have been detrimental.

Hospitalisation and stress: the stress of admission to hospital may result in anxiety or aggression (see Chapters 1 and 2). Volicier and Bohannon (1975) devised a Hospital Stress Rating Scale to assess the effects of events associated with being in hospital. Findings are mixed, but the items that are found to cause most stress are those which are related to communication issues (see hospitalisation in Chapter 2).

Hypervigilant reaction to threat: a panic response to threat that is characterised by impaired cognitive functioning, indecision and impulsivity as the frightened individual searches for a way to escape the impending threat.

Illness and stress: it is difficult to differentiate between cause and effect when discussing stress and illness. Stress can render a person more susceptible to illness, and being ill can itself be a stressful experience, which may in turn exacerbate the illness. According to Baum et al. (1984), stress can influence predisposition to illness by exposure to illness-producing conditions as well as by affecting the immune system. Stress can increase eating (particularly of high-calorie, sweet-tasting foods), smoking and abuse of alcohol and drugs, which can predispose to a range of illnesses such as hypertension, heart disease, cancer, liver disease and other organ damage.

Life events (crises or transitions): Holmes and Rahe (1967), cited in most introductory texts, devised a Social Readjustment Scale for assessing the potential stress caused by an accumulation of demanding life events or life change units (LCUs). This was derived from participants' ratings of perceived stressful events. It can be useful as a quick measure of likely stress but may be misleading as it is culture specific.

Management of stress: in relation to internal and external factors (see Figure 20.1 above), the management of stress can be seen in terms of making alterations to the:

- stressors (environmental and personal)
- perceptions (of self and events)
- response (physiological arousal and behaviour).

Changes can be effected through *relaxation training*, personal coping mechanisms, organisational strategies and the use of drugs. Interventions can be used with individuals or groups. Some of the problems with stress-related behaviour lie either in the failure of people to recognise those behaviours in themselves or in their belief that they are somehow unusual and inadequate. Sharing experiences in groups, perhaps recording behaviour on videotape, can help people to see themselves more clearly and become more able to benefit from counselling.

Cooper (1981) suggests a number of individual tactics for coping with stress:

- Know yourself
- Know your new situation
- Know other people who can help
- Learn from the past
- Look after yourself
- Let go of the past
- Set goals and make action plans
- Look for the gains you have made.

Peters (1989) suggests that stress at work can be considerably reduced if the following organisational strategies are introduced:

- Involve everyone in everything
- Use self-managing teams
- Listen, celebrate and recognise
- Spend time lavishly on recruiting

- Train and retrain
- Provide an employment guarantee
- Simplify and/or reduce the structure
- Invert the organisational chart
- Eliminate bureaucratic rules and humiliating conditions.

By inverting the organisational chart, Peters means taking the usual hierarchical pyramid diagram and turning it upside down so that managers are regarded as supporting others instead of sitting on them.

Cooper (1981), rather more realistically perhaps, identifies areas in which managers and trade unionists can help to increase understanding and reduce stress:

- knowledge of self
- personality
- motivation
- learning and teaching
- interviewing
- bargaining and negotiation
- social behaviour
- organisational behaviour
- sources of stress on managers at work
- understanding and management of personal change
- creation of change
- counselling and helping.

There is no special category of stress-reducing drugs. Treatment will depend on what combination of symptoms is present, for example anxiolytics or antidepressants for mood disturbances, beta blockers for hypertension, glucose or sucrose for hypoglycaemia, and analgesics or muscle relaxants for aches and pains. See also Chapters 2 and 13.

Perception of self: the way in which a person sees him or herself in terms of strengths and weaknesses, and the self-esteem associated with these, determines the view the person has of his or her personal resources available to cope with demands. Feelings of worthlessness or inadequacy interfere with coping. Cognitive and psychodynamic therapies seek to reveal these perceptions and point to ways of modifying them. See Chapters 6, 9, 15 and 17.

Performance: stress is commonly associated only with overarousal of physiological reactions that are seen to be harmful, and much stress reduction is centred around calming and soothing activities such as relaxation and meditation.

The inverted U-curve, or curvilinear relationship, adapted from Yerkes-Dodson (1908) (Figure 20.3), shows a fuller relationship between demands, performance and stress. It illustrates how either too much or too little in the way of perceived demands can lead to discomfort, disturbance or low performance. Stress is high when performance is low, because of either too little or too much demand. Unemployment, sensory loss and physical disability can all be stressful, not because there are too many demands, but because there are too few. Friends and relatives often try to help by taking over difficult tasks, leaving even less to strive for. Stress is at a minimum when conditions are right for the individual and performance is greatest.

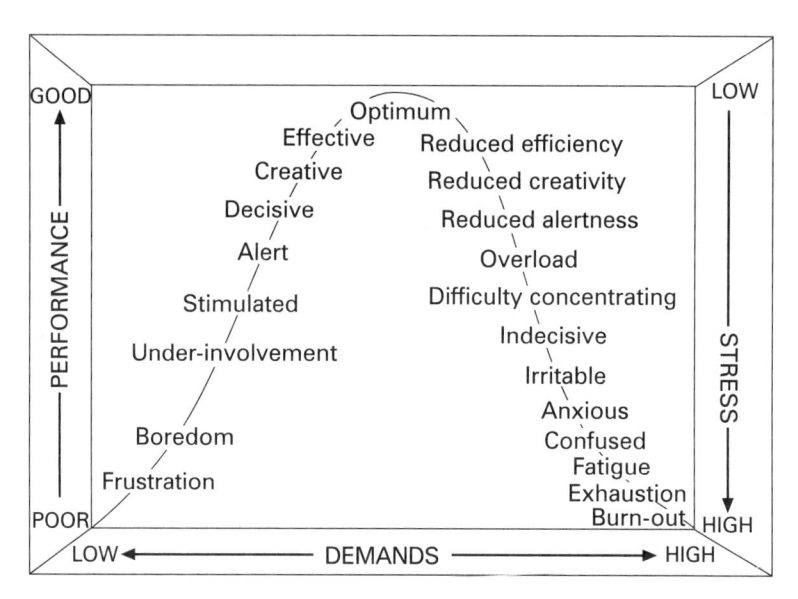

```
GOOD                                                    LOW
              Optimum
          Effective   Reduced efficiency
           Creative    Reduced creativity
          Decisive     Reduced alertness
           Alert        Overload
         Stimulated    Difficulty concentrating
       Under-involvement  Indecisive
                         Irritable
                         Anxious
         Boredom         Confused
                         Fatigue
       Frustration       Exhaustion
POOR                     Burn-out     HIGH
  LOW ←——— DEMANDS ———→ HIGH
```

PERFORMANCE (vertical axis, left) / STRESS (vertical axis, right)

Each individual functions according to a personal optimum level of demand at any particular time, for which performance would be at its peak and stress levels low. When demands are either too low or too high, performance drops and stress levels are high

Figure 20.3 Stress and performance *(modified from Yerkes-Dodson, 1908)*

It is interesting to note how attitudes and vocabulary have changed during the twentieth century. 'Nervous' used to mean well-tensioned, vigorous, like a 'nervy' or 'highly strung' horse. Nervousness was seen as a good feature, meaning an optimal balance, ready to perform well. 'Relaxed' used to mean weak, flaccid, limp, flabby, drooping, lacking vigour and feeble. In Victorian times, people considered themselves ill if they were relaxed; they needed to strive to become more nervous or nervy. Whereas we are now obsessed with the right-hand side of the inverted U-curve, previous generations were more worried about the left-hand portion.

Personality and stress: Rosenman *et al.* (1964) identified a type of person who responded in a particular way to stress and was found to be susceptible to coronary heart disease. They described such a person as having type A personality. However, as with other limited or *narrow-band* ranges of traits or types, the description is now applied to features of behaviour and is usually referred to as type A behaviour pattern (TABP) rather than personality. TABP is seen as the behaviour of a competitive, achievement-orientated person who possesses a sense of time urgency and impatience, and who is both easily aroused and hostile or angry.

The TABP profile (modified from Cooper, 1981) involves:

- doing more than one thing at a time
- scheduling more and more activities and having less time to spend on each one
- measuring success in terms of quantity
- ignoring surroundings unless they are relevant to the task
- having to be on time
- finding it difficult to sit down with nothing to do
- urging others to hurry up and finish what they are saying
- finishing others' sentences for them
- becoming impatient when watching others carry out a task
- believing that a thing will only be done correctly if done by oneself
- taking over a learner's task rather than continuing with instruction
- playing to win at every game, even with children
- becoming irritated when slow cars block traffic or when waiting in line
- gesturing a lot while talking
- nodding the head, clenching a fist or pounding table when talking
- persistently tapping the fingers or jiggling the legs
- blinking the eyes rapidly or lifting the eyebrows for emphasis
- having tense facial muscles
- speaking explosively and using obscenities.

Rosenman *et al.* (1975) confirmed their earlier findings. The Review Panel on Coronary Prone Behaviour and Coronary Heart Disease of the United States National Institutes of Health (1981: 1200) concluded that the available scientific evidence demonstrated an association between Type A behaviour and clinically apparent CHD in employed middle-aged US citizens. Since then there have been numerous studies examining the association between TABP and CHD and findings are generally inconclusive. See Johnston (1993) and Delunas (1996) for a review of studies.

An alternative profile was named as type B. The early definitions of type B indicated only an absence of type A characteristics (modified from Cooper, 1981). Other profiles identify a range from extreme type A to extreme type B.

Prior to the manifestation of coronary heart disease (CHD), type A individuals are notorious for denying their TABP tendencies and for refusing to alter this aspect of their lives. There is little evidence for successful intervention pre-CHD (Wright, 1991). Successful interventions for post-CHD patients include ongoing self-monitoring, shifting obsessive tendencies away from time urgency towards deliberate 'drifting', and changing to a different occupation (for example, Friedman and Ulmer, 1984, cited in Wright, 1991). Jenkins *et al.* (1979) have developed a questionnaire that asks questions about aspects of behaviour that may be found helpful in medical diagnosis.

Attempts to explain why type A characteristics develop include a psychodynamic approach explaining hyperactivation in terms of unresolved conflicts in childhood owing to the unachievable demands of ambitious or neurotic parents, and a behavioural approach emphasising that drive and ambition are highly rewarded qualities in Western society. As Wright (1991: 299) points out:

> It would be nice if we were able to keep 'the baby' (drive, ambition) without the 'bath water' (hyperactivation and the resulting CHD)... What is needed are ways of training ourselves and others to maintain diligence with pacing...

Maddi and Kobasa (1991) have suggested that development of *hardiness* would be one way of achieving this.

TABP is a controversial area of research. Criteria for deciding how many of the observable characteristics should be included, or the strength of these, are variable, making it difficult to compare studies. There is a wealth of research in this area, including continuing refinements to the profiles and alternative models, and the search for specific factors, rather than the general profile, that put the person most at risk.

Physiological arousal systems: two fundamental patterns of arousal are the sympathetic nervous system (SNS)-adrenal-medullary and the pituitary-adrenal-cortical systems. These are referred to as the *fight or flight mechanism* and *general adaptation syndrome* respectively. Technical advances in hormonal analysis have made it possible to go beyond these two and study a broad spectrum of hormones and endocrine systems, including the pituitary-gonadal, growth hormone, and insulin systems (Mason, 1975; Ursin et al., 1978). Based on this research, it seems that there is no single stress hormone but that all endocrine systems are responsive to psychological stress.

Work in the field of immunology suggest that the immune system, too, is responsive to psychological demands (Ader, 1980) (see psychoneuroimmunology). The physiological response to stress is best viewed as a complex and interrelated patterning of autonomic, hormonal and immune systems. See also Figures 20.1 and 20.2 above.

Post-traumatic stress disorder: it has been increasingly recognised since the 1980s that symptoms following a personal or major disaster may have psychological rather than organic origins. The DSM IV (American Psychiatric Association, 1994) includes post-traumatic stress disorder alongside anxiety and depression as a clinical syndrome (see Chapter 2). It is felt that the disorder is a normal or naturally occurring response to abnormal events. Following the witnessing or experiencing of a serious threat to life or well-being, symptoms may include:

- the initial numbing or repression of memories
- 'flashbacks' or intrusive recollections
- sudden feelings of re-experiencing the event
- recurrent dreams of the event
- the persistent avoidance of stimuli associated with the trauma
- detachment or numbing of general responsiveness
- persistent symptoms of increased arousal, exaggerated startle response and sleep disturbance
- feelings of guilt
- cognitive disturbances such as poor memory and concentration.

Treatment generally consists of a structured cognitive-behavioural programme of therapy (Scott and Stradling, 1992). See also Chapter 6. Brief counselling may be given immediately following a disaster. Those involved may be advised to seek help if symptoms appear at a later date.

For at-risk occupations, such as rescue personnel, regular briefings may be offered in order to reduce the likelihood of symptoms developing. However, these may in practice be declined or ignored by individuals who prefer to conform to a 'macho' peer group attitude. Durham *et al.* (1985) cite Laughlin (1980), who found, following a plane crash, that one third of firefighters denied any adverse effects from participating in emergency work but in fact had negative reactions and symptoms. One third felt a need to seek treatment but did not do so because of embarrassment or feeling that seeking treatment was inconsistent with self-image. The remaining third experienced no observable stress and seemed to cope well without outside help. Following more recent catastrophes, such as the Hillsborough football stadium disaster, there has been a great deal of media coverage about the way in which people involved in public services may experience symptoms.

Psychogenic illnesses: a term often confused with *psychosomatic* and used for those physical or 'bodily' conditions, such as back pain, stomach ulcer, thyroid disorder and asthma, which are thought to have been brought about by chronic emotional upset or stress rather than any recognisable medical cause or trauma.

However, this does not mean that the physical condition is imaginary or 'all in the mind'. The pain, discomfort or organic change is real. Treatment may consist of a combination of medical and psychological interventions to deal with the physical manifestations of the problem as well as the emotional precipitants. See also psychosomatic.

Psychoneuroimmunology: a study of the interrelationship between psychological, neuroendocrine and immunological factors. Research includes investigation of the effects of stressors on the immune system. For example, Cohen *et al.* (1991) found a positive correlation between the degree of stress participants experienced and their susceptibility to the common cold. In describing how the immune system responds to psychological challenge, Evans *et al.* (1997) use the terms 'upregulation' and 'downregulation' in preference to the more common terms of enhanced or suppressed immunity. They cite a number of studies suggesting that the effects of short-term acute stress and profound chronic stress can differ greatly. The immune system responds to major stressors such as bereavement, marital disharmony and caring for a relative with Alzheimer's disease with downregulation, while the immune response to short-term acute stressors, such as having to give an assessed oral presentation, is one of upregulation. Evans *et al.* (1997) suggest that these differences in immune response may be influenced by perceived coping ability rather than simply by the nature of the stressor. See also *physiological arousal systems*.

Psychosomatic: it is often thought that this means the same as psychogenic, and the term may be used in a derogatory or dismissive way when neither concept is understood. However, the psychosomatic model of health and disease does not use the term to refer to illness being caused by an emotional state but to the interrelationship of mind and body in *all* states of health and illness. Cognitive and behavioural components are as important as emotional factors in understanding the nature and progression of ill-health. The psychosomatic approach was first developed in the 1930s by Helen Flanders Dunbar. Tamm (1993: 218) cites Dunbar (1935, 1943, 1947) and discusses how the model considers that:

> diseases are developed through a continual interplay between physical and mental factors which strengthen each other by means of a complex network of feedback loops.

According to the psychosomatic model, health care is something that can be undertaken by the individual rather than being administered solely by professionals. An individual may seek help from others, such as professional services, friends and family, but needs to take responsibility for his or her own health. This can be compared with Rotter's (1954, 1966, 1975) construct of the internal *locus of control* and with the concept of *self-efficacy*. See Chapter 7.

Relaxation training: this is one of the central interventions in stress management. It can be used where there is an assumption that a disorder is stress related and has led to disruption of normal regulation of physiological systems (Schwartz, 1977). Relaxation restores normal regulation through 'cultivated low arousal', in which parasympathetic nervous system responses are dominant (Stoyva and Budzynski, 1974). There are a number of different procedures, such as:

- progressive muscle relaxation
- yoga
- meditation
- autogenic training
- biofeedback
- hypnosis or self-hypnosis
- quiet drifting, with or without specially designed music.

It is often assumed that the body mechanisms respond in the same ways in all relaxed states, but this may not be so. Muscular relaxation produces reductions of autonomic and endocrine responses, but it is not clear that meditation does (Steptoe, 1989). Biofeedback may be used in isolation or in combination with other relaxation techniques as part of a treatment package (Phillips, 1979).

Social support: Kiecolt-Glaser and Glaser (1988) found that people who are socially isolated or lonely have a decrease in immunological function. Theories that have been proposed to explained the beneficial effects of social support include:

- the buffering model, which suggests that social support blunts the effects of stress and enables the sufferer to cope more effectively
- the direct or main effects hypothesis, which suggests that social support has beneficial effects on health and well-being that are unrelated to the amount of stress being experienced.

Stress inoculation: this expression can be used in several distinct ways. It can refer to any technique that aims to prevent a *hypervigilant* reaction to an impending stressful event. This might include providing information, reassurance and recommendations about how to deal with the anticipated event so that the individual can take protective action. The term is also used for a technique of subjecting people to controlled stressful situations with the intention of preparing them for subsequent experiences. This can be done with small amounts of stimulation introduced in a graded hierarchical way similar to *progressive desensitisation*. This is continued until an individual is able to withstand highly challenging situations without undue arousal. This can be compared with the development of *hardiness*. Alternatively, a *flooding* technique may be used, in which a highly stressful situation is used, compared with which all subsequent experiences may seem relatively manageable. For example, army recruits may be required to crawl on their bellies over an open space under a constant cross-fire of bullets. The slightest upward movement or hesitation might result in injury, so this provides an extremely taxing exercise, after which genuine combat can seem relatively minor. A risk with flooding techniques is that they might lead to *sensitisation* or even *phobia* rather than the desired desensitisation.

Symptoms and signs of stress: a distinction is usually made between 'symptoms', which the sufferer notices, and 'signs', which others can use as an indication of stress. These can be conveniently grouped according to whether they are predominantly physiological or psychological. Psychological indicators can be subdivided into the three main domains of cognitive, affective and behavioural.

Physiological:
- aggravation of skin complaints (such as eczema, psoriasis)
- altered bowel habits
- altered sleep patterns
- asthma
- breathlessness or overbreathing
- changes in appetite
- changes in blood pressure
- coronary heart disease/myocardial infarction
- frequency of micturation
- headaches
- high cholesterol level
- hypoglycaemia (low blood sugar)
- increased heart rate
- loss of libido, impotence
- lower skin resistance (GSR) and sweating
- muscular pains
- palpitations
- stomach upset or indigestion
- susceptibility to infections
- ulcers.

Cognitive:
- inability to distinguish between important and inconsequential issues (*problem lumping*)
- indecisiveness
- irrational decisions
- lack of interest in planning
- loss of concentration
- preoccupation.

Affective:
- anger
- anxiety
- depression
- embarrassment
- frustration
- impatience
- irritability
- job dissatisfaction
- loss of self-esteem
- loss of tolerance
- mood swings
- sadness.

Behavioural:
- absenteeism, labour turnover
- aggression
- alcohol and drug abuse
- apathy
- changes in eating patterns
- poor performance
- poor time-keeping
- self-neglect
- signs of agitation such as nail-biting, teeth-grinding, foot-tapping, fidgeting or drumming fingers
- smoking
- social withdrawal.

Toughness: Dienstbier (1989) takes a positive attitude to stressors and stress, arguing that the proper management of stress can lead to greater toughness and improved physical and mental health.

Dienstbier (1989) considers that it is a lack of physical demands in a mechanised world that leads to:

- poor physiological endurance
- poor psychological endurance (stress tolerance)
- susceptibility to anxiety and depression
- attention and learning deficits
- susceptibility to cardiovascular diseases
- reduced immune capacity.

Greater endurance or toughness, Dienstbier argues, can be achieved through *passive toughening* (exposure to extremes of heat and cold) and *active toughening* (physical fitness). The SNS-adrenal-medullary (fight or flight) arousal system adjusts to a low base rate with fast recovery after arousal.

Dienstbier suggests that individuals with type A behaviour pattern (TABP) seem to have slower SNS-adrenal-medullary mechanism (fight or flight) recovery. However, the major health risk may be associated more with pituitary-adrenal-cortical arousal (GAS), as people with family histories of cardiovascular disease have higher cortisol levels. He concludes that although the TABP disposition has been shown to be associated with CHD, a challenge-seeking disposition is not of itself a health risk.

This concept of physiological toughness can be compared with the concept of psychological hardiness and related to the engineering concepts of resilience and stress:strain ratios. In the same circumstances, people who are tough or hardy suffer less disturbance, discomfort and ill-health.

Appendix: Using a Library

Most libraries in the UK use the Dewey Decimal Classification System. Where an alternative system is employed, guidance should be available. The Dewey system has numbers 000, 100, 200, 300 and so on for the major divisions into subject areas. A summary of the hundreds is given in Figure A.1. Within each division, subdivisions are indicated by intermediate numbers. Further subdivisions are then given by decimal points. Each extra decimal point represents a finer discrimination between topic areas.

At the time this system was devised, psychology was in its infancy. It was regarded principally as an off-shoot of philosophy and had not yet acquired its scientific credibility. For this reason, most general and introductory psychology texts are classified under 150, following philosophy. This section now also includes most cognitive psychology covering perception, memory, cognitive development and so on. Close by, books that deal with areas of psychological interest that overlap considerably with philosophy, such as mind and consciousness, are shelved under the 100s. Psychological approaches involving the paranormal, occult, telepathy and so on are given the general name of parapsychology (alongside psychology) and are also in the 100s. Communication theory and some media studies may be found in the 000s.

Social psychology developed somewhat separately from cognitive psychology and can be seen to relate more closely to other social sciences such as sociology, politics, economics and education. Hence many social and educational psychology books will be found in the 300s. This section also includes books relating to special needs. Nursing books, many of which include psychological material, are classed in 610 as medical sciences. The physiology of the brain and nervous system is in 612. The new discipline of health psychology can be found largely in 613. Therapies, including complementary therapies, may be found in 615 to 618. A short summary of some of the most useful sections is given below.

- 000 Communication theory
- 100 Philosophy and parapsychology
- 150 General and developmental psychology
- 300 Social psychology
- 360 Special needs
- 370 Education
- 610 Nursing
- 612 Brain and nervous system
- 613 Health psychology

000	**Generalities**	340	Law	680	Manufacture for specific uses	
010	Bibliographies	350	Public administration & military science	690	Buildings	
020	Library and information sciences	360	Social problems & services; associations			
030	General encyclopaedic works	370	Education	**700**	**The arts; Fine and decorative arts**	
040	Information technology	380	Commerce, communications, transportation	710	Civic & landscape art	
050	General serial publications	390	Customs, etiquette, folklore	720	Architecture	
060	General organisations & museology			730	Plastic arts; Sculpture	
070	News media, journalism, publishing	**400**	**Language**	740	Drawing & decorative arts	
080	General collections	410	Linguistics	750	Painting & paintings	
090	Manuscripts and rare books	420	English & Old English	760	Graphic arts; Printmaking & prints	
		430	Germanic languages; German	770	Photography & photographs	
100	**Philosophy & psychology**	440	Romance languages; French	780	Music	
110	Metaphysics	450	Italian, Romanian, Rhaeto-Romanic	790	Recreational & performing arts	
120	Epistemology, causation, humankind	460	Spanish & Portuguese languages			
130	Paranormal phenomena	470	Italic languages; Latin	**800**	**Literature & rhetoric**	
140	Specific philosophical schools	480	Hellenic languages; Classical Greek	810	American literature in English	
150	Psychology	490	Other languages	820	English & Old English literatures	
160	Logic			830	Literatures of Germanic languages	
170	Ethics (Moral philosophy)	**500**	**Natural sciences & mathematics**	840	Literatures of Romance languages	
180	Ancient, medieval, Oriental philosophy	510	Mathematics	850	Italian, Romanian, Rhaeto-Romanic	
190	Modern western philosophy	520	Astronomy & allied sciences	860	Spanish & Portuguese literatures	
		530	Physics	870	Italic literatures; Latin	
200	**Religion**	540	Chemistry & allied sciences	880	Hellenic literatures; Classical Greek	
210	Philosophy & theory of religion	550	Earth sciences	890	Literatures of other languages	
220	Bible	560	Palaeontology; Paleozoology			
230	Christianity & Christian theology	570	Life sciences; Biology	**900**	**Geography & history**	
240	Christian moral & devotional theology	580	Plants	910	Geography & travel	
250	Christian orders & local church	590	Animals	920	Biography, genealogy, insignia	
260	Social & ecclesiastical theology			930	History of ancient worlds to ca.499	
270	History of Christianity & Christian church	**600**	**Technology (Applied sciences)**	940	General history of Europe	
280	Christian denominations & sects	610	Medical Sciences; Medicine	950	General history of Asia; Far East	
290	Comparative religion & other religions	620	Engineering & allied operations	960	General history of Africa	
		630	Agriculture & related technologies	970	General history of North America	
300	**Social sciences**	640	Home economics & family living	980	General history of South America	
310	Collections of general statistics	650	Management & auxiliary services	990	General history of other areas	
320	Political science	660	Chemical engineering			
330	Economics	670	Manufacturing			

Figure A.1 Outline of the Dewey Decimal Classification

615   Complementary therapies
616–618 Psychotherapy, counselling, substance abuse family and play therapies

The chief problem for librarians lies in deciding the best place for a particular book. The tendency is to go by title and general impressions of content. This means that books may be differently classified in different libraries. It also means that books of related content may be in quite separate sections. Cognitive therapy may be found either with cognitive psychology under 150 or as therapy under 616. Books on stress, for example, may be found variously in 155, 158, 361, 610, 613, 616 or 658, depending on whether the emphasis appears to be general, lifespan, social, biological, medical, nursing or survival.

Journals are normally located separately from books and tend to be shelved in alphabetical order and by date. The most recent issues may be displayed in a reading area.

If the title or author of a book or article is known, it can be located quickly and easily via the library cataloguing system. Bibliographies and computer databanks can be used for tracking down books and articles relating to topic areas. Three useful CD ROM data banks for psychology and health psychology are PSYCHLIT, CINAHL and MEDLINE.

Given sufficient time, browsing along shelves is often the most successful way of finding relevant material. Some of the best research has been triggered by serendipity or chance finding.

BIBLIOGRAPHY

Abraham C. and Shanley E. (1992) *Social Psychology for Nurses, Understanding Interaction in Health Care*. London: Edward Arnold.

Adam K. and Oswald I. (1983) Protein synthesis, bodily renewal and the sleep–wake cycle, *Clinical Science*, **65**: 561–7.

Adams B. (1986) Models of the processes and purposes of communication, *Social Science Teacher*, **15**(2): 55–60.

Adams B. (1989) Colour Physics in the Curriculum: A Comparison of the Ways in which Colour Theory is Taught in Art and Science. MSc dissertation, Reading University.

Ader R. (1980) Psychosomatic and psychoimmulogic research, *Psychosomatic Medicine*, **42**(3): 307–21.

Adler A. (1927) *The Practice and Theory of Individual Psychology*. New York: Harcourt Brace Jovanovich. (See also Gross,1996.)

Adorno T.W., Frenkey-Brunswick E., Levinson D.J. and Sanford R.N. (1950) *The Authoritarian Personality*. New York: Harper & Row. (See also Gross, 1996.)

Ajzen I. (1988) *Attitudes, Personality and Behaviour*. Milton Keynes: Open University Press.

Ajzen I. (1991) Theory of planned behaviour, *Organizational Behaviour and Human Decision Processes*, **50**: 179–211.

Ajzen I. and Fishbein M. (1980) *Understanding Attitudes and Predicting Social Behaviour*. Englewood Cliffs, NJ: Prentice Hall. (See also Hayes, 1994; Niven, 1994; Gross, 1996.)

Aldiss B.W. (1970) *The Shape of Further Things: Speculations on Change*. London: Faber.

Alexander C.N., Zucker L.G. and Brady C.L. (1970) Experimental expectations and autokinetic experiences: consistency theories and judgment convergence, *Sociometry*, **33**: 108–22.

Alexander F.M. (1969) *Resurrection of the Body*. New York: University Books.

Allis S. (1992) Less pain more gain, *Time*, 19 October.

Allport G.W. (1937) *Personality: A Psychological Interpretation*. New York: Holt, Reinhart & Winston. (See also Atkinson *et al.*, 1996; Gross, 1996.)

Allport G.W. (1947) *The Use of Personal Documents in Psychological Science*. London: Holt, Rinehart & Winston. (See also Gross, 1996.)

Allport G.W. (1954) *The Nature of Prejudice*. Reading, MA: Addison-Wesley. (See also Cardwell *et al.*, 1996; Gross, 1996.)

Allport G.W. (1962) The general and the unique in psychological science. In Lazarus R.S. and Option E.M. Jr (1967) *Personality: Selected Readings*. Harmondsworth: Penguin.

Allyn J. and Festinger L. (1961) The effectiveness of unanticipated persuasive communications. *Journal of Abnormal and Social Psychology*, **62**: 35–40. (See also Wright *et al.*, 1970.)

American Psychiatric Association (1994) *Diagnostic and Statistical Manual of Mental Disorders*, 4th edn. Washington DC: American Psychiatric Association. (See also Cardwell *et al.*, 1996; Gross, 1996.)

Anderson C.A. (1987) Temperature and aggression: effects on quarterly, yearly and city rates of violent and nonviolent crime, *Journal of Personality and Social Psychology*, **52**: 1161–73.

Anderson J.R. (1985) *Cognitive Psychology and its Implications*, 2nd edn. New York: Freeman.
Annas G. (1974) Rights of the terminally ill patient, *Journal of Nursing Administration*, **4**: 403. (See also Broome, 1994.)
Appleby S. (1996) *The Box of Secret Thoughts*. London: Bloomsbury.
Archer J. (1991) The influence of testosterone on human aggression, *British Journal of Psychology*, **82**: 1–28.
Argyle M. (1983) *The Psychology of Interpersonal Behaviour*. Harmondsworth: Penguin. (See also Cardwell *et al.*, 1996; Gross, 1996.)
Argyle M. and Trower P. (1979) *Person to Person*. London: Harper & Row.
Aronson E. (1992) *The Social Animal*, 6th edn. San Francisco: W.H. Freeman and Co. (See also Hayes, 1994; Niven, 1994; Atkinson *et al.*, 1996; Cardwell *et al.*, 1996; Gross, 1996.)
Aronson E. and Osherow N. (1980) Co-operation, prosocial behaviour and academic performance: experiments in the desegregated classroom. In Bickman L. (ed.) *Applied Social Psychology Annual*, Vol. 1. Beverly Hills, CA.: Sage. (See also Gross, 1996.)
Atkinson R.L. and Shiffrin R.M. (1968) Human memory: a proposed system and its control processes. In Spence K.W. and Spence J.T. (eds) *The Psychology of Learning and Motivation*, Vol. 2. London: Academic Press.
Atkinson R.L. and Shiffrin R.M. (1971) The control of short-term memory, *Scientific American*, **224**: 82–90. (See also Atkinson *et al.*,1996; Cardwell *et al.*, 1996; Gross, 1996.)
Atkinson R.L., Atkinson R.C., Smith E.E., Bem D.J. and Nolen-Hoeksema S. (1996) *Hilgard's Introduction to Psychology*, 12th edn. London: Harcourt Brace Jovanovich.
Ausubel D.P. (1968) *Educational Psychology: A Cognitive View*. New York: Holt, Rinehart & Winston.
Ayer A.J. (1963) *The Concept of a Person and Other Essays*. London: Macmillan.
Baddeley A. (1982) *Your Memory: A User's Guide*. Harmondsworth: Penguin. (See also Hayes, 1994; Atkinson *et al.*, 1996.)
Baddeley A. (1990) *Human Memory: Theory and Practice*. London: Lawrence Erlbaum.
Baddeley A.D. and Hitch G. (1974) Working Memory. In Bower G.A. (ed.) *Recent Advances in Learning and Motivation*, 8. New York: Academic Press. (See also Hayes, 1994; Atkinson *et al.*, 1996; Cardwell *et al.*, 1996; Gross, 1996.)
Baldwin E. (1990) Sexuality and breast cancer, *Midwife, Health Visitor and Community Nurse*, **26**(10): 385–6.
Bales R.F. (1950) *Interaction Process Analysis: A Method for the Study of Small Groups*. Chicago: University of Chicago Press. (See also Brown, 1988; Gross, 1996.)
Bandler R. and Grinder J. (1975) *The Structure of Magic*. Palo Alto, CA: Science and Behaviour Books.
Bandler R. and Grinder J. (1976) *The Structure of Magic II*. Palo Alto, CA: Science and Behaviour Books.
Bandura A. (1965) Influence of models' reinforcement contingencies on the acquisition of imitative responses, *Journal of Personality and Social Psychology*, **1**: 589–95. (See also Cardwell *et al.*, 1996.)
Bandura A. (1969) *Principles of Behaviour Modification*. New York: Holt, Rinehart & Winston.
Bandura A. (1977) *Social Learning Theory*. Englewood Cliffs, NJ: Prentice Hall. (See also Hayes, 1994.)
Bannister D. (1971) *Inquiring Man: The Theory of Personal Constructs*. (See also Hayes, 1994.)
Bannister D. and Fransella F. (1986) *Inquiring Man: The Theory of Personal Constructs*, 3rd edn. Harmondsworth: Penguin. (See also Gross, 1996.)
Barlow H., Blakemore C. and Weston-Smith M. (1990) *Images and Understanding*. Cambridge: Cambridge University Press.

Barlow H.B. and Mollon J.D. (eds) (1982) *The Senses*. Cambridge: Cambridge University Press.
Barnett K. (1972) A theoretical construct of the concepts of touch as they relate to nursing, *Nursing Research*, **21**: 102–10.
Baron-Cohen S. (1989) The autistic child's theory of mind: a case of specific developmental delay, *Journal of Child Psychology and Psychiatry*, **30**: 85–297. (See also Cardwell *et al.*, 1996.)
Barraclough J. (1994) *Cancer and Emotion: A Practical Guide to Psycho-oncology*, 2nd edn. Chichester: John Wiley & Sons.
Barron F. (1965) The psychology of creativity. In *New Directions in Psychology II*. London: Holt, Rinehart & Winston.
Bartlett F.C. (1932) *Remembering*. Cambridge: Cambridge University Press.
Bartlett F.C. (1958) *Thinking*. New York: Basic Books.
Baum A., Singer J. and Baum C.S. (eds) (1984) *A Handbook of Psychology and Health*. Hillsdale, NJ: Erlbaum Associates.
Becker M.H. (1974) The health belief model and personal health behaviour, *Health Education Monographs*, **2**: 324–508.
Becker M.H. and Maiman L.A. (1975) Socio-behavioural determinants of compliance with health and medical care recommendations, *Medical Care*, **13**: 10–24.
Bee H. (1997) *The Developing Child*, 8th edn. London: Addison-Wesley. (See also Niven, 1994; Atkinson *et al.*, 1996; Cardwell *et al.*, 1996; Gross, 1996.)
Bee H.L. and Mitchell S.K. (1984) *The Developing Person*. New York: Harper & Row. (See also Cardwell *et al.*, 1996; Gross, 1996.)
Beech J.R. and Harding L. (1990) (eds) *Testing People; A Practical Guide to Psychometrics*. Windsor: NFER-NELSON.
Beecher H.K. (1956) Relationship of significance of wound to pain experience, *Journal of the American Medical Association*, **161**: 1609-13.
Beecher H.K. (1959) *Measurement of Subjective Responses: Quantitative Effects of Drugs*. Oxford: Oxford University Press.
Beezley-Mrazek P. and Kempe C.H. (1981) *Sexually Abused Children on their Families*. Oxford: Pergamon Press.
Bem D.J. (1970) *Beliefs, Attitudes and Human Affairs*. Belmont, CA: Brooks Cole. (See also Atkinson *et al.*, 1996; Gross, 1996.)
Bem S.L. (1981) Gender schema theory: a cognitive account of sex-typing, *Psychological Review*, **88**: 354–64. (See also Atkinson *et al.*, 1996; Cardwell *et al.*, 1996.)
Benson J. and Falk A. (eds) (1996) *The Long Pale Corridor: Contemporary Poems of Bereavement*. Newcastle: Bloodaxe Books.
Berkowitz L. (1962) *Aggression: A Social Psychological Analysis*. New York: Academic Press. (See also Cardwell *et al.*, 1996; Gross, 1996.)
Berkowitz L. (1983) The experience of anger as a parallel process in the display of impulsive 'angry' aggression. In Geen R.G. and Donnerstein E.I. (eds) *Aggression: Theoretical and Empirical Reviews, 2: Issues in Research*. New York: Academic Press.
Berkowitz L. (1993) *Aggression, Its Causes, Consequences and Control*. New York: McGraw-Hill. (See also Gross, 1996.)
Berlo D.K. (1960) *The Process of Communication: An Introduction to Theory and Practice*. London: Holt, Rinehart & Winston.
Berne E. (1964) *Games People Play*. Harmondsworth: Penguin.. (See also Hayes, 1994.)
Bion W.R. (1961) *Experiences in Groups and Other Papers*. London: Routledge.
Blakemore C. (1988) *The Mind Machine*. London: BBC Publications. (See also Gross, 1996.)
Blumer H. (1969) *Symbolic Interactionism: Perspective and Method*. Englewood Cliffs, NJ: Prentice Hall.
Bourbonnais F. (1981) Pain assessment: development of a tool for the nurse and the patient, *Journal of Advanced Nursing*, **6**: 277–82.
Bowie M. (1991) *Lacan*. London: Fontana.

Bowlby J. (1951) *Maternal Care and Mental Health*. Geneva: World Health Organisation. (See also Cardwell *et al.*, 1996; Gross, 1996.)
Bowlby J. (1953) *Child Care and the Growth of Love*. Harmondsworth: Penguin. (See also Cardwell *et al.*, 1996: Gross, 1996.)
Bowlby J. (1961) The process of mourning, *International Journal of Psychoanalysis*, **44**: 317.
Bowlby J. (1969) *Attachment and Loss, I: Attachment*. London: Hogarth. (See also Hayes, 1994; Niven, 1994; Cardwell *et al.*, 1996; Gross, 1996.)
Bowlby J. (1973) *Attachment and Loss II: Separation, Anxiety and Anger*. London: Hogarth. (See also Hayes, 1994; Niven, 1994; Atkinson *et al.*, 1996; Cardwell *et al.*, 1996; Gross, 1996.)
Bowlby J. (1980) *Attachment and Loss III: Loss, Sadness and Depression*. London: Hogarth. (See also Hayes, 1994; Niven, 1994; Cardwell *et al.*, 1996.)
Bowlby J. (1988) *A Secure Base: Clinical Applications of Attachment Theory*. London: Tavistock/Routledge. (See also Gross, 1996.)
Bradley J.C. and Edinberg M.A. (1990) *Communication in the Nursing Context*, 3rd edn. Norwalk, CT: Appleton & Lange.
Bransford J.D. and Stein B.S. (1993) *The Ideal Problem Solver: A Guide for Improving Thinking, Learning and Creativity*, 2nd edn. New York: W.H. Freeman.
Breakwell G.M. (1989) *Facing Physical Violence*. Leicester: BPS Books.
Brechin A. and Swain J. (1987) *Changing Relationships: Shared Action Planning with People with a Mental Handicap*. London: Harper & Row.
Breggin P. (1993) *Toxic Psychiatry: Drugs and Electroconvulsive Therapy: The Truth and the Better Alternatives*. London: Fontana.
British Association of Counselling (1989) *Code of Ethics and Practice for Counselling Skills*. Rugby: BAC.
British Association of Counselling (1990) *BAC Code of Ethics and Practice for Counsellors*. Rugby: BAC.
Broadbent D.E. (1958) *Perception and Communication*. London: Pergamon Press. (See also Hayes, 1994; Atkinson *et al.*, 1996; Gross, 1996.)
Bromley D.B. (1966) *The Psychology of Human Ageing*. Harmondsworth: Penguin. (See also Hayes, 1994; Gross, 1996.)
Broome A.K. (1994) *Health Psychology – Processes and Applications*, 2nd edn. London: Chapman & Hall.
Brown R. (1988) *Group Processes*. Oxford: Basil Blackwell.
Bruner J.S. (1960) *The Process of Education*. Cambridge, MA: Harvard University Press.
Bruner J.S. (1964) The course of cognitive growth, *American Psychologist*, **19**: 1–15. (See also Hayes, 1994.)
Bruner J.S. (1966) *Towards a Theory of Instruction*. Cambridge, MA: Harvard University Press. (See also Gross, 1996.)
Bruner J.S. (1971) *The Relevance of Education*. London: George Allen & Unwin.
Bryant P. (1982) *Piaget: Issues and Experiments*. Leicester: BPS.
Buckman R. (1988) *I Don't Know What to Say: How to Help and Support Someone Who is Dying*. London: Macmillan Papermac.
Bunton R. and Macdonald G. (eds) (1992) *Health Promotion: Disciplines and Diversity*. London: Routledge.
Burnard P. (1994) *Counselling Skills for Health Professionals*, 2nd edn. London: Chapman & Hall.
Burnard P. and Morrison P. (1991) Client-centred counselling: a study of nurses' attitudes, *Nurse Education Today*, **11**: 104–9.
Burt K. (1995) The effects of cancer on body image and sexuality, *Nursing Times*, **91**(7): 36–7.
Burton G. and Dimbleby R. (1995) *Between Ourselves*, 2nd edn. London: Edward Arnold.
Buss A.H. (1961) *The Psychology of Aggression*. New York: John Wiley & Sons. (See also Gross, 1996.)

Buss A.H. and Plomin R. (1975) *A Temperament Theory of Personality Development.* New York: John Wiley and Sons. (See also Niven, 1994; Atkinson *et al.*, 1996.)

Butler J.M. and Haigh G.V. (1954) Changes in the relation between self-concepts and ideal concepts consequent upon client-centred counseling. In Rogers C.R. and Dymond R.F. (eds) *Psychotherapy and Personality Change.* Chicago: University of Chicago Press.

Buzan T. (1988) *Use Your Head.* London: Pan.

Calder N. (1970) *The Mind of Man.* London: BBC Publications.

Calev A., Gaudino E.A., Squires N.K., Zervas I.M. and Fink M. (1995) ECT and non-memory cognitions: a review, *British Journal of Clinical Psychology,* **34**(4): 505–15.

Calisch A. (1989) Eclectic blending of theory in the supervision of art psychotherapists, *The Arts in Psychotherapy,* **16**: 37–43.

Cannon W.B. (1929) *Bodily Changes in Pain, Hunger, Fear and Rage.* Boston: Branford. (Original work published in 1915.) (See also Hayes, 1994; Atkinson *et al.*, 1996.)

Cardwell M., Clark L. and Meldrum C. (1996) *Psychology for A Level.* London: Harper-Collins.

Carey, P. (1988) *Oscar and Lucinda.* London: Faber.

Carlsmith J.M. and Anderson C.A. (1979) Ambient temperatures and the occurrence of collective violence: a new analysis, *Journal of Personality and Social Psychology,* **37**: 337–44.

Carrie L.E.S., Simpson P.J. and Popat M.T. (1996) *Understanding Anaesthesia,* 2nd edn. London: Butterworth Heinemann.

Cattell R.B. (1965) Personality structure: the larger dimension. In Lazarus R.S. and Option E.M. Jr (1967) *Personality: Selected Readings.* Harmondsworth: Penguin. (See also Hayes, 1994; Atkinson *et al.*, 1996; Gross, 1996, for other references.)

Chalmers D. J. (1995) The puzzle of conscious experience, *Scientific American.* Dec. 62–8.

Child D. (1986) *Psychology and the Teacher,* 4th edn. London: Cassell.

Clarkson P. and Gilbert M. (1990) Transactional Analysis. In Dryden W. (ed.) *Individual Therapy, A Handbook.* Milton Keynes: Open University Press.

Clegg C. (1986) *Biology for Schools and Colleges,* 2nd edn. London: Heinemann Educational.

Clegg F. (1982) *Simple Statistics: A Course Book for the Social Sciences.* Cambridge: Cambridge University Press.

Cohen S., Tyrrell D.A.J. and Smith A.P. (1991) Psychological stress and susceptibility to the common cold, *New England Journal of Medicine,* **325**: 606–12.

Collier J., Pattison H.M., MacKinlay D.R.E. and Watson A.R. (1993) Pain in Children: Myths and Attitudes of Health Care Professionals. Paper presented to the Special Group in Health Psychology Conference, Nottingham.

Collins A.M. and Quillian M (1969) Retrieval time for semantic memory, *Journal of Verbal Learning and Verbal Behaviour,* **8**: 240–7.

Collins A.M. and Quillian M (1972) How to make a language user. In Tulving E. and Donaldson W. (eds) *Organisation of Memory.* New York: Academic Press.

Concise Oxford Dictionary (1982) 7th edn. Oxford: Clarendon Press.

Conner M., Martin E., Silverdale N. and Grogan S. (1996) Dieting in adolescence: an application of the theory of planned behaviour, *British Journal of Health Psychology,* **1**(4): 315–25.

Cooper C.L. (ed.) (1981) *Psychology and Management: A Text for Managers and Trade Unionists.* London: British Psychological Association/Macmillan Press.

Cornsweet T.N. (1970) *Visual Perception.* New York: Academic Press.

Cox D.F. and Bauer R.A. (1964) Self-confidence and persuasability in women, *Public Opinion Quarterly,* **28**: 453–66. (See also Wright *et al.,* 1970.)

Craik F. and Lockhart R. (1972) Levels of processing. *Journal of Verbal Learning and Verbal Behaviour,* **11**: 671–84. (See also Atkinson *et al.,* 1996, Gross, 1996.)

Crammond W.A. (1970) Psychotherapy of the dying patient, *British Medical Journal,* **15**(4): 389–93.

Crowe M. and Ridley J. (1990) *Therapy with Couples*. Oxford: Blackwell.
Curzon L.B. (1985) *Teaching in Further Education. An Outline of Principles and Practice*, 3rd edn. London: Holt, Rinehart & Winston.
Cytovic R.E. (1994) *The Man Who Tasted Shapes*. London: Abacus.
Dalgleish T. and Rosen K. (1996) Rhythm and blues: the theory and treatment of seasonal affective disorder, *British Journal of Clinical Psychology*, **35**: 163–82.
Damasio A.R. (1994) *Descartes' Error*. London: Picador.
Dance F.E. and Larson C.E. (1976) *The Functions of Human Communication, A Theoretical Approach*. New York: Holt, Rinehart & Winston.
Danish S.J. and D'Augelli A.R. (1982) *Helping Skills, II: Life Development Intervention*. New York: Human Sciences Press. (See also Niven, 1994.)
Davies A. (1983) Back on their feet: behavioural techniques for elderly patients – 1. *Nursing Times*, 19 October, 49–51.
Davis H. and Fallowfield L. (1991) *Counselling and Communication in Health Care*. Chichester: John Wiley & Sons.
de Bono E. (1971) *The Use of Lateral Thinking*. Harmondsworth: Penguin. (See also Gross, 1996.)
de Certeau M. (1984) *The Practice of Everyday Life*. London: University of California Press.
Deliege I. and Sloboda J. (eds) (1996) *Musical Beginnings: Origins and Development of Musical Competence*. Oxford: Oxford University Press.
Delunas L.R. (1996) Beyond Type A: hostility and coronary heart disease – implications for research and practice, *Rehabilitation Nursing*, **21**(4): 196–201.
Dennet D.C. (1991) *Consciousness Explained*. London: Allen Lane/Penguin.
Department of Health (1991) *Welfare of Children and Young People in Hospital*. London: HMSO.
Department of Health (1992) *The Health of the Nation*. London: HMSO.
de Shazer S. (1985) *Key Solutions in Brief Therapy*. New York: W.W. Norton.
de Shazer S. (1986) Brief therapy: focused solution development, *Family Process*, **25**: 207–21.
Dickson D. (1993) *Rewarding People: Skill of Responding Positively*. London: Routledge & Kegan Paul.
Dienstbier R.A. (1989) Arousal and physiological toughness: implications for mental and physical health, *Psychology Review*, **96**(1): 84–100.
Dixon N. (1987) *Our Own Worst Enemy*. London: Fontana.
Dollard J., Doob L., Miller N.E., Mowrer O.H. and Sears R.R. (1939) *Frustration and Aggression*. New Haven, CT: Yale University Press. (See also Hayes, 1994; Gross, 1996.)
Donaldson M. (1978) *Children's Minds*. London: Fontana. (See also Hayes, 1994; Niven, 1994; Cardwell *et al.*, 1996; Gross, 1996.)
Donaldson M. (1992) *Human Minds*. Harmondsworth: Penguin.
Drabman R.S. and Thomas M.H. (1974) Does media violence increase children's tolerance of real-life aggression? *Developmental Psychology* **10**: 418–21. (See also Cardwell *et al.*, 1996; Gross, 1996.)
Drever J. (1964) *A Dictionary of Psychology*, rev. edn. Harmondsworth: Penguin.
Dryden W. (ed.) (1990) *Individual Therapy, A Handbook*. Milton Keynes: Open University Press. (See also Cardwell *et al.*, 1996.)
Dryden W. (1992) (ed.) *Integrative and Eclectic Therapy, A Handbook*. Milton Keynes: Open University Press.
Dryden W. and Rentoul R. (1991) *Adult Clinical Problems*. London: Routledge.
Duffy (1996) *Stopping for Death*. London: Penguin/Viking.
Durham T.W., McCammon S.L. and Allison E.J. Jr (1985) The psychological impact of disaster on rescue personnel, *Annals of Emergency Medicine*, **14**: 664–8.

Eagly A. and Chaiken S. (1975) An attribution analysis of the effect of communication characteristics on opinion change: the case of communicator attractiveness, *Journal of Personality and Social Psychology*, **32**: 136–44.
Ebbinghaus H. (1885) *On Memory*. Leipzig: Duncker.
Edwards A.L. (1957) *Techniques of Attitude Scale Construction*. New York: Appleton-Century Croft.
Edwards B. (1992) *Drawing on the Right Side of the Brain, How to Unlock Your Artistic Talent*. London: Souvenir Press.
Ekman P. and Oster H. (1979) Facial expressions of emotion, *Annual Review of Psychology*, **30**: 527–54.
Elliot G.R. and Eisdorfer C. (eds) (1982) *Stress and Human Health*. New York: Springer. (See also Monat and Lazarus, 1991.)
Ellis A. (1973) *Humanistic Psychotherapy*. New York: McGraw Hill. (See also Gross, 1996.)
Ellis A. and Grieger R. (1977) *Handbook of Rational Emotive Therapy*. New York: Julian Press. (See also Cardwell *et al.*, 1996.)
Enright D.J. (1983) *The Oxford Book of Death*. Oxford: Oxford University Press.
Erikson E.H. (1979) *Identity and the Life Cycle: A Reissue*. New York: Norton. (See also Cardwell *et al.*, 1996; Gross, 1996.)
Erikson E.H. (1982) *The Life Cycle Completed*. New York: Norton.
Escher M.C. (1967) *The Graphic Work of M.C. Escher*. Translated from the Dutch by John E. Brigham. London: Macdonald & Co.
Evans P. (1991) Symbol Clash, *Listener*, January 3, 7.
Evans P. and Deehan G. (1988) *The Keys to Creativity*. London: Grafton Books.
Evans P., Clow A. and Hucklebridge F. (1997) Stress and the immune system, *Psychologist*, **10**(7): 303–7.
Ewing T.N. (1942) A study of certain factors involved in changes of opinion, *Journal of Social Psychology*, **16**: 63–8. (See also Wright *et al.*, 1970.)
Eysenck H.J. (1947) *Dimensions of Personality: A Record of Research Carried Out in Collaboration with H.T. Himmelweit*. London: Kegan Paul. (See also Hayes, 1994.)
Eysenck H.J. (1962) *Know your Own IQ*. Harmondsworth: Penguin/Pelican.
Eysenck H.J. (1985) Personality, cancer and cardiovascular disease: a causal analysis, *Personality and Individual Differences*, **6**: 535–56.
Eysenck H.J. (1994) Cancer, personality and stress: prediction and prevention, *Advances in Behaviour Research and Therapy*, **16**(3): 167–215.
Eysenck H.J. and Wilson G. (1976) *Know Your Own Personality*. Harmondsworth: Penguin/Pelican.
Fantz R.L. (1961) The origin of form perception, *Scientific American*, **204**(5): 66–72.
Farabaugh N.F. (1988) Menopause or midlife changes, *Midwife, Health Visitor and Community Nurse*, **24**(1): 29–32.
Fazio R.H. and Zanna M.D. (1978) Attitudinal qualities relating to the strength of the attitude–behaviour relation, *Journal of Experimental and Social Psychology*, **14**: 398–408. (See also Gross, 1996.)
Fellows B. (1988) The use of hypnotic susceptibility scales. In Heap M. (ed.) *Hypnosis, Current Clinical Experimental and Forensic Practices*. London: Croom Helm.
Ferrant F.M., Ostheimer G.W. and Covino B.G. (eds) (1990) *Patient Controlled Analgesia*, 2nd edn. Oxford: Blackwell Scientific.
Feshbach S. (1964) The function of aggression and the regulation of the aggressive drive, *Psychological Review*, **71**: 257–62. (See also Gregory, 1987; Gross, 1996.)
Festinger L. (1957) *A Theory of Cognitive Dissonance*. New York: Harper & Row. (See also Hayes, 1994; Niven, 1994; Atkinson *et al.*, 1996; Gross, 1996.)
Fields H.L. and Levine J.D. (1984) Placebo analgesia – a role for endorphins? *Trends in Neurosciences*, **7**: 271–3.
Fiske J. (1990) *Introduction to Communication Studies*, 2nd edn. London: Routledge.
Fontana D. (1990) *Your Growing Child: From Birth to Adolescence*. London: Fontana.

Fordyce W.E. (1976) *Behavioural Methods of Chronic Pain and Illness.* St Louis: C.V. Mosby.
Foucault M. (1978) *History of Sexuality,* Vol. 1. New York: Pantheon.
Fransella F. (1990) Personal construct theory. In Dryden W. (ed.) *Individual Therapy, A Handbook.* Milton Keynes: Open University Press. (See also Gross, 1996.)
French J.R. and Raven B. (1959) The bases of social power. In Cartwright D. (ed.) Studies in social power, *Journal of Applied Communication,* **11**(2): 23–5.
French P. (1994) *Social Skills for Nursing Practice,* 2nd edn. London: Chapman & Hall.
Freud S. (1924) *A General Introduction to Psychoanalysis.* New York: Washington Square Press. (See also Cardwell *et al.*, 1996.)
Freud S. (1938) *Psychopathology of Everyday Life.* Harmondsworth: Penguin/Pelican.
Fromm E. (1941) *Escape from Freedom.* New York: Rinehart.
Fromm E. (1947) *Man for Himself.* New York: Holt, Rinehart & Winston.
Fromm E. (1956) *The Art of Loving.* New York: Harper & Row.
Geen R.G. (1990) *Human Aggression.* Milton Keynes: Open University Press. (See also Gross, 1996.)
Gill D. and Adams B. (1992) *ABC of Communication Studies.* London: Nelson.
Gilling D. and Brightwell R. (1982) *The Human Brain.* London: Orbis Publishing/BBC.
Glaser B.G. and Strauss A.L. (1965) *Awareness of Dying.* Chicago: Aldine.
Glaser B.G. and Strauss A.L. (1967) *The Discovery of Grounded Theory: Strategies for Qualitative Research.* Chicago: Aldine.
Glass D.C. and Singer J.E. (1972) *Urban Stress: Experiments on Noise and Social Stressors.* New York: Academic Press. (See also Atkinson *et al.*, 1996.)
Glassman W.E. (1979) The biological approach. In Medcof J. and Roth J. (eds) *Approaches to Psychology.* Milton Keynes: Open University Press.
Gleick J. (1988) *Chaos.* London: Sphere.
Green C. and McCreery C. (1989) *Apparitions.* Oxford: Institute of Psychophysical Research.
Green S. (1994) *Principles of Biopsychology.* Hove: Lawrence Erlbaum Associates.
Greenberg M. and Littlewood R. (1995) Post-adoption incest and phenotype matching: experience, personal meanings and biosocial implications, *British Journal of Medical Psychology,* **68**(1): 29–44.
Gregory R.L. (1971) *The Intelligent Eye.* London: Weidenfeld & Nicolson.
Gregory R.L. (1981) *Mind in Science: A History of Explanations in Psychology and Physics.* Harmondsworth: Penguin. (See also Gross, 1996.)
Gregory R.L. (ed.) (1987) *The Oxford Companion to the Mind.* Oxford: Oxford University Press.
Gregory R.L. (1990) How do we interpret images? In Barlow H., Blakemore C. and Weston-Smith M. (eds) *Images and Understanding.* Cambridge: Cambridge University Press.
Gregory S., Shawcross C.R. and Gill D. (1985) The Nottingham ECT study: a double-blind comparison of bilateral, unilateral and simulated ECT in depressive illness, *British Journal of Psychiatry,* **146**: 520–4.
Gross R. (1992) *Psychology, the Science of Mind and Behaviour,* 2nd edn. London: Hodder & Stoughton.
Gross R. (1996) *Psychology, the Science of Mind and Behaviour,* 3rd edn. London: Hodder & Stoughton.
Guilford J.P. (1967) *The Nature of Human Intelligence.* New York: McGraw Hill. (See also Cardwell *et al.*, 1996; Gross, 1996.)
Hall E.T. (1969) *The Hidden Dimension: Man's Use of Space in Public and Private.* Bodley Head. (See also Gill and Adams, 1992; Gross, 1996.)
Hannigan T.J. (1982) *Mastering Statistics.* London: Macmillan.
Harlow H.F. (1959) Love in infant monkeys. In *Frontiers of Psychological Research: Readings from Scientific American.* London: WH Freeman & Co. (See also Hayes, 1994; Niven, 1994; Gross, 1996.)
Harvey S. and Hales-Tooke A. (1972) *Play in Hospital.* London: Faber & Faber.

Hayes N. (1994) *Foundations of Psychology – An Introductory Text*, London: Routledge.
Hayward I. (1975) *Information: A Prescription Against Pain*. London: Royal College of Nursing.
Hebb D.O. (1949) *Organization of Behaviour: A Neuropsychological Theory*. New York: John Wiley & Sons. (See also Hayes, 1994.)
Heider F. (1958) *The Psychology of Interpersonal Relations*. New York: John Wiley & Sons.
Heider F. and Simmel M. (1944) An experimental study of apparent behaviour, *American Journal of Psychology*, **57**: 243–59.
Heim A. (1954) *The Appraisal of Intelligence*. London: Methuen (1970 edn NFER). (See also Hayes, 1994, for other references.)
Hein E.C. and Nicholson M.J. (eds) (1994) *Contemporary Leadership Behaviour: Selected Readings*, 4th edn. London: Lippincott.
Hendin H. (1964) *Suicide and Scandinavia*. New York: Grune & Stratton. (See also Retterstol, 1990.)
Heron (1957) The pathology of boredom. In *Frontiers of Psychological Research: Readings from Scientific American*. London: WH Freeman. (See also Gross, 1996.)
Hershenson M., Munsinger H. and Kessen W. (1965) Preference for shapes of intermediate variability in the newborn human, *Science*, **147**: 630–1.
Hindmarch C. (1993) *On the Death of a Child*. Oxford: Radcliffe Medical Press.
Hinton J. (1972) *Dying*, 2nd edn. Harmondsworth: Penguin. (See also Gross, 1996.)
Hinton J.M. (1980) Whom do dying patients tell? *British Medical Journal*, **281**: 1328–30.
Hinton J.M. (1984) Coping with terminal illness. In Fitzpatrick R., Hinton J.M., Newman S. *et al.* (eds) *The Experience of Illness*. London: Tavistock.
Hirschorn P. (1979) The behaviourist approach. In Medcof J. and Roth J. (eds) *Approaches to Psychology*. Milton Keynes: Open University Press.
Hobson R.P. (1993) *Autism and the Development of Mind*. Hove: Lawrence Erlbaum Associates.
Hohmann G.W. (1966) Some effects of spinal cord lesions on experienced emotional feelings, *Psychophysiology* **3**: 143–56. (See also Pitts and Phillips, 1991; Atkinson *et al.*, 1996; Gross, 1996.)
Hohmann G.W. (1975) Psychological aspects of treatment and rehabilitation of the spinal injured person, *Clinical Orthopaedics*, **112**: 81–8. (See also Davis and Fallowfield, 1991.)
Hollin C.R. and Howells K. (1989) An introduction to concepts, models and techniques. In Howells K. and Hollin C.R. (eds) *Clinical Approaches to Violence*. Chichester: John Wiley & Sons.
Holmes T.H. and Rahe R.H. (1967) The social readjustment rating scale, *Journal of Psychosomatic Research*, **11**: 213–18. (See also Hayes, 1994; Atkinson *et al.*, 1996; Gross, 1996.)
Holt R.R. (1962) Individuality and generalisation in the psychology of personality. In Lazarus R.S. and Option E.M. Jr (1967) *Personality: Selected Readings*. Harmondsworth: Penguin.
Homans G.C. (1961) *Social Behaviour: Its Elementary Forms*. New York: Harcourt Brace Jovanovich.
Hopson B. (1981) Response to papers by Schlossberg, Brammer and Abrego. *Counselling Psychology*, **9**: 36–9. (See also Niven, 1994.)
Horgan M. and Choonara I. (1996) Measuring pain in neonates: an objective scale, *Paediatric Nursing*, **8**(10): 24–7.
Horne J. (1988) *Why We Sleep: The Functions of Sleep in Humans and Other Mammals*. Oxford: Oxford University Press.
Horney K. (1942) *Self-analysis*. New York: Norton.
Horney K. (1945) *Our Inner Conflicts*. New York: Norton.
Houde R.W. (1982) Methods for measuring clinical pain in humans, *Acta Anaesthesiologica Scandinavica* (supplement 74): 25–9.

Hovland C.I. and Weiss W. (1951) The influence of source credibility on communication effectiveness, *Public Opinion Quarterly*, **15**: 635–50. (See also Gross, 1996.)

Howe G (1990) *Schizophrenia – A Fresh Approach*, 2nd edn. London: David & Charles.

Huczynski A. and Buchanan D. (1991) *Organisational Behaviour: An Introductory Text*, 2nd edn. New York: Prentice Hall. (See also Gross, 1996.)

Hunter I.M.L. (1957) *Memory*. Harmondsworth: Penguin. (See also Hayes, 1994.)

Insko C.A. (1967) *Theories of Attitude Change*. New York: Appleton-Century-Croft.

Isaacson J., Walker H., Hayes S., and Legg D. (1982) Post pump psychosis, *Critical Care Nurse*, Jan/Feb: 14–16.

James W. (1890) *Principles of Psychology*. New York: Holt. (See also Hayes, 1994; Gross, 1996.)

Janis I.L. (1982) *Groupthink: Psychological Studies of Policy Decisions and Fiascos*, 2nd edn. Boston: Houghton Mifflin. (See also Niven, 1994; Gross, 1996.)

Janis I.L. and King B. (1954) The influence of role-playing on opinion change, *Journal of Abnormal and Social Psychology*, **49**: 211–18. (See also Wright *et al.*, 1970.)

Janis I.L. and Mann L. (1965) Effectiveness of emotional role-playing in modifying smoking habits and attitudes, *Journal of Experimental Personality Research*, **1**: 84–90. (See also Gross, 1996.)

Jenkins C.D., Zyzansk S.J. and Rosenman R.H. (1979) *The Jenkins Activity Survey for Health Prediction*. New York: Psychological Corporation.

Jenner S. (1993) *QED: The Family Game*. London: BBC Education.

Johnson D.W. and Johnson F.P. (1994) *Joining Together: Group Theory and Group Skills*, 5th edn. Boston: Allyn & Bacon.

Johnston D.W. (1993) The current status of the coronary prone behaviour pattern, *Journal of the Royal Society of Medicine*, **86**(7): 406–9.

Jones E.E. (1979) The rocky road from acts to dispositions, *American Psychologist*, **34**: 107–17. (See also Cardwell *et al.*, 1996.)

Jones E.E. and Nisbett R.E. (1971) *The Actor and the Observer: Divergent Perceptions of the Causes of Behaviour*. Morristown, NJ: General Learning Press. (See also Cardwell *et al.*, 1996; Gross, 1996.)

Jouve N.W. (1980) *Baudelaire. A Fire to Conquer Darkness*. London: Macmillan.

Jung C.G. (ed.) (1964) *Man and his Symbols*. London: Picador. (See also Hayes, 1994; Gross, 1996.)

Jung C.G. (1983 edn) *Memories, Dreams and Reflections*. London: Fontana. (See also Gross, 1996.)

Kahney H. (1993) *Problem Solving: Current Issues*, 2nd edn. Buckingham: Open University Press.

Kalish R.A. and Reynolds D.K. (1976) *Death and Ethnicity: A Psychocultural Study*. University of South California, Los Angeles (unpublished manuscript). (See also Broome, 1994.)

Kanner A.D., Coyne J.C., Schaeffer C. and Lazarus R.S. (1981) Comparison of two models of stress measurement: daily hassles and uplifts versus major life events, *Journal of Behavioural Medicine*, **4**: 1–39.

Kaplan S.G. and Wheeler E.G. (1983) Survival skills for working with potentially violent clients, *Social Casework*, **64**: 339–46.

Kasl S.V. and Cobb S. (1966) Health behaviour, illness behaviour and sick-role behaviour, *Archives of Environmental Health*, **12**: 246–66, 531–41. (See also Niven, 1994.)

Kelly G.A. (1955) *The Psychology of Personal Constructs*. New York: Norton. (See also Hayes, 1994; Atkinson *et al.*, 1996; Cardwell *et al.*, 1996; Gross, 1996.)

Kennell J.H., Voos D.K. and Klaus M.H. (1979) Parent–infant bonding. In Osofsky J.D. (ed.) *Handbook of Infant Development*. New York: John Wiley & Sons. (See also Gross, 1992; Bee, 1997.)

Kermis M.D. (1983) *The Psychology of Human Aging: Theory, Research and Practice*. Boston: Allyn & Bacon.

Kerns R.D., Turk D.C. and Rudy T.E. (1985) The West Haven–Yale Multidimensional Pain Inventory (WHYMPI), *Pain*, **23**: 345–56.
Kerr J. (1986) Multidimensional health locus of control, adherence, and lowered diastolic blood pressure, *Heart and Lung*, **15**: 87–92.
Kerr W. and Thompson M. (1972) Acceptance of disability of sudden onset in paraplegia, *International Journal of Paraplegia*, **10**: 94–102. (See also Pitts and Phillips, 1991.)
Kesey K. (1976) *One Flew Over the Cuckoo's Nest*. London: Picador/Pan.
Kiecolt-Glaser J.K. and Glaser R. (1988) Psychological influences on immunity: implications for AIDS, *American Psychologist*, **43**: 892–8.
Kiger A.M. (1995) *Teaching for Health*, 2nd edn. Edinburgh: Churchill Livingstone.
Kinzel A.F. (1970) Body buffer zone in violent prisoners, *American Journal of Psychiatry*, **127**: 59–64.
Kleiner A. (1987) Amplitude and phase spectra as indices of infants' pattern preferences, *Infant Behaviour and Development*, **10**: 49–59.
Kohler W. (1925) *The Mentality of Apes*. New York: Harcourt Brace Jovanovich. (See also Hayes, 1994; Atkinson *et al.*, 1996; Gross, 1996.)
Kreuger W.C.F. (1929) The effect of overlearning on retention, *Journal of Experimental Psychology*, **12**: 71–8.
Kubler-Ross E. (1970) *On Death and Dying*. London: Tavistock. (See also Cardwell *et al.*, 1996.)
Kuhn M.H. and McPartland T.S. (1954) An empirical investigation of self-attitudes, *American Sociological Review*, **19**: 68–76; **47**: 647–52.
Lacan J. (1977) *Ecrits. A Selection*. Translated by Alan Sheridan. London: Tavistock Norton.
Laing R.D. (1967) *The Politics of Experience and the Bird of Paradise*. Harmondsworth: Penguin. (See also Gross, 1996.)
Lamb M.H. (1995) Effects of cancer on sexuality and fertility of patients, *Seminars in Oncology Nursing*, **11**(2): 6–7.
La Piere R.T. (1934) Attitudes versus action, *Social Forces*, **13**: 230–7.
Lasagna L. (1970) Physicians' behaviour toward the dying patient. In Brim O.G., Freeman H.E., Levine S. and Scotch N.A. (eds) *The Dying Patient*. New York: Russell Sage Foundation. (See also Broome, 1994.)
Latane B. (1981) The psychology of social impact, *American Psychologist*, **36**: 343–56. (See also Atkinson *et al.*, 1996.)
Latane B. and Wolf S. (1981) The social impact of majorities and minorities, *Psychological Review*, **88**: 438–53. (See also Gross, 1996.)
Lazarus A.A. (1981) *The Practice of Multi-modal Therapy: Systematic, Comprehensive and Effective Therapy*. New York: McGraw Hill.
Lazarus R.S. (1966) *Psychological Stress and the Coping Process*. New York: McGraw-Hill. (See also Niven, 1994; Gross, 1996.)
Lazarus R.S. (1976) *Patterns of Adjustment*, 3rd edn. New York: McGraw Hill.
Lazarus R.S. (1982) Thoughts on the relations between emotion and cognition, *American Psychologist*, **37**: 1019–24. (See also Hayes, 1994; Gross, 1996.)
Lazarus R.S. and Cohen J.B. (1977) Environmental stress. In Altman L. and Wohlwill J.F. (eds) *Human Behaviour and the Environment: Current Theory and Research*, Vol. 2. New York: Plenum.
Lazarus R.S. and Folkman S. (1984) *Stress, Appraisal and Coping*. New York: Springer-Verlag. (See also Niven, 1994; Atkinson *et al.*, 1996; Gross, 1996.)
Lazarus R.S. and Option E.M. Jr (1967) *Personality: Selected Readings*. Harmondsworth: Penguin.
Lefebvre M.F. (1981) Cognitive distortion and cognitive errors in depressed psychiatric and low back pain patients, *Journal of Consulting and Clinical Psychology*, **49**: 517–25.
Leiber J. (1991) *An Invitation to Cognitive Science*. Oxford: Basil Blackwell.

Leventhal H., Nerentz D.R. and Steels D.J. (1984) Illness representations and coping with health threats. In Baum A, Singer J. and Baum C.S. (eds) *A Handbook of Psychology and Health*. Hillsdale, NJ: Erlbaum Associates.

Levine F.M. and de Simone L.L. (1991) The effects of experimenter gender on pain report in male and female subjects, *Pain*, **44**: 69–72.

Lewis C.S. (1940) *The Problem of Pain*. London: Century Press.

Linton S.J. and Gotestam K.G. (1983) A clinical comparison of two pain-scales: correlation remembering chronic pain and measure of compliance, *Pain*, **17**: 57–65.

Livingstone W.K. (1943) *Pain Mechanisms: A Physiologic Interpretation of Causalgia and its Related States*. New York: Macmillan. (See also Niven, 1994.)

Loeser J.D. and Fordyce W.E. (1983) Chronic pain. In Carr J.E. and Dengerink H.A. (eds) *Behavioural Science in the Practice of Medicine*. New York: Elsevier Biomedical. (See also Niven, 1994.)

Loftus E.F. and Palmer J.C. (1974) Reconstruction of automobile destruction: an example of the interaction between language and memory, *Journal of Verbal Learning and Verbal Behaviour*, **13**: 585–89.

Lorenz K. (1966) *On Aggression*. London: Methuen. (See also Hayes, 1994; Atkinson et al., 1996; Gross, 1996.)

Lucariello J. (1987) Spinning fantasy: themes, structure, and the knowledge base, *Child Development*, **58**(2): 434–42.

Lucock M.P. and Morley S. (1996) The health anxiety questionnaire, *British Journal of Health Psychology*, **1**: 137–150.

Lyn B. (1984) The detection of injury and tissue damage. In Wall P.D. and Melzack R. (eds) *Textbook of Pain*, 2nd edn. Edinburgh: Churchill Livingstone. (See also Niven, 1994.)

McCaffery M. (1968) *Nursing Practice Theory Related to Cognitive, Bodily Pain and Man–Environment Interactions*. Los Angeles: University of California.

McCaffery M. (1983) *Nursing the Patient in Pain*. London: Harper & Low/Lippincott.

McCarthy R.A. and Warrington E.K. (1990) *Cognitive Neuropsychology, A Clinical Introduction*. London: Academic Press.

Maccoby E.E. (1980) *Social Development: Psychological Growth and the Parent–Child Relationship*. New York: Harcourt Brace Jovanovich.

McGarrigle J. and Donaldson M. (1974) Conservation accidents, *Cognition*, **3**: 341–50. (See also Donaldson, 1978; Bryant, 1982.)

McGhie A. and Russell S.M. (1962) The subjective assessment of normal sleep patterns, *Journal of Mental Science*, **108**: 642.

McGinn C. (1993) *The Problem of Consciousness*: Oxford: Blackwell.

Mackean D.G. (1973) *Introduction to Biology*, 5th edn. London: John Murray.

MacKellaig J.M. (1987) A study of the psychological effects of intensive care with particular emphasis on patients in isolation, *Intensive Care Nursing*, **2**: 176–85.

McLeod J. (1993) *An Introduction to Counselling*. Buckingham: Open University Press.

Maddi S.R. and Kobasa S.C. (1991) The development of hardiness. In Monat A. and Lazarus R. S. *Stress and Coping*, 3rd edn. New York: Columbia University Press.

Manning M., Heron J. and Marshall T. (1978) Styles of hostility and social interactions at nursery, at school and at home. In Hersov L.A. and Berger M. (eds) *Aggression and Antisocial Behaviour in Childhood and Adolescence*. Oxford: Pergamon Press.

Marks I.M. (1986) *Behavioural Psychotherapy: Maudsley Pocket Book of Clinical Management*. Bristol: Wright.

Marquis B. L. and Huston C.J. (1996) *Leadership Roles and Management Functions in Nursing: Theory and Application*, 2nd edn. Philadelphia: J.B. Lippincott.

Marris, P. (1986) *Loss and Change*. London: Routledge & Kegan Paul.

Maslach C. and Jackson S.E. (1986) *Maslach Burnout Inventory*. California: Consulting Psychologists Press. (See also Niven, 1994, for related references.)

Maslow A. (1962) *Towards a Psychology of Being*. New York: van Nostrand. (See also Cardwell *et al.*, 1996; Gross, 1996.)
Mason J.W. (1975) Emotion as reflected in patterns of endocrine integration. In Levi L. (ed.) *Emotions: Their Parameters and Measurement*. (See also Monat and Lazarus, 1991.)
Masters W.H. and Johnson V.E. (1966) *Human Sexual Response*. Boston: Little, Brown.
Mathews K.E. and Cannon L.K. (1975) Environmental noise level as a determinant of helping behaviour, *Journal of Personality and Social Psychology*, **32**: 571–7.
Mayo S. (1996) Symbol, metaphor and story; the function of group art therapy in palliative care, *Palliative Medicine*, **10**: 209–16.
Mead G.H. (1934) *Mind, Self and Society*. Chicago: University of Chicago Press. (See also Gross, 1996.)
Melzack R. (1973) *The Puzzle of Pain*. New York: Basic Books. (See also Hayes, 1994; Niven,1994; Atkinson *et al.*, 1996.)
Melzack R. (1975) The McGill pain questionnaire: major properties and scoring methods, *Pain*, **1**: 277–99.
Melzack R. and Dennis S.G. (1978) Neurophysiological foundations of pain. In Sternbach R.A. (ed.) (1978) *The Psychology of Pain*. New York: Raven Press.
Melzack R. and Wall P.D. (1965) Pain mechanisms: a new theory. *Science*, **150**: 971–79. (See also Niven, 1994.)
Melzack R. and Wall P.D. (1982) *The Challenge of Pain*. Harmondsworth: Penguin. (See also Hayes, 1994; Niven, 1994.)
Merskey H. (1979) Pain terms: a list with definitions and notes on usage, *Pain*, **6**: 249–52.
Messenger J.B. (1979) *Nerves, Brain and Behaviour*. London: Edward Arnold.
Messer D. and Meldrum C. (eds) (1995) *Psychology for Nurses and Health Care Professionals*. London: Prentice Hall/Harvester Wheatsheaf.
Milgram S. (1963) Behavioral study of obedience, *Journal of Abnormal and Social Psychology*, **67**: 371–8. (See also Hayes, 1994; Atkinson *et al.*,1996; Cardwell *et al.*, 1996; Gross, 1996.)
Milgram S. (1965) Liberating effects of group pressure, *Journal of Personality and Social Psychology*, **1**: 127–34. (See also Gross, 1996.)
Milgram S. (1974) *Obedience to Authority: An Experimental View*. New York: Harper & Row. (See also Hayes, 1994; Niven, 1994; Atkinson *et al.*, 1996; Cardwell *et al.*, 1996; Gross, 1996.)
Miller G.A. (1956) The magical number seven plus or minus two: some limits on our capacity for processing information, *Psychological Review*, **63**: 81–97. (See also Simon, 1974; Hayes, 1994; Atkinson *et al.*,1996; Cardwell *et al.*, 1996.)
Miller G.A. (1962) *Psychology: The Science of Mental Life*. Harmondsworth: Penguin.
Miller L., Rustin M., Rustin M. and Shuttleworth J. (eds) (1989) *Closely Observed Infants*. London: Duckworth.
Miller S.M. (1987) Monitoring and blunting: validation of a questionnaire to asses style of information-seeking under threat, *Journal of Personality and Social Psychology*, **52**(2): 345–3.
Miller S.M. (1989) Coping style in hypertensive patients: nature and consequences, *Journal of Consulting and Clinical Psychology*, **57**(3): 333–7.
Miller S.M. and Mangan C. (1983) Interacting effects of information and coping style in adapting to gynaecological stress: should the doctor tell all? *Journal of Personality and Social Psychology*, **45**(1): 223–5.
Millon T. and Everly G.S. Jr (1985) *Personality and its Disorders: A Biosocial Approach*. Chichester: John Wiley & Sons.
Milne D. (1993) *Psychology and Mental Health Nursing*. Basingstoke: BPS/Macmillan.
Milner B., Corkin S. and Teuber H.L. (1968) Further analysis of the hippocampal amnesic syndrome: 14-year follow-up study of H.M, *Neuropsychologia*, **6**: 215–34.
Mollon J.D. (1990) The tricks of colour. In Barlow H., Blakemore C. and Weston-Smith M. *Images and Understanding*. Cambridge: Cambridge University Press.

Monat A. and Lazarus R. S. (1991) *Stress and Coping*, 3rd edn. New York: Columbia University Press.

Montgomery S.A. (1990) *Anxiety and Depression*. Petersfield: Wrightson Biomedical Publishing.

Moon, E.G. and Karb, V.B. (1993) Psychotropic Medication. In Rawlins R.P., Williams S.R. and Beck C.K. (eds) *Mental Health – Psychiatric Nursing: A Holistic Life-cycle Approach*, 3rd edn. St Louis: C.V. Mosby.

Moos R.H. (1986) *Coping With Life Crises: An Integrated Approach*. New York: Plenum. (See also Niven, 1994.)

Moreno J.L. (1946) *Psychodrama*, Vol. 1. New York: Beacon House.

Morgan C.T. and King R.A. (1971) *Introduction to Psychology*. London: McGraw Hill.

Morris B. (1987) *Anthropological Studies of Religion*. Cambridge: Cambridge University Press.

Morris D. (1978) *Manwatching: A Field Guide to Human Behaviour*. St Albans: Triad/Panther.

Moyer K.E. (1976) *The Psychobiology of Aggression*. New York: Harper & Row. (See also Gross, 1996.)

Mueller C.W. (1983) Environmental stressors and aggressive behaviour. In Geen R.G. and Donnerstein E.I. (eds) *Aggression: Theoretical and Empirical Reviews*, Vol. 2: *Issues in Research*. New York: Academic Press.

Murgatroyd S. (1985) *Counselling and Helping*. Leicester/London: BPS/Routledge.

Murstein B.I. (1972) Physical attractiveness and marital choice, *Journal of Personality and Social Psychology*, **22**(1): 8–12. (See also Cardwell et al., 1996; Gross, 1996.)

Myers D. and Lamm H. (1975) The group polarization phenomenon, *Psychological Bulletin*, **83**: 602–27. (See also Gross, 1996.)

Naidoo J. and Wills J. (1994) *Health Promotion. Foundations for Practice*. London: Baillière Tindall.

Naish P.L.N. (1986) *What is Hypnosis? Current Theories and Research*. Milton Keynes: Open University Press.

Napier R.W. and Gershenfeld, M.K. (1989) *Groups: Theory and Experience*, 4th edn. Boston: Houghton Mifflin.

Neisser U. (1976) *Cognition and Reality*. San Francisco: W.H. Freeman. (See also Cardwell et al., 1996; Gross, 1996.)

Newcomb T. (1953) An approach to the study of communication acts, *Psychological Review*, **60**: 393–404.

Newman B.M. and Newman P.R. (1991) *Development Through Life*. London: Brooks/Cole.

Nichols G. (1984) *The Fat Black Woman's Poems*. London: Virago.

Nisbett R.E. and Ross L. (1980) *Human Inference: Strategies and Shortcomings of Social Judgement*. Englewood Cliffs, NJ: Prentice-Hall. (See also Hayes, 1994; Atkinson et al., 1996.)

Nisbett R.E., Caputo C., Legant P. and Maracek J. (1973) Behaviour as seen by the actor and as seen by the observer, *Journal of Personality and Social Psychology*, **27**: 154–65.

Niven N. (1994) *Health Psychology, An Introduction for Nurses and Other Health Care Professionals*, 2nd edn. London: Churchill Livingstone.

Nordholm L. (1980) Beautiful patients are good patients: evidence for the physical attractiveness stereotype in first impressions of patients, *Social Science and Medicine*, **14**: 81–3.

North C. (1987) *Welcome Silence, My Triumph Over Schizophrenia*. London: Arrow Books.

Novaco R.W. (1975) *Anger Control: The Development and Evaluation of An Experimental Treatment*. Lexington, MA: D.C. Heath. (See also Niven, 1994.)

Novaco R.W. (1978) Anger and coping with stress. In Foreyt J.P. and Rathjen D.P. (eds) *Cognitive Behavior Therapy*. New York: Plenum Press.

Novaco R.W. and Welsh W.N. (1989) Anger disturbances: cognitive mediation and clinical prescriptions. In Howells K. and Hollin C. (eds) *Clinical Approaches to Violence*. Chichester: John Wiley & Sons.

Olds J. (1956) Pleasure centres in the brain. In *Frontiers of Psychological Research: Readings from Scientific American*. London: W.H. Freeman. (See also Gross, 1996.)

Olds J. and Milner P. (1954) Positive reinforcement produced by electrical stimulation of septal area and other regions of the rat brain, *Journal of Comparative and Physiological Psychology*, **47**: 419–27. (See also Gross, 1996.)

Ornstein R.E. (ed.) (1973) *The Nature of Human Consciousness: A Book of Readings*. New York: W.H. Freeman.

Osgood C., Suci G.J. and Tannenbau P.H. (1957) *The Measurement of Meaning*. Urbana IL.: University of Illinois Press. (See also Gill and Adams, 1992.)

Oswald I. (1966) *Sleep*. Harmondsworth: Penguin.

Oswald I. (1984) *Sleep*, 4th edn. Harmondsworth: Penguin. (See also Cardwell *et al.*, 1996; Gross, 1996.)

Paritsis N.C. and Stewart D.J. (1983) *A Cybernetic Approach to Colour Perception*. London: Gordon & Breach.

Parkes C.M. (1996) *Bereavement*, 3rd edn. London: Routledge. (See also Hayes, 1994; Niven, 1994; Gross, 1996.)

Parliamentary Office of Science and Technology (1996) *Common Illegal Drugs and Their Effects*. London: POST.

Partlett M. and Page F. (1990) Gestalt therapy. In Dryden W. (ed.) *Individual Therapy, A Handbook*. Milton Keynes: Open University Press.

Partridge E. (1958) *Origins. An Etymological Dictionary of Modern English*. London: Routledge.

Peck D. and Whitlow D. (1975) *Approaches to Personality Theory*. London: Methuen.

Penfield W. (ed.) (1958) *Neurological Bases of Behaviour*. Boston: Little, Brown. (See also Cardwell *et al.*, 1996; Gross, 1996.)

Perls F.S. (1969) *Gestalt Therapy Verbatim*. New York: Bantam.

Peters T. (1989) *Thriving on Chaos: Handbook for a Management Revolution*. London: Pan Books.

Philips H.C. and Jahanshahi M. (1986) The components of pain behaviour report, *Behaviour Research and Therapy*, **24**: 117–25. (See also Pitts and Phillips, 1991.)

Phillips, J.R. (1990) The different views of health, *Nursing Science Quarterly*, **3**(3): 115–22.

Phillips K.C. (1979) Biofeedback as an aid to autogenic training. In Stoll B.A. (ed.) *Mind and Cancer Prognosis*. Chichester: John Wiley & Sons. (See also Pitts and Phillips, 1991.)

Phillips K. (1991) Biofeedback. In Pitts M. and Phillips K. *The Psychology of Health, An Introduction*. London: Routledge .

Piaget J. (1989) *The Language and Thought of the Child*. London: Routledge (original publication 1926.)

Piaget J. (1990) *The Child's Conception of the World*. Distributed by Eurospan Group (original publication 1929.)

Piaget J. and Inhelder B. (1956) *The Child's Conception of Space*. London: Routledge & Kegan Paul.

Piercy M. (1976) *Woman on the Edge of Time*. London: Women's Press.

Pinel J.P.J. (1997) *Biopsychology*, 3rd edn. London: Allyn & Bacon.

Pitts M. (1991) Personality. In Radford, J. and Govier, E. (eds) *A Textbook of Psychology*, 2nd edn. London: Routledge.

Pitts M. and Phillips K. (1991) *The Psychology of Health, An Introduction*. London: Routledge.

Platzer H. (1988) Ageing in men and the crisis of middle age, *Nursing*, **26**: 963–5.

Polit D.F. and Hungler B.P. (1995) *Nursing Research: Principles and Methods*, 5th edn. Philadelphia: J.B. Lippincott.

Price B. (1986) Mirror, mirror on the wall. . ., *Nursing Times*, **24**: 30–2.

Price B. (1990) *Body Image – Nursing Concepts and Care*. London: Prentice Hall.

Pritchard C. (1995) *Suicide – The Ultimate Rejection? A Psycho-social Study*. Buckingham: Open University Press.

Prochaska J.O., DiClemente C.C. and Norcross J.C. (1992) In search of how people change: applications to addictive behaviours, *American Psychologist*, **47**: 1102–14.

Rabbitt P.M.A. and Winthorpe C. (1988) What do old people remember? The Galton Paradigm reconsidered. In Grunberg M.M., Morris P.E. and Sykes R.N. (eds) *Practical Aspects of Memory*, Vol. 2. Chichester: John Wiley & Sons.

Radcliffe-Brown A.R. (1952) *Structure and Function in Primitive Society*. London: Cohen & West.

Randall P. (1997) *Adult Bullying: Perpetrators and Victims*. London: Routledge.

Rankin P.M. and O'Carroll P.J. (1995) Reality discrimination, reality monitoring and disposition towards hallucination, *British Journal of Clinical Psychology*, **34**: 517–28.

Rapoport R. and Rapoport R. (1980) *Growing Through Life*. London: Harper & Row.

Rau M.T. (1993) *Coping with Communication Challenges in Alzheimer's Disease*. San Diego: Singular Publishing Group.

Retterstol N. (1990) *Suicide, A European Perspective*. Cambridge: Cambridge University Press.

Richards D.A. and McDonald B. (1990) *Behavioural Psychotherapy: A Handbook for Nurses*. London: Heinemann Nursing.

Robbie E. (1988) Neuro-linguistic programming. In Rowan J. and Dryden W. (eds) *Innovative Therapy in Britain*. Milton Keynes: Open University Press.

Robinson J.O. (1972) *The Psychology of Visual Illusion*. London: Hutchinson University Library. (See also Gross, 1996.)

Robinson J.O. (1996) An Emotional View of Cognition. Unpublished manuscript.

Robinson R. (1992) Sex and sexuality, *Cancer Topics*, **9**(2): 13–14.

Rogers C.R. (1961) *On Becoming a Person*. Boston: Houghton Mifflin. (See also Hayes, 1994; Atkinson *et al.*, 1996; Gross, 1996.)

Rogers C.R. (1965) *Client-centred Therapy*. Boston: Houghton Mifflin. (See also Cardwell *et al.*, 1996.)

Rogers C.R. (1975) Empathic: an appreciated way of being, *Counselling Psychologist*. **5**(2): 2–10.

Rogers C.R. (1980) *A Way of Being*. Boston: Houghton Mifflin.

Rogers R.W. (1975) A protection motivation theory of fear appeals and attitude change, *Journal of Psychiatry*, **91**: 93–114.

Rokeach M. (1960) *The Open and Closed Mind*. New York: Basic Books. (See also Hayes, 1994; Gross, 1996.)

Rokeach M. (1968) *Beliefs, Attitudes and Values*. San Francisco: Jossey-Bass. (See also Atkinson *et al.*, 1996; Gross, 1996.)

Rosenberg M.J. and Hovland C.I. (1960) Cognitive, affective and behavioural components of attitude. In Rosenberg M.J., Hovland C.I., McGuire W.J., Abelson R.P. and Brehm J.W. (eds) *Attitude Organization and Change: An Analysis of Consistency Among Attitude Components*. New Haven, CT: Yale University Press. (See also Hayes, 1994; Gross, 1996.)

Rosenblum L.A. and Harlow H.F. (1963) Approach-avoidance conflict in the mother surrogate situation, *Psychological Reports*, **12**: 83–5.

Rosenman R.H., Friedman M., Straus R. *et al.* (1964) A predictive study of coronary heart disease, *Journal of the American Medical Association*, **189**: 103–10.

Rosenman R.H., Brand R.J., Jenkins C.D. *et al.* (1975) Coronary heart disease in the western collaborative group study, *Journal of the American Medical Association*, **233**: 872–7. (See also Hayes, 1994; Atkinson *et al.*, 1996; Gross, 1996.)

Rosenstock I.M. (1974) The health belief model and preventative health behaviour, *Health Education Monographs*, **2**: 354–86. (See also Niven, 1994.)

Rosenteil A.K. and Keefe F.J. (1983) The use of cognitive coping strategies in chronic low back pain patients. Relationship to client characteristics and current adjustment, *Pain*, **17**: 33–44.

Ross L. (1977) The intuitive psychologist and his shortcomings. In Berkowitz L. (ed.) *Advances in Experimental and Social Psychology*, Vol. 10. New York: Academic Press.

Roth S. and Cohen L.J. (1986) Approach, avoidance and coping with stress, *American Psychologist*, **41**: 813–19.

Rotter J.B. (1954) *Social Learning and Clinical Psychology*. Englewood Cliffs, NJ: Prentice Hall.

Rotter J.B. (1966) Generalized expectancies for internal versus external control of reinforcement, *Psychological Monographs*, **30**(1): 1–26. (See also Hayes, 1994; Gross, 1996.)

Rotter J. (1975) Some problems and misconceptions related to the construct of internal versus external control of reinforcement, *Journal of Consulting and Clinical Psychology*, **43**: 56–67.

Rowan J. (1988) Primal integration therapy. In Rowan J. and Dryden W. (eds) *Innovative Therapy in Britain*. Milton Keynes: Open University Press.

Rowe D. (1983) *Depression, The Way Out of Your Prison*. London: Routledge.

Rule B.G., Taylor B.R. and Dobbs A.R. (1987) Priming effects of heat on aggressive thoughts, *Social Cognitions*, **5**: 131–43.

Rumsey N. (1991) Counselling and disfigurement. In Davis H. and Fallowfield L. *Counselling and Communication in Health Care*. Chichester: John Wiley & Sons.

Runco M.A. and Albert R.S. (1990) *Theories of Creativity*. London: Sage.

Ruse M. (1990) *Homosexuality*. Oxford: Basil Blackwell.

Rutter M. (1979) *Maternal Deprivation Reassessed*. Harmondsworth: Penguin.

Ryckman R.M. (1989) *Theories of Personality*, 4th edn. Pacific Grove, California: Brooks/Cole.

Ryle A. and Cowmeadow P. (1992) Cognitive-analytic therapy (CAT.) In Dryden W. (ed.) *Integrative and Eclectic Therapy: A Handbook*. Milton Keynes: Open University Press.

Sacks O. (1984) *A Leg To Stand On*. London: Duckworth.

Sacks O. (1985) *The Man who Mistook his Wife for a Hat*. London: Pan. (See also Hayes, 1994.)

Sacks O. (1989) *Seeing Voices: A Journey into the World of the Deaf*. Los Angeles, California: University of California Press.

Sacks O. (1991) *Awakenings*. London: Pan.

Sander L. and Thompson P. (1989) *Epilepsy: A Practical Guide to Coping*. Marlborough: Crowood Press.

Sarafino, E. (1990) *Health Psychology: Biopsychosocial Interactions*. New York: John Wiley & Sons.

Saunders C. (1966) Management of terminal illness, *Hospital Medicine*, **5**(8): 22. (See also Broome, 1994.)

Schaffer R. (1977) *Mothering*. London: Fontana. (See also Cardwell *et al.*, 1996; Gross, 1996; Bee, 1997.)

Schank R.C. (1982) *Dynamic Memory*. New York: Cambridge University Press. (See also Atkinson *et al.*, 1996; Cardwell *et al.*, 1996; Gross, 1996.)

Schneidman E.S. (1978) Some aspects of psychotherapy with dying persons. In Garfield C.A. (ed.) *Psychological Care of the Dying Patient*. New York: McGraw Hill. (See also Broome, 1994.)

Schramm W. (1970) *Men, Messages and Media*. New York: Harper & Row.

Schramm W. (1982) *Men, Women, Messages and Media*, 2nd edn. New York: Harper & Row.

Schreiber F.R. (1974) *Sybil: The True Story of a Woman Possessed by Sixteen Separate Personalities*. Harmondsworth: Penguin.

Schwartz G.E. (1977) Psychosomatic disorders and biofeedback: a psychobiological model of disregulation. In Maser J.D. and Seligman M.E.P. (eds) *Psychopathology: Experimental Models*. San Francisco: W.H. Freeman.

Schwarzer R. (ed.) (1992) *Self-efficacy: Thought Control of Action*. Washington DC: Hemisphere.

Scott J., Williams J.M.G. and Beck A.T. (1991) *Cognitive Therapy in Clinical Practice*. London: Routledge.
Scott M.J. and Stradling S.G. (1992) *Counselling for Post-Traumatic Stress Disorder*. London: Sage. (See also Cardwell *et al.*, 1996.)
Sear J.W. (1992) General anaesthesia and local anaesthetics. In Grahame-Smith D.G. and Aronson J.K. (eds) *Oxford Textbook of Clinical Pharmacology and Drug Therapy*. Oxford: Oxford University Press.
Searle J. (1989) *Minds, Brains and Science*. Harmondsworth: Penguin.
Seligman M.E.P. (1975) *Helplessness: On Depression, Development and Death*. San Francisco: W.H. Freeman. (See also Hayes, 1994; Niven, 1994; Atkinson *et al.*, 1996; Gross, 1996.)
Selye H. (1956) *The Stress of Life*. New York: McGraw-Hill. (See also Hayes, 1994; Niven, 1994; Cardwell *et al.*, 1996.)
Selye H. (1974) *Stress Without Distress*. Toronto: McClelland & Stewart.
Shannon C.E. and Weaver W. (1949) *The Mathematical Theory of Communication*. Urbana IL.: University of Illinois Press. (See also Gill and Adams, 1992.)
Shorter Oxford English Dictionary (1983) 3rd edn. London: Book Club Associates.
Silverstone L. (1993) *Art Therapy the Person-Centred Way*. London: Autonomy Books.
Simon H.A. (1974) How big is a chunk?, *Science*, **183**: 482–8.
Simpkins J. and Williams J.I. (1987) *Advanced Human Biology*. London: Unwin Hyman.
Skevington S.M. (1984) *Understanding Nurses*, Chichester: John Wiley & Sons.
Skevington S.M. (1995) *Psychology of Pain*. Chichester: John Wiley & Sons.
Slade P. (1995) *Child Play: Its Importance for Human Development*. London: Jessica Kingsley.
Slater A. (1989) Visual memory and perception in early infancy. In Slater A. and Bremner G. (eds) *Infant Development*. Hove: Lawrence Erlbaum Associates.
Sperling G. (1960) The information available in brief visual presentation. *Psychological Monographs*, **74**: 1–29.
Sperling G. (1963) A mode for visual memory tasks, *Human Factors*, **5**: 19–31.
Spielberger C.D. (1977) *Stress and Anxiety*, Vol. 4. Washington, DC: Hemisphere.
Spielberger C.D., Gorsuch R.L. and Lushene R. (1968) *Self-evaluation Questionnaire*. Palo Alto, CA: Consulting Psychologists Press.
Spielberger C.D., Krasner S.S. and Solomon E.P. (1988) The experience, expression and control of anger. In Janisse M.P. (ed.) *Health Psychology: Individual Differences and Stress*. New York: Springer-Verlag.
Springer S.P. and Deutsch G. (1989) *Left Brain, Right Brain*. New York: W.H. Freeman.
Springer S.P. and Deutsch G. (1993) *Left Brain, Right Brain*, 2nd edn. New York: W.H. Freeman.
Srivastava L. (1995) *Proceedings of the National Academy of Sciences*, **92**: 2785.
Stayton D.J. and Ainsworth M.D.S. (1973) Individual differences in infant response to brief, everyday separation as related to other infant and maternal behaviours, *Developmental Psychology*, **9**: 226–35. (See also Gross, 1996.)
Steiner I.D. (1972) *Group Process and Productivity*. New York: Academic Press.
Stephenson W. (1953) *The Study of Behaviour: Q Technique and its Methodology*. Chicago: University of Chicago Press. (See also Wright *et al.*, 1970.)
Steptoe A. (1989) Psychophysiological interventions in behavioural medicine. In Turpin G. (ed.) *Handbook of Clinical Psychophysiology*. Chichester: John Wiley & Sons. (See also Pitts and Phillips, 1991.)
Stern W. (1912) *The Psychological Methods of Testing Intelligence* (translated by G.M. Whipple, Baltimore, MD: Warwick & York, 1914.)
Sternbach R.A. (1968) *Pain: A Psychophysiological Analysis*. New York: Academic Press. (See also Niven, 1994.)
Sternberg R.J. (1995) *In Search of the Human Mind*. London: Harcourt Brace.

Stevens R. (1975) The functions of communication. In *Communication. Social Sciences, A Foundation Course: Making Sense of Society D101 Block 3 Units 7,8,9 and 10*. Milton Keynes: Open University Press.
Stoyva J. and Budzynski T. (1974) Cultivated low arousal – an anti-stress response? In DiCara L.V. (ed.) *Recent Advances in Limbic and Autonomic Nervous System Research*. New York: Plenum. (See also Pitts and Phillips, 1991.)
Stratton P. and Hayes N. (1993) *A Student's Dictionary of Psychology*, 2nd edn. London: Edward Arnold.
Stroebe M.S., Stroebe W. and Hanson R. (eds) (1993) *Handbook of Bereavement*. New York: Cambridge University Press.
Stroebe W. and Stroebe M.S. (1995) *Social Psychology and Health*. Buckingham: Open University Press.
Stuart-Hamilton I. (1991) *The Psychology of Ageing, An Introduction*. London: Jessica Kingsley.
Stuart-Hamilton I. (1994) *The Psychology of Ageing, An Introduction*, 2nd edn. London: Jessica Kingsley.
Suinn R.M. (1990) *Anxiety Management Training: A Behaviour Therapy*. New York: Plenum.
Sully P. (1996) The impact of power in therapeutic relationships, *Nursing Times*, **41**: 40–1.
Sutherland V.J. and Cooper C.L. (1990) *Understanding Stress: A Psychological Perspective for Health Professionals*. London: Chapman & Hall.
Tajfel H. and Fraser C. (1978) *Introducing Social Psychology*. Harmondsworth: Penguin.
Talbot L. (1995) *Principles and Practice of Nursing Research*. New York: C.V. Mosby.
Tamm M.E. (1993) Models of health and disease, *British Journal of Medical Psychology*, **66**: 213–28.
Tan S.Y. (1982) Cognitive and cognitive-behavioural methods for pain control: a selective review, *Pain*, **12**: 201–28.
Teigen K.H. (1994) Yerkes–Dodson: a law for all seasons, *Theory and Psychology*, **4**(4): 525–47.
The Review Panel on Coronary Prone Behaviour and Coronary Heart Disease (1981) Coronary prone behaviour and coronary heart disease: a critical review, *Circulation*, **63**: 1199–215.
Thelan L.A., Davie J.K., Urden L.D. and Lough M.E. (1994) *Critical Care Management*, 2nd edn. New York: C.V. Mosby.
Thomas A. and Chess S. (1977) *Temperament and Development*. New York: Brunner Mazel. (See also Niven, 1994.)
Thomson R. (1959) *The Psychology of Thinking*. Aylesbury: Pelican.
Thorndike E.L. (1931) *Human Learning*. New York: Century.
Thurstone L.L. (1948) *Primary Mental Abilities*. Chicago: Chicago University Press. (See also Hayes, 1994; Niven, 1994; Gross, 1996.)
Ticklenberg J.R. and Ochberg F.M. (1981) Patterns of adolescent violence. In Hamburg D.A. and Trudeau M.B. (eds) *Biobehavioural Aspects of Aggression*. New York: Alan Liss.
Tizard B. and Rees J. (1975) A comparison of the effects of adoption, restoration to the natural mother and continued institutionalisation on the cognitive development of four-year old children, *Child Development*, **45**: 92–9. (See also Gross, 1996.)
Towle V.L., Sutcliff E. and Sokol S. (1985) Diagnosing functional visual deficits with the P300 component of the visual evoked potential, *Archives of Ophthalmology*, **103**: 47–50.
Triandis H.C. (1971) *Attitude and Attitude Change*. London: John Wiley & Sons.
Tuckman B.W. and Jensen M.A.C. (1977) Stages of small-group development revisited, *Group and Organizational Studies*, **2**(4): 419–27.
Tulving E. (1972) Episodic and semantic memory. In Tulving E. and Donaldson W. (eds) *The Organization of Memory*. New York: Academic Press.

Tulving E. (1985) How many memory systems are there? *American Psychologist*, **40**: 385–98.
Turk D.C., Meichenbaum D. and Genest M. (1983) *Pain and Behavioural Medicine: A Cognitive–Behavioural Perspective*. New York: Guilford.
Turk D.C., Wack J.T. and Kerns R.D. (1985) An empirical examination of the 'pain-behaviour' construct, *Journal of Behavioural Medicine*, **8**: 119–30.
Tursky B. (1976) The development of a pain perception profile: a psychological approach. In Weisenberg M. and Tursky B. (eds) *New Perspectives in Therapy and Research*. New York: Plenum Press.
Twaddle V. and Scott J. (1991) Depression. In Dryden W. and Rentoul R. *Adult Clinical Problems*. London: Routledge.
Twycross R.G. (1975) *The Dying Patient*. London: Christian Medical Fellowship.
Ursin H., Baade E. and Levine S. (eds) (1978) *Psychobiology of Stress: a Study of Coping Men*. New York: Academic Press. (See also Niven, 1994.)
Vaillant G. (1977) *Adaptation to Life*. Boston: Little, Brown.
van Wynsberghe D., Noback C.R. and Carola R. (1995) *Human Anatomy and Physiology*, 3rd edn. New York: McGraw Hill.
Volicier B.J. and Bohannon M.W. (1975) A hospital rating scale, *Nursing Research*, **24**: 352–9.
Wadeson H. (1980) *Art Psychotherapy*. Chichester: John Wiley & Sons.
Wall P.D. and Melzack R. (eds) (1984) *Textbook of Pain*, 2nd edn. Edinburgh: Churchill Livingstone.
Wallas G. (1926) *The Art of Thought*. New York: Harcourt Brace.
Walster E. and Festinger L. (1962) The effectiveness of 'overheard' persuasive communication, *Journal of Abnormal and Social Psychology*, **65**: 395–402. (See also Hayes, 1994.)
Walster E., Aronson V. and Abrahams D. (1966) On increasing the persuasiveness of a low prestige communicator, *Journal of Experimental Psychology*, **2**: 325–42. (See also Hayes, 1994; Gross, 1996.)
Warrington E.K. and Shallice T. (1969) The selective impairment of auditory verbal short-term memory, *Brain*, **92**: 885–96.
Warrington E.K. and Shallice T. (1972) Neuropsychological evidence of visual storage in short-term memory tasks, *Quarterly Journal of Experimental Psychology*, **14**: 30–40.
Wason P.C. and Johnson-Laird P.N. (1968) *Thinking and Reasoning*. Harmondsworth: Penguin. (See also Atkinson *et al.*, 1996.)
Wattley L. A. and Muller D. J. (1984) *Investigating Psychology: A Practical Approach for Nursing*. London: Harper & Row.
Watts F. (1992) Applications of current cognitive theories of the emotions to the conceptualization of emotional disorders, *British Journal of Clinical Psychology*, **31**(2): 153–67.
Waugh N.C. and Norman D.A. (1965) Primary memory, *Psychological Review*, **72**: 89–104. (See also Atkinson *et al.*, 1996; Gross, 1996.)
Webb C. (1985) *Sexuality, Nursing and Health*, Chichester: John Wiley & Sons.
Webb C. (1994) *Living Sexuality*, London: Scutari Press.
Weinstein N. (1988) The precaution adoption process, *Health Psychology*, **7**: 355–86.
Weinstein N.D. and Sandman P.M. (1992) A model of the precaution adoption process: evidence from home radon testing, *Journal of Health Psychology*, **11**(3): 170–80.
Weitz S. (ed.) (1979) *Nonverbal Communication, Readings with Commentary*, 2nd edn. New York: Oxford University Press.
Welch S. and Booth A. (1975) The effect of crowding on aggression, *Sociological Symposium*, **14**: 105–27.
Wells G.L. and Loftus E.F. (1984) *Eyewitness Testimony: Psychological Perspectives*. Cambridge: Cambridge University Press. (See also Cardwell *et al.*, 1996; Gross, 1996.)

Whittaker J.O. and Meade R.D. (1967) Sex and age variables in persuasability, *Journal of Social Psychology*, **73**: 47–52. (See also Wright *et al.*, 1970.)

Williams D. (1992) *Nobody Nowhere*. London: Corgi Books/Bantam.

Williams J.M.G., Watts F.N., Macleod C. and Matthews A. (1988) *Cognitive Psychology and Emotional Disorders*. Chichester: John Wiley & Sons.

Wingard L.B., Brody T.M., Larner J. and Schwartz A. (1991) *Human Pharmacology*. New York: Mosby Year Book.

Winnicott (1960) The theory of the parent–infant relationship, *International Journal of Psychoanalysis*, **41**: 585–95. (See also Miller *et al.*, 1989.)

Woodgate R. and Kristjanson L. (1995) Young children's behaviour responses to acute pain: strategies for getting better, *Journal of Advanced Nursing*, **22**: 2.

Worchel S. and Teddle C. (1976) The experience of crowding: a two-factor theory, *Journal of Personality and Social Psychology*, **34**: 30–40.

Worden J.W. (1991) *Grief Counselling and Grief Therapy. A Handbook for the Mental Health Practitioner*, 2nd edn. London: Routledge.

World Health Organisation (1992) *The ICD-10 Classification of Mental Behavioural Disorders: Clinical Descriptions and Diagnostic Guidelines*. Geneva: WHO.

Wright B. (1996) *Sudden Death: A Research Base for Practice*, 2nd edn. London: Churchill Livingstone.

Wright D.S., Taylor A., Davies D.R. *et al.* (1970) *Introducing Psychology: An Experimental Approach*. Harmondsworth: Penguin.

Wright, L. (1991) The Type A behaviour pattern and coronary artery disease: quest for the active ingredients and the elusive mechanism. In Monat A. and Lazarus R.S. (eds) *Stress and Coping*, 3rd edn. New York: Columbia University Press.

Yerkes R.M. and Dodson J.D. (1908) The relation of strength of stimulus to rapidity of habit-formation, *Journal of Comparative and Neurological Psychology*, **18**: 459–82. (See also Teigen, 1994.)

Zander A. (1982) *Making Groups Effective*. San Francisco: Jossey Bass.

Zarkowska E. and Clements J. (1994) *Problem Behaviour and People with Severe Learning Disabilities: The STAR Approach*, 2nd edn. London: Chapman & Hall.

Zborowski M. (1969) *People in Pain*. San Francisco: Jossey-Bass. (See also Niven, 1994.)

Ziesler A.A. (1993) Art therapy: a meaningful part of cancer care, *Journal of Cancer Care*, **2**: 107–11.

INDEX

A

A-beta fibres, 196, 198, 200
accommodation (Piaget), 251
acetylcholine, 2, 73
acoustic code, 163
acoustic store, 163
acronym, 163
action potential, 57, 64, 72, 73, 76, 197, 202, 208, 225
activity trace, 163
acupuncture, 196
A-delta fibres, 194, 196, 200, 207
adherence, 227
adjuvants, 196
Adler, Alfred, 265
adolescence, 228
adrenaline, 320, 324
adrenocorticotrophic hormone (ACTH), 321, 325
adult bullying, *see* bullying
advance organisers, 101
advocacy, 300
affect, 81
 definition of, 79, 80
 negative, 9, 12, 90
 positive, 91
 see also emotion
affective, 81
affective aggression, 4, 5, 9
affective disorders, 81
 see also individual disorders
affective domain, 30, 79, 80
after-image, 210
aggression, 1–14, 17
 as a reaction to trauma, 14
 behavioural approach, 2
 biopsychological approach 2, 71, 82
 classification of, 1, 7–8, 11, 12, 14
 cognitive approach, 3, 8
 definitions of, 1
 environmental antecedents to, 9–10
 ethological approach, 2, 6, 7–8
 expression of, 1, 3, 7, 9, 10, 11, 12, 13, 14
 frustration–aggression hypothesis, 10
 in children, 8
 in the workplace, 1
 intent, 12
 psychodynamic approach, 2, 3, 11
 reinforcement of, 2, 3, 7
 social learning theory approach, 2–3
agitation, 18, 22
agonistic, 4
Alexander technique, 321
alienation, 300
alter ego *see* principle of opposites
altruism, 269, 300
Alzheimer's disease, 2, 163, 180, 211
ambivalance, 30
amnesia, 163,
amygdala, 4, 62, 71, 82
anaesthesia, 178
analysis, 251
analysis of variance (ANOVA), 281
analytical psychology (Jung), 268
anger, 4
 as a factor in illness, 111, 186
 as a response to loss, 150
 expression of, 89
anger arousal
 model of, 4, 5
anger management, 4, 9, 11
anima, 269–70
animism, 229
animus, 269–70
anorexia nervosa, 52, 228, 270
anticathexis, 270
anticipation, 270
anxiety, 6, 24
 abnormal, 17
 assessment, 19–20
 behavioural approach, 16, 26
 biopsychosocial approach, 16
 cognitive approach, 17
 conditioned, 21
 definitions of, 15–16
 humanistic approach, 17
 psychodynamic approach, 17, 21, 24, 26, 266, 267
 social learning theory approach, 17, 26
 treatment of, 16, 18, 20, 48
anxiety and health problems, 24–5
anxiety depression syndrome, 16
anxiety disorders, 17, 18, 21, 25–6
anxiety management, 19
anxiety neurosis, 19
apparitions, 178, 179
appeasement gesture, 6
appraisal
 primary, 13
 secondary, 14
apprehension, 19
arbitrary inference, 81
archetypes, 269, 270, 271
arguments, 6
 and family therapy, 6, 12, 13
 appraisal of, 84
 inducement of, 11
 intractable, 12
arousal
 and anxiety, 15, 19
 appraisal of, 84–5
 physiological systems, 16, 320–1, 323–5, 330, 335
artificial intelligence, 81–2, 86
art therapy, 125–6,
 art psychotherapy, 270
 person-centred, 119, 123, 125–6
 use of bridges and links in, 119,
asceticism, 270
aspirin, 197
assault, 6
assault cycle, 6
assaulter, 7
assertiveness, 7, 9, 14
assertiveness training, 7, 19
assimilation, 251–2
attachment and bonding, 150–1
attention
 and information and perception, 217, 219, 220
 processing, 90
 selective attention, 220–1
attitude change, 30, 36
 and health behaviour, 105, 107–8
 see also persuasion
attitude object, 30,
attitude questionnaire, 30
attitudes, 28–39
 behaviour and, 29, 30, 31, 34, 114
 cognitive, affective and behavioural components of, 29–30, 34
 definitions, 28
 development of, 31
 dimensions of, 31
 measurement of, 30, 31
 reasons for holding, 29
 three-component model of, 29–30
attribution, 101, 230
attribution processes
 actor–observer effect, 233
 animism, 229
 false consensus, 232–3
 false consistency, 233
 fundamental attribution error, 233
 halo/horns effect, 234–5
 primacy/recency effects, 239,
 self-fulfilling prophesy, 233, 240
 stereotyping, 300
attribution theory, 108, 227
auditory location, 210–11
auditory pathways in the brain, 67, 69
autism, 178–9, 217
autogenic relaxation training, 321
autohypnotic, 179
autokinetic effect, 220, 300–1
autonomic nervous system, 73, 176
autophany, 179
autoscopy, 179
avoidance as a response to loss, 151
avoidance learning, 42, 48, 51, 52
axons, 60, 73

B

backward span procedure, 164, 172
Bales interaction process analysis, 301
bargaining for goals, 152
baseline observations, 281
behaviour, 43
 instrumental, 12
 precipitated by loss, 153, 156,
behaviour change
 barriers to, 101, 102
 benefits of, 101, 102
 risk behaviour, 101–3
behaviour therapy, 4, 42, 45
 assessing suitability for, 45
 aversion therapy, 42
 behaviour modification, 17, 43–4, 54, 258

360

INDEX   361

behaviour shaping, 44–5
exposure, 19, 47, 48, 50
flooding, 47–8
implosion, 47, 48
paradoxical techniques, 6,12,
progressive desensitisation, 17, 26, 47, 48, 50–1
response prevention, 42, 52–3
behavioural analysis, 43
behavioural contract, 43, 44
behaviourism, xiv, xxii, 40–55
assumptions underpinning, 41
contrasted with psychodynamic approaches, 264–5
definitions, 40
belief, 82–3
benzodiazepines, 18, 20–1, 183
bereavement
definition of, 147
see also loss
biofeedback, 57, 63, 73
Bion, Wilfred, 265, 271
biopsychology, xiv, xv, 56–77
bipolar disorder, 18, 21, 85
black box, 46
blocking, 271
body boundaries, 230–1
body image, 231,
altered, 228–9
aspects of, 239
hairstyle and, 234
make-up, 237
body language, 132
and leakage, 137, 144
responding to, 90
Bowlby, John, 265–6
brain, 58–60
aggression and, 59
basal nuclei, 57, 62
cells, 58, 60, 62, 66, 73
electrical impulses within, 57, 60, 63, 64, 74
function of, 60
hemispheric specialisation, 66–70
learning and, 59, 60
number of nerve cells in, 58
structure of, 4, 57, 58–9, 62, 66–70, 71, 75, 82, 88, 166, 169, 220
topography, 76

brain damage, 60–1, 63, 71, 169
brain scans, 61,
see also under individual names
brain surgery
split brain, 75–6
Broca's area (speech), 58, 70
broken information games, 301
Bruner, Jerome, 249–50,
developmental theory, 249, 255, 257, 261, 262
Bryant, Peter, 250–1
bullying, 3, 11, 307
burn-out, 321–2

C
camouflage, 231
cancer-prone personality (type C), 111, 150
catastrophe theory see chaos theory
catharsis, 3, 6, 89, 271, 276
catharsis hypothesis, 7
cathexis, 271
central executive system, 162, 164, 168, 172
central nervous system, 57, 72
see also brain
central tendency, 281–2, 287
cerebellum, 59, 169
cerebral cortex, 57, 58, 82, 171
cerebral hemispheres, 59, 66–70
cerebrovascular accident, 7, 60, 70
C fibres, 194, 198, 200, 207
chaining, 46
chaos theory, 83–4
character, 226–7, 231
chi-square measure of association, 282
chromosome, 61, 65, 70, 74, 75
chromosome mutations, 61–2
chronic conditions, 103
circadian rhythms, 180, 187
clairvoyance, 179
client–carer relationships, 119–20
client-centred therapy, see person-centred therapy
coercion, 8

cognitive appraisal, 80, 84
in aggression, 3, 4, 8
of pain, 198
cognitive appraisal theory, 84–5
cognitive-behaviour therapy, 45, 85–6
assessment techniques, 85
assumptions underpinning, 85
cognitive development, 249–51, 252
Bruner's theory of, 249, 255, 257, 261, 262
Piaget's theory of, 251, 252, 253, 255, 256, 261
cognitive dissonance, 31, 252, 307
cognitve distortions, 86, 92
arbitrary inference, 81
catastrophising, 83
dichotomous reasoning, 87
excessive reliance on the words 'should' and 'must', 88
selective abstraction, 93
cognitive domain, 79, 80
cognitive impairment, 87
cognitive labelling, 8
cognitive psychology, 78–94, 246–62
cognition and emotion, 79
definitions, 78–9
see also problem solving, reasoning, thinking
cognitive science, 86
cognitive styles, 252
enactive 249, 255, 260
iconic, 249, 257, 260
symbolic, 249, 256, 260, 262,
cognitive therapy, 4, 17, 86–7,
assumptions underpinning, 80, 84
cognitive restructuring, 19, 80, 86, 88
thought stopping, 24
see also entries for separate therapies
collective unconscious, 271
colour constancy, 211
colour of surroundings, 212

colour vision, 65, 212–13
variations in, 213–14
coma, 179
communication
approaches to, 129
barriers to, 130–2
codes, 128, 132–3
definitions of, 128–9
facilitation of in families, 6
faulty patterns of and schizophrenia, 187
form of, 130, 135, 136
medium used for, 137
networks, 308–9
oral, 139
phatic, 139
purposes of, 141
with children, 133
see also verbal communication and non-verbal communication
communication categories, 132
extrapersonal, 132, 133
in a group, 135–6, 301, 314
interpersonal, 130, 132, 136
intrapersonal, 130, 132, 136–7
mass media, 132
medio, 132, 137
communication process, 129, 130
channels, 132
decoding, 133
encoding, 133
feedback, 135
models of, 140–1
signs and signals, 144–5
communication skills, 133
comparative psychology, 47
compensation, 271, 275
complementary colours, 214
complementary interventions, 17
complementary therapies, 73, 196, 200–1, 320, 321
complex, 271
electra, 273
oedipus, 274–5
compliance, 302
compulsions, 21, 24
treatment of, 53
computerised axial tomography (CT scan), 61, 62, 71, 176
conative domain, 79, 80

concept, 171, 252
concrete operations, 249, 252–3
conditioned response, 46, 47
conditioned stimulus, 46, 47
conditioning, 16, 42, 44, 98
  classical, 16, 21, 41, 46–7, 204
  operant, 17, 21, 31, 41, 43, 49–50, 204
  of gender-linked characteristics, 234
confabulation, 164
conflict, 6, 302
conformity, 302, 310
confusion, 4
confusional state, 179
congenital insensitivity to pain, 198
consciousness, 174–190, 266
  altered state of, 175, 177, 178, 179, 180, 182–3, 184, 185–7, 191
  approaches to, 176–8, 181
  definitions of, 174–5, 263–4
  Freud's theory of, 177, 264
  preconscious, 276
  subconscious, 277
  unconscious, 263–4, 266, 268, 271
consensus, 302
conservation, 253
constancy
  colour, 211
  identity, 217
  perceptual, 219
  shape, 223
  size, 222, 223
container for emotions, 265, 271
context dependence (forgetting), 164
contingency table, 282
control group, 282
control processes, 164
coping
  appraisal-focused, 103
  emotion-focused, 103
  personal competency model of, 104
  problem-focused, 103
  responses, 104
  styles, 203, 322
  tasks, 104
coronary heart disease, vulnerability to, 111
corpus callosum, 59, 70, 75
correlation, 282
  Spearman's rho, 294

correlation coefficient, 282
counselling, 65
  aim of, 116
  supervision, 125
  styles, 116–17
counselling skills, 120–1
  active listening, 3, 118–19, 121, 126
  code of ethics and practice for, 120
  concreteness, 120
  confrontation, 120
  empathic listening, 121
  empathy-building statements, 119, 122–3
  immediacy, 123
  mirroring, 119
  questioning technique, 142–3
counterconditioning, 47, 50
countertransference, see transference
creative arts,
  expression of emotion and, 4, 89
  loss and, 152–3
creativity, 253–4
  definition of, 247
critical illness
  signs of not coping with, 104–5
cross-sectional study, 282–3
crowds, 302–3
crystallised intelligence, 171, 258
cue dependence (forgetting), 164
cybernetics, 86, 87

D
daily hassles, 322
dark adaptation, 214–15
data, 283
data collection methods
  experiment, 284
  focus group interview, 284–5
  focused (semistructured) interview, 284
  participant observation, 289
  questionnaire, 286, 291–2
death
  awareness of, 151–2
  sudden, 158–9
death wish, 3, 271
debriefing, 303
decision-making, 94
  and emotions, 81

within groups, 303–4, 306
defence mechanisms, 21, 271
  anger as, 3, 10, 150, 306
  anxiety and, 6, 18, 24, 26, 269
  following loss, 150, 153, 157
  see also individual names
degrees of freedom, 283
delirium, 179
delusions, 186
dementia, 7, 170–80
  pseudo-, 185
dendrites, 60, 73
denial, 153, 272–3
deoxyribonucleic acid (DNA), 61
depersonalisation, 232
depression, 9, 14, 21–3, 25, 27
  approaches to the study of, 16–17
  assessment of, 19
  classification, 22
  definitions of, 15–16
  learned helplessness and, 108
  pseudodementia and, 185
  treatment of, 16, 18, 62–1, 86
desensitisation, 2, 9
development
  cognitive, 249, 251, 252, 253, 255, 256, 257, 261, 262
  psychosexual, 276–7
  psychosocial, 266
deviates, 303
deviation score, 283
diabetes, 7
didactic, 105
discovery learning, 98, 249, 254
discrimination, 31–2, 37, 39
dispersion, 283
  mean deviation, standard deviation, 287, 294
  range, 292
  variance, 297
displacement, 273
  and aggression, 4, 6, 9, 10, 11
  and anger, 150
  and anxiety, 24
distancing, 153
distraction
  and aggression, 9
  in pain management, 199, 204
distribution
  bimodal, 281
  frequency, 285

normal (Gaussian), 281, 287–8
diurnal rhythms, 180, 191
diversionary strategies, 9
DNA, 61
Donaldson, Margaret, 250
dopamine, 62, 73
  levels in schizophrenia, 186
dorsal horns, 199, 200, 202
double-blind design, 283, 284
Down's syndrome, 61
dreaming, 180–1, 191
dreams
  and repressed material, 177, 181, 266
  lucid, 184
drug therapy,
  for anxiety, 18, 19, 20–1
  for depression, 18
  for insomnia, 183–4
  for pain, 197, 201, 202, 205
  psychotropic drugs, 185–6
dysfunctional cognition, 87
dyslexia, 68

E
ecsomatic experiences, 185
ECT, 62–3
EEG, xxiii, 63, 176
  wave traces in sleep, 188
efforts after meaning, 165
ego, 126, 266, 273
egocentricity, 255, 261
eidetic image, 165
electra complex, 273
electroconvulsive therapy see ECT
electroencephalogram see EEG
emotion, 87
  basic emotions, 4, 15, 82
  cognition and, 79–80, 87–8
  cognitive appraisal theory of, 84–5
  container for, 265, 271
  definition of, 78–80
  expression of, 6, 88–9
  psychological perspectives of, 80
  see also affect

emotional colour, 80, 87–8, 94
emotional maturity scale, 121
empathic pain, 199
empathy, 9, 117, 121–2, 124, 240, 274
empiricists, xx
empowerment, 123
enactive representation (Bruner), 249, 255
and problem-solving, 260
encoding
in communication process, 133
in memory storage, 165, 168
endorphins, 194, 196, 199, 200, 202
engineering model of stress, 318
epilepsy, 7, 181, 184
episodic memory 162, 165
equilibrium, 255
Erikson, Erik, 266
Eros, 3, 274, 275
ethnography, xv
ethological approach
aggression, 2, 6, 7–8, 15
ethology, xiv
eugenics, 63–4
eustress, 323
euthanasia, 153
evoked potentials, 63, 64
exercise, 4, 321
pain tolerance and, 199
expectation of aggression, 10
experimental conditions, 284
experimenter effect, 283, 284
see also Hawthorne effect
expertise, 255
exposure, 19
extinction of behaviour, 46, 47, 51, 52, 54
eye contact and gaze, 133
eye witness testimony, 165

F
facial expressions, 134–5
factor analysis, 284
faith healing, 199
false awakening, 182
false memory syndrome, 165–6
family therapy, 17
fantasy
guided 123, 126

play, 255–6
fear, 4, 23,
and perceptions, 80
anticipatory, 48
as a conditioned response, 47, 50
effects on health behaviour, 105, 112
field theory, xxii
fight or flight mechanism, 73, 318, 323–4
finding behaviour, 153
fixity, 261
flashbulb memory, 166
fluid intelligence, 258
forgetting, 162, 166
context dependence, 164
cue dependence, 164
curve of, 164
decay, 164
gestalt theory of, 166
interference, 162, 167
motivated, 162, 171
overlearning and, 169
partial reports, 169
state dependence, 172
formal operations, 256
free association, 273
free-floating anxiety, 23
Freud, Sigmund, xxi, 264, 266, 271, 273, 274, 275, 276, 277
Freudian slip, 273
Fromm, Eric, 266–7
frustration, 4, 6, 10, 12
frustration–aggression hypothesis, 10
fugue, 166

G
GABA, 20, 73, 183
galvanic skin response, 63, 64
gamma rays see X-rays
gate control theory, 194, 195, 196, 200
gender, 233
pain tolerance and, 200
gender identity, 233–4
general adaptation syndrome, 318, 325
generalised anxiety, 23
genes, 61, 65, 70, 75
dominant, 65, 66
heterozygous, 70, 74
homozygous, 70, 74
recessive, 64, 65, 66
genetic counselling, 65
genetic disorders
Down's syndrome, 61
Klinefelter's syndrome, 75
Turner's syndrome, 75
genetic engineering, 66
genetics, 61, 63

genotype, 66, 77
genuineness, 123, 124
gestalt psychology, 89
gestalt theory
of forgetting, 166
of perception, 216–17
gestalt therapy, 89–90
glia, 66
grief, 155
anticipatory, 150
definition of, 147
models of, 148–9, 156–8
poems of, 154
unresolved, 159
grief therapy, 155
ground rules, 303
grounded theory, 149, 286
group
decision-making, 303–4, 306
development, 304–5
dynamics, 305
effectiveness, 305
initiation rituals, 307
membership, 306
norms, 309
polarisation, 306
processes, 307–8
roles, 313
group of displacements and reversibility, 256, 261
group therapy, 4, 17, 200
groups
analysing interaction within, 301, 314
behaviour within, 265
cohesion within, 301–2
definitions of, 299
self-help, 313
groupthink, 307
guilt and self-blame, 155

H
hallucinations, 178, 179, 182, 184,
explanation for, 181, 186, 187
in schizophrenia, 182, 186–7
negative, 185
sensory deprivation and, 215, 222
hardiness, 318, 325
Hawthorne effect, 285
health,
approaches to, 98–9
assumptions about, 96
definition, 95
dimensions of, 96–7
lifestyle and, 96, 98
personality patterns in, 108, 109, 111

health action process approach, 101, 105–6
health anxiety, 105, 106
health behaviour
barriers to behaviour change, 101, 102
benefits of behaviour change, 101, 102
cues to action, 105, 106
definition of, 95
intention to engage in, 108, 113–14
models explaining adoption of, 99–101, 102, 105–6, 106–7, 112, 113–14
teleological approach to, 113
health belief model 99, 105, 106–7
health beliefs, 96, 106
health education, 95, 107
health education programme, 107
Health of the Nation, 108
health promotion, 96, 98, 102
strategies, 96
health psychology
definition of, xxiv
health risk behaviour
fear and, 105
persistence of, 110
stages of change, 101–3
targets for change, 108
hearing, 209, 217
hemianopia, 219
hemispheric specialisation in the brain, 66–70
heterozygote fitness, 70
heuristic strategies, 256
hierarchical network model (memory), 166
hierarchy construction, 48, 50
hierarchy of needs, 41, 53, 110, 113, 221
hippocampus, 62, 71, 166
Hippocrates, xviii
history of psychology, xviii–xxiv
homosexuality, 42
hormones,
and aggression, 2, 10, and physiological arousal, 332, 321, 325
as a determinant of sex, 74–5
production of, 59

Horney, Karen, 267–8, 275
hospitalisation
 responses to, 10, 23, 325
hostile aggression, *see* affective aggression
humanistic counselling *see* person-centred therapy
humanistic psychology, xiv, xxii, 115–27, 289
 definitions of, 116
 philosophy underpinning, 115, 117, 124
humour, 6, 11
hypervigilant reaction to threat, 325
hypnobate, 182
hypnogogic, 182
hypnopompic, 182
hypnosis, xxi, 63, 73, 179, 182–3,
 memories and, 163, 165–6
 pain management and, 200–1
hypnotherapy, 183
hypnotic, 183
hypnotic state, 184
hypnotics, 183–4
hypochondria, 105, 106, 108
hypothalamus, 4, 59, 71, 82
hypothesis, 285
hypotheticodeductive, 285

I
ibuprofen, 201
iconic
 imagery, 136, 251
 memory, 166
 representation (Bruner), 249, 257, 260
id, 126, 266, 274, 275
ideal-self, 235, 240
identification, 274
ideographic, 285–6
illness
 factitious, 105
 psychogenic, 105
 severity of, 113
 susceptibility to, 113
illness behaviour
 definition, 95
illusions, 217–18
 distortions, 215
 fictions (embedded figure), 216
 Müller-Lyer, 219
 Necker cube, 219
image (person perception), 235
imagery, 166, 201
guided, 123
iconic, 136
implicit personality theory, 236, 238
incest, 315
individual programme planning, 307
individuation, 274
inferences, 166
information processing, 90, 177
 bottom-up, 83, 90,
 parallel, 90, 91, 224,
 serial, 90, 93
 top-down, 93–4,
inheritance, 66, 74
 of eye colour or other single-gene characteristic, 65
inhibition *see* interference
inhibitions towards aggression, 2
insight (in problem-solving), 257, 260
insomnia, 184, 190
instinct, 274
instrumental aggression, 8, 12, 14
intellectualisation, 142, 274
intelligence, 171, 257–8
 artificial, 81–2
interference (theory of forgetting), 162, 167
intergenerational transmission of aggression *see* violence, cycle of
intergroup relations, 308
interpersonal perception, 226–8, 236
 errors in, 232 *see also* attribution processes
introspection, xxi, xxii
ITU syndrome, 222

J
jealousy, 12
Jung, Carl Gustav, xxi–xxii, 268, 269, 270, 271, 273, 274, 275, 276,

K
kinaesthesia, 218, 221
Klein, Melanie, 268, 271
Klinefelter's syndrome, 75

L
labelling, 32–3, 300
Lacan, Jaques, 268–9
language, 137
and cognitive development, 249
and the unconscious mind, 268
centres in the brain, 67–8, 70–1
consciousness and, 177
constraints, 93
development of, 71, 256, 262
register, 131, 143
semantics, 143
lateral thinking, 258
law, 286
leadership, 308
leading questions, 142
and memory, 167
learned helplessness, 17, 108, 195
learning,
 behavioural approach to, 41, 42, 46–7
 definition of, 108
 deductive, 101, 254
 factors affecting, 108–9
 inductive, 257
 objectives, 109
 overlearning and forgetting, 169
 paired-associate, 169
 styles, 98, 254
 transfer of, 173
 vicarious, 55
learning theory, 49
libido, 268, 274
lifespan development, personal competency model of, 104
lifestyle
 health beliefs and, 95–6, 98–9, 107,
 hypnotherapy and, 183
Likert scale, 30, 286–7
limbic system, 4, 62, 71, 82, 88
 amnesia and, 163
listening
 active, 3, 118–19, 121, 126
 dichotic, 215
local anaesthetics, 202
localised anxiety, 23
locus of control, 109
longitudinal study, 287
long-term memory, 162, 167–8
 episodic, 162, 165
 flashbulb, 166
 pattern recognition, 169
 procedural, 162, 169–70
 remote memory, 162, 171
 semantic, 162, 166, 171
 structural change and, 172–3
loss, 147–159
 acceptance of impending threat, 149–50
 coping strategies following, 104
 poems of, 154
 precipitants of, 148
 readjustment following, 156
 responses to, 150, 151, 153, 155, 156
 theories of, 148

M
magnetic resonance imaging (MRI), 61, 71, 176
malice, 12
mandala, 274
manipulation, 33
Mann-Whitney U test, 287
massage, 202
McGill pain questionnaire, 204–5
means–end analysis, 255, 258
mediation, 308
memory, 160–73
 approaches to, 161–2
 brain damage and, 61
 control processes, 164
 definitions of, 160
 dynamic theory of, 164–5
 electrical stimulation studies, 165
 impairment, 63, 163, 165, 166
 levels of processing model, 162, 167
 multistore model, 162, 168–9
 prospective, 170
 strategies to improve, 161, 170 *see also* mnemonics
 structural components, 172
 triggers, 173
 see also long-term, sensory, short-term, and working memory, forgetting and remembering
memory distortions in the elderly, 168
 false memory syndrome, 165–6
 leading questions and, 167
 malleability, 168

INDEX

memory as reconstruction, 168
  see also remembering
memory storage,
  acoustic store, 163
  encoding, 163, 165,
  iconic store, 166
  modality-specific, 168
memory tests, 161,
  backward span, 164, 172
  free recall, 166
  ordered recall, 169
  serial probe technique, 171–2
  serial reproduction, 172
menarche, 237
menopause, 237
metabolism, 59
metachoric experiences, 184
metacognition, 248, 259
metacommunication, 138
metamemory, 168
micrograph, 71
mid-life and menopause, 237
migraine, 24
mind *see* consciousness
mind–body dualism, 176
miscarriage, 155
mnemonics, 168
  acronym, 163
  chunking, 164
  initial letter sentences, 166
  key word technique, 167
model, 287
modelling, 49
  aggression, 2,
  attitudes, 31,
  health behaviours, 98–9, 114
  social learning theory and, 54, 55
mood 90
  see also emotions
mood disorders *see* affective disorders
morphine, 202
motion parallax, 215, 218–19
motivation, 109–10
mourning 155–6
  definition of, 147
  tasks of, 156
Munchausen's syndrome, 105, 233
myoclonic jerk, 184–5

N

narcolepsy, 185
nature–nurture debate

aggression, 2
personality, 231
needs
  hierarchy of, 41, 53, 110, 113, 221
  motivation and, 110
  neurotic (Horney), 267
nerve fibres, 71–2
  and pain, 194, 196, 198
nervous system, xx, 72–3
  autonomic nervous system, 73, 176
  central nervous system, 57, 72
  motor and sensory pathways, 66–8
  parasympathetic nervous system, 59, 73
  peripheral nervous system, 57, 72, 82
  sympathetic nervous system, 59, 73, 320
neurolinguistic programming, 87, 90–1, 119, 130, 218, 268
  primary representation, 90, 91, 128
  secondary representation, 90, 92–3, 128
neurones, 58, 60, 62, 66, 73
  axons, 60, 73
  dendrites, 60, 73
neuropsychology *see* biopsychology
neurosis, 19, 23, 24, 267
neurotic, 24
neurotic needs, 267
neurotransmitters, 73
  and drug therapy, 185
  see also individual names
nociceptors, 202, 205
noise,
  and aggression, 12
  as a barrier to communication, 131
nominal data, 287
nomothetic, 286, 287
non-steroidal anti-inflammatory drugs, 202
non-verbal communication, 138–9
  eye contact and gaze, 133
  facial expression, 134–5
  orientation, 139

paralanguage, 139, 146, 217
proximity, 141
silence, 145
touch and bodily contact, 145–6
noradrenaline, 18, 73, 191
null hypothesis, 288

O

obedience, 309
object concept, 259, 261
objective viewpoint, 288
obsessions, 24
  treatment of, 86
obsessive-compulsive disorder, 17, 21, 24, 53
obsessive-compulsive personality, 24
oedipus complex, 274–5
ontological insecurity, 237
operational definition, 288–9
opiate, 202
opinion, 3
opiod, 197, 202, 206
opiod peptides, 202
opium, 202
ordinal data, 289
out-of-body experience, 179, 185
outliers, 281, 289
overlearning and forgetting, 169

P

pain, 192–207
  and aggression, 7, 12
  anticipatory, 204
  approaches to, 195–6
  avoidance, 43
  children and, 198
  congenital insensitivity to, 198
  context of, 198
  definitions of, 192–3
  empathic, 199
  perception of, 193
  post-herpetic, 206
  psychogenic, 206
  puzzle or paradox of, 194
  referred, 194, 206
  threshold, 25, 196, 205
  tolerance, 205, 232, 236
pain assessment, 197
  assessment scales, 197–8
  multiple-baseline approach, 202
  pain questionnaires, 204–5

pain behaviour, 202–3
  cultural differences and, 199, 200
  gender and, 200
pain-carrying fibres, 194, 196, 198, 200, 203,
pain management, 194, 195, 196 203–4
  acupuncture, 196
  behavioural techniques, 204
  distraction, 199, 204
  drugs, 197, 201, 202, 205
  early assumptions underpinning, 193–4
  exercise, 199
  faith healing, 199
  group counselling, 200
  hypnotism, 200–1
  imagery, 201, 204
  massage, 202
  multimodal programmes, 195, 202, 204
  patient-controlled analgesia, 205
  transcutaneous electrical nerve stimulation (TENS), 207
  use of counterirritants, 198–9
pain stages
  acute, 195, 196
  chronic, 195, 196, 203
pain theories
  gate control theory of, 194, 195, 196, 200
  linear model of, 193, 201
  pattern theory of, 193, 205
  specificity theory of, 193, 194, 206–7
panic, 25
panic attack, 18, 25
panic disorder, 25
paracetamol, 205
paradigm, 289
paradoxical pain, 205
paradoxical prescription, 12, 89
paralanguage, 139, 146, 217
parallel processing, 90, 91
parametric and non-parametric tests, 289
  analysis of variance (ANOVA), 281
  Mann-Whitney U test, 287
  t-tests, 295

Wilcoxon test, 297
paranormal, 185
parasympathetic nervous system, 59, 73
parenting skills, 309–10
parenting styles, 310
Parkinson's disease, 57, 62, 180
participant, 289
pattern recognition, 169
peer group, 2, 310
peer influence, 310
penis envy, 275
perception, 208–225
 and fear, 80
 approaches to, 210
 colour of surroundings, 212
 coloured lights and, 211
 constancies, 211, 217, 219, 222, 223
 definitions of, 208–9
 disorders of, 182, 215, 217–18, 219
 figure–ground reversal, 216
 Gestalt theory of, 216–17
 habituation, 217, 220
 of colour, 88
 of depth, 215
 of faces, 215–16
 sensory loss and, 211, 213, 215, 217, 219
 subliminal, 223
perceptual neglect, 219
perceptual set, 219–20
perceptual skills, 237
peripheral nervous system, 57, 72, 82
perseveration, 169
persona, 275
personal construct theory, 92, 237–8
personal construct therapy, 124
personal constructs, 92
personal growth, 124
personal space, 10, 13
personality, 226–8, 238–9
 authoritarian, 36, 125, 230
 definitions of, 226–7
 extroversion, 232
 hardiness, 318, 325
 introversion, 236
 locus of control, 109
 multiple, 184
 psychoanalytic theories of, 265, 266, 267, 273, 274, 277
 traits, 228, 244,
 type A, 111, 318, 328–30
 type B 329

type C (cancer-prone), 111, 150
types, 111, 150, 242, 245, 265, 318, 328–30
personality and stress, 325, 328–30
personality disorder, 7
personality patterns in health, 111
person-centred therapy, 115,
 basic principles, 117–18
 definitions of, 115
 features of, 118
 responsibility for self, 125
 Rogers' approach to, 117–18, 121–2, 123, 124
 use of art in, 125–6
 see also counselling skills
persuasion, 34–6
 and fear, 33, 105
 communication variables in, 33–4, 37, 38
 message (text) variables, 33
 receiver (consumer) variables, 37
 sender (producer) variables, 38
 using rhetoric, 37
phantom pain, 182, 206
phenomenological psychology see humanistic psychology
phenomenology, 289–90
phenomenon, 289
phenotype, 74
philosophy
 influence on psychology, xviii–xxi
phobias, 19, 21, 23, 25, 26, 50–1
 agoraphobia, 18, 26, 50
 treatment, 17, 18, 47, 48, 50–1
phonological loop, 162, 169, 172
Piaget, Jean, 249
 theory of cognitve development, 251, 252, 253, 255, 256, 261
pineal body, 190–1
placebo effect, 111
placebo medication, 206
play, 259
 approaches to, 248
 fantasy, 255–6

in hospital, 249, 250
pleasure principle, 274, 275
population (research), 290
positron emission tomography, xxiv, 61, 73–4, 176
post-traumatic stress disorder, 22, 25, 26, 330–1
power, 3, 12, 310–12, 315
power struggle, 13,
precaution adoption model, 102
preconscious, 276
prejudice, 36–7, 39
prevention of disease, 112
primal integration therapy, 276
principle of opposites, 184, 276
problem, 260
problem behaviour, 312
problem-lumping, 91
problem solver
 definition of, 247
problem-solving, 83, 93, 247, 257, 258, 260
 abilities, 251
 transfer effects, 262
 see also reasoning, thinking
procedural memory, 169–70
projection, 150, 276
projective techniques, 276, 277, 278
proprioception, 220
prospective studies, 294
protection motivation theory, 100, 112
pseudodementia, 185
psyche, 276
psychoanalysis, xxi, xxii, 265, 276
psychoanalytic theory (Freud), 264
psychodrama, 276
psychodynamic psychology, xv, 263–78
 formative years and, 273
 theorists, 265–9
psychodynamic therapy, 4, 263
 free association, 273
 primal integration therapy, 276
 projective techniques, 276
psychogenic illnesses, 331
psychological processes
 classification of, 79

psychology
 definition of, xxiv
 history of, xviii–xxiv
 main perspectives, xiv–xvi
psychometric tests, 290
psychometrics, 290
psychoneuroimmunology, 331
psychosexual stages, 276–7
psychosis, 24
psychosocial theory (Erikson), 266
psychosomatic, 331–2
psychotropic drugs, 185–6
punishment, 41, 51

Q
Q technique, 239
questions, 142–3

R
rank order, 292
rate, 292
rational-emotive therapy, 87, 92
rationalisation, 91–2, 142
raw data, 292
reaction formation, 277
reality orientation, 170
reasoning, 247
 deductive, 101, 254
 dichotomous, 254, 268
 inductive, 257
recall, 170
reciprocity negotiation, 13
recognition, 170
redintegration, 170
reductionism, 176, 210, 292
reflective practice, 261
Reformation, the, xix–xx
registers, 131, 143
regression, 277
rehabilitation, 112
rehearsal (in STM), 162, 170
reinforcement, 41, 44, 51–2, 54
 intermittent, 41, 48
 of aggression, 2, 3
 of attitudes, 31
 of health behaviour, 98
 positive and negative, 43, 52
 schedules, 41, 47, 52, 53
 time out from, 51, 55
relationship inventory, 124
relaxation, 50, 332
relearning, 170

relearning savings, 170
reliability, 292–3
remembering
  accessibility of stored information, 163
  availability of stored information, 163
  confabulation, 164
  forms of, 162
  recall, 170
  recognition, 170
  redintegration, 170
  relearning, 170
  retrieval, 171
reminiscence, 165, 171
remote memory, 162, 171
REM sleep, 186, 187, 188
  deprivation of, 190
  dreaming and, 180–1
repertory grid, 92, 238
repression, 9, 162, 171, 177, 181, 277
research, 279–97
research methodology
  grounded theory, 149, 286, 295
  qualitative, 285, 290–1, 295
  quantitative, 285, 291, 295
research process, 293–4
resting potential, 74
retention of learned material, 171
reticular activating system, 191
retrieval, 171
  see also remembering
retrospective studies, 294
reward, 53–4
rights and obligations (in groups), 312–13
Rogers, Carl, xxii, 115, 117, 121, 122, 123, 124, 127
role conflict, 121, 313
role models see modelling
role play, 9
Rorscharch psychodiagnostic test, 276, 277

S
sample, 285, 294
scapegoating, 36
schema, 171, 252, 261
schizophrenia, 7, 62, 84, 186–7, 217
scientific psychology
  criteria for scientific studies, 280
  definitions of, 279
searching behaviour, 156

seasonal affective disorder, 26, 191
self-actualisation, xxii, 89, 110, 113, 124, 274
self-concept, xxii, 96, 226–8, 239–40
  and group membership, 313
  components of, 240
  during adolescence, 228
self-efficacy, 112–13, 125
  and maintenance of health behaviours, 96, 99, 106, 107, 113, 125
self-esteem, 6, 12, 32, 110, 240
  and persuasability, 37
  body image and, 228–9
self-fulfilling prophecy, 32
self-harm, 11, 12, 233
self-help groups, 313
self-image, 240
  definition of, 227
  see also body image
semantic memory, 162, 166, 171
sensation, 221
senses, 91, 221–2
  see also individual senses
sensitisation, 54
sensorimotor, 249, 255, 256, 261
sensory deprivation, 222–3
sensory impairment
  communication and, 132
  dreams and, 180
  perception and, 211, 213, 215, 217, 219, 222
sensory memory, 162, 163, 171
  activity trace, 163
sensory overload, 222–3
sensory systems/channels, 132
serial probe technique, 171–2
serial processing, 90, 93
serial reproduction, 172
seriation, 261
serotonin, 18, 26, 73, 74, 191
set
  in problem-solving, 261
  perceptual, 219
sex, 74
sexual abuse, 316
sexuality, 240–2

ambisexual, 229
bisexual, 230
cross-dressing, 232
definition of, 241
homosexual identity, 235
homosexuality, 235
poem about, 243
transsexual, 244–5
transvestite, 232, 245
shared action planning, 313
shock, 156
short-term memory, 162, 172
  capacity, 164
  duration, 164
  iconic store, 166
  span, 172, 173
  see also working memory
sick role behaviour,
  definition, 95
  pain and, 195
sign language, 143–4
signal detection theory, 93
signs and signals, 144
skilled activity, 261
slave systems (memory), 162, 172
sleep, 187–8
  cycles, 188–90
  deprivation, 190
  duration, 184, 190
  EEG wave traces in, 188
  orthodox, 185
  paralysis, 190
  REM sleep, 180–1, 186, 187, 188, 190
  stages of, 188–9
  thoughts during, 130
sleep disorders
  insomnia, 184
  narcolepsy, 185
sleep switching mechanism, 190–1
sleep walking, 191
sleepy sickness, 191
smell (olfaction), 223
social consensus, 314
social exchange theory, 314
social learning theory, 54–5
social psychology, xv, xvi, 298–316
  definitions of, 298–9
  see also groups
social roles, 242
sociograms, 314
solution-focused therapy, 87, 93
sound
  auditory location, 210–11
span (memory), 172

speech disorders, 70–1
state and trait anxiety, 23, 27
state and trait effects, 26–7
state dependence (memory), 172
statistical tests,
  parametric, 281, 289, 295
  nonparametric, 287, 289, 297
statistics and psychometrics, 279–97
  definition of, 280
  descriptive statistics, 283
  inferential, 286
status, 315
stereotype, 33, 38–9
stereotyping, 300
stimulus
  aversive, 42
stimulus overload
  and aggression, 14
stimulus–response theories, 41, 46, 49–50
stress, 317–35
  and performance, 327–8
  and personality, 325, 328–30
  anxiety and, 321
  appraisal, 13, 14
  approaches to, 318–20
  complementary therapies and, 320
  definitions of, 317
  engineering model of, 318
  eustress, 323
  factors, 9, 318, 319
  fight or flight mechanism, 73, 318, 323–4
  general adaptation syndrome, 318, 325
  physiology, 320–1, 323–5, 330, 335
  social support, 332
  symptoms and signs of, 333–4
  toughness, 334–5
stress and illness, 326
  post-traumatic stress disorder, 22, 25, 26, 330–1
  psychogenic illnesses, 331
stress inoculation, 4, 333
stress management, 326–7
  aerobic exercise and, 321

Alexander technique, 321
autogenic relaxation training, 321
  perception of self and, 327
  relaxation training, 332
  see also coping
stress measurement
  hospital stress rating scale, 325
  social readjustment scale, 149, 326
stressors
  daily hassles, 322
  environmental, 322–3
  life events, 326
stroke
  see cerebrovascular accident
subconscious, 277
subjective norm, 315
subjective viewpoint, 294
subjects, 295
sublimation, 273, 275
subliminal perception, 223
substantia gelatinosa, 200, 207
sudden infant death syndrome, 155
suicide, 159
  and aggression, 8, 11, 14
  phases preceding, 14
suicide risk and aggression, 14
superego, 126, 266, 277
suppression, 277
syllogism, 254, 261–2
symbolic interactionism, 285, 295
symbolic representation (Bruner), 249, 256, 262,
  and problem-solving, 260
sympathetic nervous system, 59, 73, 320
synaesthesia, 223–4
synapse, 71, 76
synthesis, 262

T
taboos, 315–16
taste (gustation), 224
teaching
  definition of, 113
  styles, 98, 105
teleology, 113
temperament, 226–7, 242, 244
  dimensions of, 242, 244
thalamus, 57, 59, 71, 220
Thanatos, 3, 271
thematic apperception test, 276, 278
theory, 295
theory of planned behaviour, 100, 113
theory of reasoned action, 100, 113–14
therapeutic approaches, xvi,
  behaviour therapies, 40–55
  cognitve behaviour, 78–94
  complementary therapies, 73, 196, 200–1, 320, 321
  humanistic approaches, 115–27
  hypnotherapy, 183
  physical interventions, 56–77
  psychodynamic, 263–78
thesis, 295
thinking
  abstract, 251
  convergent, 253
  definition of, 247–8
  divergent, 255
  lateral, 258
  ways of, 247–8
thoughts
  and emotions, 79, 80
  emotionally coloured, 80
token economy, 54, 55
tolerable aggression, 14
touch, 209, 224–5
  as a form of communication, 145–6, 224

haptic, 209, 224
passive, 224
toughness, 318
transactional analysis, 126–7
transcutaneous electrical nerve stimulation (TENS), 207
transfer effects, 262
transference, 127, 278
traps, 14
t-tests, 295
Turner's syndrome, 75
twins, 76, 77
type A behaviour pattern, 111, 318, 328–30
type B pattern 329
type C personality (cancer-prone), 111, 150

U
unconditional positive regard, 124, 127
unconditioned response, 55
unconditioned stimulus, 55
unconscious (mind)
  collective (Jung), 271
  definitions of, 263–4

V
validity, 295–7
value, 39, 94
variable, 297
  dependent, 283, 284, 285, 286, 288
  independent, 283, 284, 285, 286, 288
  qualitative, 290
  quantitative, 290
variance, 297
  see also dispersion
verbal aggression, 14
verbal communication, 146
verbal memory, 173
vestibular sense, 221, 225
violence
  classification of, 8
  cycle of, 9

exposure to, 3, 9
high temperatures and, 10
vision, 209, 225
  binocular disparity, 211
  colour, 65, 212–13
  colour vision variations, 213–14
  dark adaptation, 214–15
  following brain surgery, 75–6
  impossible figures, 218
  pathways in the brain, 66, 68
  visual neglect, 219
  visuospatial sketchpad, 162, 172, 173, 257
vitamin B12
  and autism, 178
vocal, 146
voice, 146

W
weapons effect, 14
Wernicke's area (speech), 58, 70–1
white light, 213, 214
Wilcoxon test, 297
Winnicott, Donald, 269
working memory, 173
  central executive system, 162, 164, 168, 172
  phonological loop, 162, 169, 172
  phonological suppression, 169
  slave systems, 162, 172
  visuospatial sketchpad, 162, 172, 173, 257

X/Y/Z
X-rays, 77
yoga, 73
zygote, 77